Forms of Brief Therapy

Edited by

Simon H. Budman

HARVARD COMMUNITY HEALTH PLAN
AND HARVARD MEDICAL SCHOOL

Foreword by Mardi J. Horowitz, MD

THE GUILFORD PRESS

NEW YORK, LONDON

To the Best Form of Long-Term Therapy
Susan, Gabrielle, and Shari

© 1981 The Guilford Press, New York
A Division of Guilford Publications, Inc.

Printed in the United States of America

Last digit is print number   9   8   7   6

Library of Congress Cataloging in Publication Data

Main entry under title:

Forms of brief therapy.

Includes bibliographies and indexes.
1. Psychotherapy, Brief.   I. Budman, Simon.
RC480.55.F67   616.89'14   81-2779
AACR2
ISBN 0-89862-900-4 p

CONTRIBUTORS

Michael J. Bennett, MD, Harvard Community Health Plan and Department of Psychiatry, Harvard Medical School, Boston, Massachusetts

Arnon Bentovim, MB, BS, FRCPsych, Department of Psychological Medicine, The Hospital for Sick Children, and the Tavistock Clinic, London, England

Bernard L. Bloom, PhD, Department of Psychology, University of Colorado at Boulder, Boulder, Colorado

Simon H. Budman, PhD, Harvard Community Health Plan and Department of Psychiatry, Harvard Medical School, Boston, Massachusetts

Jack D. Burke, Jr., MD, Applied Biometrics Research Branch, Division of Biometry and Epidemiology, National Institute of Mental Health, Bethesda, Maryland

Barbara Sabin Daley, RN, MS, Harvard Community Health Plan, Cambridge, Massachusetts

James M. Donovan, PhD, Harvard Community Health Plan and Department of Psychiatry, Harvard Medical School, Boston, Massachusetts

Alan S. Gurman, PhD, Department of Psychiatry, University of Wisconsin Medical School, Madison, Wisconsin

James P. Gustafson, MD, Department of Psychiatry, University of Wisconsin, Madison, Wisconsin

Leston L. Havens, MD, Department of Psychiatry, Harvard Medical School at the Massachusetts Mental Health Center, Boston, Massachusetts

Neil S. Jacobson, PhD, Department of Psychology, University of Washington, Seattle, Washington

Warren Kinston, BSc (Hons.), MB, BS, MRCPsych, Brunel Institute of Organization and Social Studies, Brunel University, Uxbridge, Middlesex, England

Geraldine Suzanne Koppenaal, RN, MS, Harvard Community Health Plan, Cambridge, Massachusetts

James Mann, MD, Division of Psychiatry, Boston University School of Medicine, Boston, Massachusetts

Christine M. McElroy, BA, Department of Mental Health, Harvard Community Health Plan, Boston, Massachusetts

Herbert Pardes, MD, National Institute of Mental Health, Rockville, Maryland

Harold Alan Pincus, MD, National Institute of Mental Health, Rockville, Maryland

James E. Sabin, MD, Harvard Community Health Plan, Wellesley, Massachusetts, and Department of Psychiatry, Harvard Medical School, Boston, Massachusetts

Peter E. Sifneos, MD, Department of Psychiatry, Beth Israel Hospital and Harvard Medical School, Boston, Massachusetts

Hans H. Strupp, PhD, Department of Psychology, Vanderbilt University, Nashville, Tennessee

Robert L. Weiss, PhD, Department of Psychology, University of Oregon, Eugene, Oregon

Henry S. White, MD, Department of Psychiatry, Harvard Medical School at the Massachusetts Mental Health Center, Boston, Massachusetts

G. Terence Wilson, PhD, Graduate School of Applied and Professional Psychology, Rutgers University, Piscataway, New Jersey

M. J. Wisneski, MD, Harvard Community Health Plan and Department of Psychiatry, Harvard Medical School, Boston, Massachusetts

FOREWORD

As psychoanalysis became a longer and longer form of treatment, attempts at shorter forms of psychotherapy were made. Waves of effort occurred before World War II and involved Ferenczi, Rank, and others. During World War II, major efforts were made to relieve combat neuroses as quickly as possible and to return soldiers to duty. Lindemann, Caplan, Balint, Alexander, French, Malan, Sifneos, and others added other waves of effort. The recent decade witnessed a revitalized interest in brief therapy. The revitalization was partly scientific, based upon publications by innovative clinicians, and partly economic, based upon the limitations imposed by third-party payments for delivery of mental health services. For these reasons and others, an almost explosive array of new or rediscovered treatment-technique packages appeared during the 1960s and 1970s. Many of the more faddish varieties have vanished from the scene. This book is timely, for it describes a spectrum of promising contemporary approaches to brief therapy.

The mind works as a series of interlocking and transactive processes at many levels of operation. We do not yet have a good general psychology of these processes, but rather fragments of theory, each illuminating parts of a domain. Every phenomenon, a symptom for example, is the result of interactive functions. An effort to change one thing, to pull on one thread, entangles the whole cloth. Recognition of overdetermination and the importance of unconsciously proceeding mental functions led psychoanalysts from shorter therapies, aimed at resolving neurotic symptoms by exposure of conflict, to longer therapies, aimed at mutative change of immature structures and organizers of mental processes. This approach to change required giving up an agreed-upon aim of relieving target symptoms as rapidly as possible, and resulted in a sense of timelessness of procedures. Brief therapies are called "brief" because they substitute time for timelessness.

This attitude of timelessness and the aim at structural change are appropriate to psychoanalysis. But in the 1950s, psychoanalysis became a model upon which less arduous efforts were based. Many of the techniques for once-a-week, more focused therapy were based upon the practical techniques evolved for elaboration and resolution of a transference neurosis in the four- or five-times-a-week psychoanalysis. The aura of timelessness was carried over, and the aims of once- or twice-a-week therapy were often left vague far into the treatment, far longer than required by efforts to obtain sufficient information for clinical formulation. Indeed, clinical formulation in psychotherapies may have been dominated by historical reconstructions, with insufficient attention to relating intervention strategies to patterns of desired change in the present and future.

The effect of timelessness was allied with the establishment of the most far-reaching goals, often never explicitly stated in the communication between the patient and the therapist. I am not speaking of psychoanalysis, but a variety of psychoanalytically oriented psychotherapies offered during the period in question to ever wider patient populations. The residual effect may still be noted in training settings. When students are asked about their supervision, one finds that this central aspect of training seldom involves explicit statements of the goals of the treatment. Probing questions, addressed to trainees, may elicit startling illusions about what is "supposed to take place" as a result of their interventions, illusions that continue for years. I have noted such illusions in behavioral therapy trainees as well.

Re-entry of the concept of time into therapy reawakens concern for formulating what the therapy is to accomplish. What is the set of problems and strengths? What can be done? What are the positive and negative sequelae? How and when will changes come about? We do not yet have the answers to these questions, but *Forms of Brief Therapy,* in examining diverse strategies, and examining the time they take as an expense factor, helps us sharpen our concern for them, a concern that may invigorate observations in both "brief" and "long" therapies.

Brief therapy is, in a sense, an attitude. It is a position statement about the balance between goals and the processes to be used to achieve them. There is great ferment because clinicians concerned about brief therapy do not agree about these goals, these processes, and the likely results. Their questions are challenging and exciting, even if the answers are not yet available. As I have already indicated, such questions may illuminate the issue of therapeutic change and the methodology for its evaluation in *general*. Then, later on, we can pass beyond the "testimonial" and "boasting" phases of how the therapy marketplace works, to an era that goes beyond brand names to a general and scientific theory. We will select the optimal therapy for a given case, and I daresay we will not add "brief" or "long" to describe the type of treatment.

The ideal of such a reorganization of theories of psychopathology and therapeutics will be to relate a treatment approach to the specific kind of complaint, to a specific explanation of the pathology and the available strengths, to a theory of how change takes place, and to the individual's style of coping and defense. Such an ordering has not yet taken place. In several chapters of this book, however, the presentation of a developmental model may be a very useful step in helping us think about the kind of relationship which patients may find most catalytic for change. Some of the excitement revolves around the fairly simple device already mentioned—of setting a time limit explicitly or implicitly, rather than allowing the kind of timelessness appropriate to psychoanalysis to be overextended into fields where it may be inappropriate, since the goals are not the same.

Forms of Brief Therapy covers many areas of interest, and the reader will end with his or her eyes wide open to the vast range of viewpoints. The editor, Simon Budman, is to be complimented for assembling a fascinating volume whose many exciting themes will stimulate subsequent systematic investigation.

Mardi J. Horowitz
University of California

PREFACE

In October of 1975, when I arrived at the Harvard Community Health Plan (HCHP), my bias was that brief therapy could be useful to some small part of the population, but that truly helpful therapy goes on for years. Throughout my training as a clinical psychologist, I had heard repeatedly that whenever the patient made the first move to terminate, this clearly indicated resistance or "running away from therapy." Over a period of time, I became quite skilled at treating patients for ever extended periods and came to think that early terminations represented transference cures, with rapid changes being inevitably doomed to later relapse. Beginning to work at HCHP jogged my thinking dramatically.

At that time, the Plan was still a fledgling health maintenance organization which had previously struggled for survival and had now demonstrated its staying power. In the first years of its existence, HCHP had "controlled" mental health costs by restricting treatment to the healthiest part of the population, with the "release valve" of referral-out for private (fee-for-service) therapy of those who needed more extended therapeutic work. Several months after I began at the Plan, various legislative changes in Massachusetts and decisions within HCHP brought about a lifting of restrictions regarding who could receive mental health care, and at the same time, it became necessary to treat all mental health patients without making outside referrals.

As is true of most settings where brief therapy approaches have become important, necessity became the mother of invention. Confronted with the task of caring for an ever growing, highly sophisticated (psychologically oriented) population, the staff began to think long and hard about how much we could expand the parameters of brief treatment. Since I had had considerable experience and training in short-term psychoeducational groups (with new parents, medical patients, etc.) and with encounter groups, Mike Bennett, then Director of Mental Health, was quite supportive of my early attempts to develop a short-term group therapy program. To our colleagues in the fee-for-service community, for whom short-term individual treatment was heresy enough, considering the possibility of short-term group treatment for a large number of patients was unimaginable.

In part to assuage our anxiety (and perhaps guilt), a group of HCHP mental health clinicians began meeting on a regular basis to discuss the short-term group therapy program. These clinicians diligently met for nearly two years and became the first GRIP (Group for Research in Psychotherapy) workshop. Happily, our early attempts at expanding and testing the limits of brief therapy were most encouraging. A bright, well-trained, flexible, and enthusiastic staff spearheaded these efforts. By early 1979, with the experience of having treated literally thousands of patients in short-term individual, group, and marital treatment, we felt the time to be right to share some of what we had learned with others. It was out of this interest that the Harvard Community Health Plan conference on brief individual and group therapy grew. *Forms of Brief Therapy* is, in turn, the offspring of that conference.

I hope that this book will address many needs and a wide audience. There is material here for the clinician, theoretician, and researcher. Those who have had many years of more traditional clinical training can hopefully consider applications of brief treatment to what they now do. The student can bring an unbiased eye to brief treatment and look at it as an increasingly sought after and essential set of treatment modalities.

As is invariably true in putting together a book, there are many to be thanked and appreciated. First, my fond thanks to the mental health staff of the Kenmore Center of HCHP. Rather than the competitive, dog-eat-dog atmosphere which I had previously found in some academic settings, the Plan provided a warm and supportive ambience, which truly was and is the essence of our "group practice" model and our ability to be thoughtfully innovative. In particular, Mike Bennett, Mary Clifford, and Don Wertlieb have been most available to share ideas, critique papers, and be helpful friends. Thanks to John Ludden, Associate Medical Director of the Kenmore Center, for knowing and nurturing a good idea (the brief therapy conference) when he saw one, and to Bob Lurie, Vice President of HCHP, for the same reason. As a person with a great deal of previous editing experience, Alan Gurman has been of tremendous assistance to me over the course of this project, as has Seymour Weingarten, Editor-in-Chief of The Guilford Press.

Last, but most certainly not least, I wish to thank Susan, my wife, and Gabrielle and Shari, my daughters—Susan for her great interest, support, and advice, and Gabrielle and Shari for just being there.

Simon H. Budman
Boston, Massachusetts

CONTENTS

Chapter 1. **Introduction** 1
SIMON H. BUDMAN

    References 4

Chapter 2. **Brief Therapy in the Context of National Mental Health Issues** 7
HERBERT PARDES AND HAROLD ALAN PINCUS

    The Historical Context of Mental Health Care in the
        United States 7
    The Development of Brief Treatments 12
    Future Implications of the Development of Brief Treatments 17
    References 21

Section I
Individual Brief Therapy: Dynamic Models

Chapter 3. **The Core of Time-Limited Psychotherapy: Time and the Central Issue** 25
JAMES MANN

    The Importance of Time 27
    Defining the Central Issue 33
    Conclusion 42
    References 42

Chapter 4. **Short-Term Anxiety-Provoking Psychotherapy: Its History, Technique, Outcome, and Instruction** 45
PETER E. SIFNEOS

    Criteria for Selection of Suitable Patients 46
    Technique 47
    The Outcome 48
    The Instruction of STAPP 49
    An Example of Typical Interviews 49
    Conclusion 79
    References 80

Chapter 5. **The Complex Secret of Brief Psychotherapy in the
Works of Malan and Balint** 83
JAMES P. GUSTAFSON

   From Intuitive to Conceptual Mastery 83
   The Counteroffer 85
   Breaking the Traditional Bonds of Psychoanalysis 90
   The Potential for Planning Brief Psychotherapy in
      Advance of Treatment 94
   The Current Methods of Selection and Technique 102
   Reinterpretation of the Intuitive Mastery in Malan's Case Examples 107
   The Neglected Study of Technique 112
   The Remarkable Contributions Reviewed 120
   Acknowledgments 122
   Notes 122
   References 127

Section II
Individual Brief Therapy: Alternative Models

Chapter 6. **Behavior Therapy as a Short-Term
Therapeutic Approach** 131
G. TERENCE WILSON

   Introduction 131
   Clinical Illustrations of Short-Term Behavior Therapy 133
   The Broad Applicability of Behavior Therapy 140
   Technical Characteristics of Behavior Therapy as Short-Term
      Treatment 141
   How Effective Is Behavior Therapy? 151
   Evaluating the Outcome of Short-Term Therapy 152
   Summary 161
   References 161

Chapter 7. **Focused Single-Session Therapy: Initial Development
and Evaluation** 167
BERNARD L. BLOOM

   The Frequency of Single-Session Episodes of Care 169
   Early Termination and Client Satisfaction 171
   The Effectiveness of a Single Therapeutic Session 173
   Focused Single-Session Therapy: A Preliminary Report 180
   Focused Single-Session Therapy: A Case Example 190
   Concluding Remarks 213
   References 214

Section III
Theoretical Issues in Forms of Brief Therapy

Chapter 8. Toward the Refinement of Time-Limited Dynamic Psychotherapy   219
HANS H. STRUPP

    Patient Selection   221
    Therapeutic Goals   225
    Therapeutic Technology   227
    Future Directions   233
    References   241

Chapter 9. Choosing a Method of Short-Term Therapy: A Developmental Approach   243
HENRY S. WHITE, JACK D. BURKE, JR., AND LESTON L. HAVENS

    Introduction   243
    Approaches to Short-Term Dynamic Psychotherapy   244
    Matching Method and Patient   253
    Conclusion   266
    Acknowledgment   266
    References   267

Section IV
Planned Short-Term Group Therapy

Chapter 10. Short-Term Group Psychotherapy: Historical Antecedents   271
JAMES E. SABIN

    Introduction   271
    Kurt Lewin   273
    Emergence of the National Training Laboratoˉies   275
    From T-Groups to the Encounter Movement   277
    From Encounter Groups to Short-Term Group Psychotherapy   279
    References   281

Chapter 11. The Crisis Group: Its Rationale, Format, and Outcome   283
JAMES M. DONOVAN, MICHAEL J. BENNETT, AND CHRiSTINE M. MCELROY

    The Format and Management of the Group   284
    Review of the Literature   287
    Our Outcome Study   289
    The Curative Parameters of the Group   297
    Conclusion: Limitations and Strengths of the Group   301
    References   303

Chapter 12. **An Adult Developmental Model of Short-Term Group Psychotherapy**   305
SIMON H. BUDMAN, MICHAEL J. BENNETT, AND M. J. WISNESKI

    Young Adult Groups   308
    Midlife Groups   320
    Later Midlife Groups   332
    Conclusions   340
    Acknowledgments   340
    References   341

Chapter 13. **The Treatment of Women in Short-Term Women's Groups**   343
BARBARA SABIN DALEY AND GERALDINE SUZANNE KOPPENAAL

    Review of the Literature   344
    Women's Psychotherapy Groups versus Consciousness-Raising
      Groups   347
    How Women Are Referred to Groups   348
    Short-Term Women's Therapy Groups   349
    Conclusion   355
    Acknowledgment   356
    References   356

Section V
Marital and Family Therapy as Brief Treatment

Chapter 14. **Creating a Focus for Brief Marital or Family Therapy**   361
WARREN KINSTON AND ARNON BENTOVIM

    Introduction   361
    The Initial Attempt: Method, Results, Aftermath   363
    Focal Hypothesis   365
    What Is a Focus?   367
    Forms of Meaning   369
    Failure to Create a Focal Hypothesis   380
    Stress and Meaning   381
    Conclusion   383
    References   385

Chapter 15. **Behavioral Marital Therapy as Brief Therapy**   387
ROBERT L. WEISS AND NEIL S. JACOBSON

    Contrasting BMT with Other Therapies   388
    Current Examples of BMT Approaches   396
    BMT: Brief Therapy by Design   408
    References   412

Chapter 16. **Integrative Marital Therapy: Toward the Development of an Interpersonal Approach** 415
ALAN S. GURMAN

    The Myth of Brief Individual Psychotherapy 416
    The Countermyth of Brief Marital Therapy 417
    Time-Limited Marital Therapy: When Means Have Little Meaning 419
    Toward the Development of an Integrative Marital Therapy 420
    Three Approaches to Marital Therapy 422
    Some Conceptual and Technical Principles for an Integrated
        Approach to Marital Therapy 428
    Conclusion 452
    Acknowledgments 453
    References 453

Section VI
Conclusion

Chapter 17. **Looking toward the Future** 461
SIMON H. BUDMAN

    Unifying Elements in Brief Therapies 461
    Other Forms of Brief Therapy 463
    The Future of Brief Therapy 463
    Conclusions 466
    References 466

Index 469

CHAPTER 1
INTRODUCTION

Simon H. Budman

Forms of Brief Therapy examines the area of brief treatment in broad brush strokes. I have included contributions which cover individual, group, and marital therapies, as well as the psychodynamic and behavioral perspectives. In many ways, brief therapy is hardly new or uncommon. Brief treatment, when it is defined as therapy of less than 25 sessions' duration, represents the standard practice of outpatient mental health intervention in this country (Pardes & Pincus, Chapter 2, this volume), the types of therapy most often examined as part of psychotherapy or behavior therapy research (Smith, Glass, & Miller, 1980), as well as the usual length of many of the "newer" therapies, for example, Gestalt, TA, Rolfing, and so on.

If all of us have been doing it for years, is that not sufficient? Is not a lengthy examination of short-term treatment simply an exercise in semantics? I think not. What, in fact, is relatively new and uncommon is the growing interest in planned, defined, short-term, and often time-limited treatment. A broad survey of planned brief therapy allows a distillation, clarification, refinement, and further synthesis of the area.

In their contribution, Pardes and Pincus (Chapter 2) consider brief therapy within the context of national mental health issues. It is certain to this observer that if and when national health insurance with mental health coverage arrives on the scene, the backbone of such a program will have to be short-term therapy.

The next three chapters represent an overview of what are currently the major psychodynamic approaches to brief treatment. Although all these approaches have their roots in psychoanalytic thinking, their respective foci differ considerably. As Gustafson (Chapter 5) so eloquently clarifies, even within the Tavistock group, Malan and Balint appear to

SIMON H. BUDMAN. Harvard Community Health Plan and Department of Psychiatry, Harvard Medical School, Boston, Massachusetts.

1

diverge in some rather important areas of practice and conceptualization.

Mann's (Chapter 3) formulation of time as the central issue in time-limited psychotherapy, his "prescription" of 12 sessions, as well as his specificity regarding the required elements in setting the focus of such treatment, could conceivably provide psychotherapy researchers with a rich opportunity to study the specific elements in psychoanalytic psychotherapy, such as the establishment of an alliance and termination.

Short-term anxiety-provoking psychotherapy represents a major modification of current analytic practice, in that Sifneos (Chapter 4) builds his approach on the interpretation of the impulse *before* the defense. Like Mann, Sifneos's treatment has a clear focus, in this case Oedipal issues. Unlike Mann, however, Sifneos sees his approach as having (at least at this point) utility for a small and carefully specified population.

Wilson (Chapter 6) looks at behavior therapy as brief treatment. His examination of this issue is most enlightening. Among other important points, we find that behavioral treatment is growing in length from its early (and briefer) days. A similar lengthening phenomenon is described by Marmor (1979) for dynamic psychotherapy over the course of its history. One wonders about the degree to which all therapies become longer —because, as Wilson states, "more complex problems are dealt with" (i.e., a patient-induced phenomenon)—and the degree to which many therapists may be highly resistant to briefer therapy. From both an economic and an emotional perspective, planned brief therapy is far more demanding of the therapist. Obviously, the therapist, too, goes through the process of terminating treatment. At what cost remains to be clarified. Moreover, in the cold, cruel world of economic realities, it is far easier for a therapist to know that a given hour is indefinitely filled, rather than that for every x number of weeks, there exists some greater or lesser degree of financial uncertainty. Wilson goes on to explicate the importance of homework and other types of specific task setting, which are part of behavioral treatments, and which he sees as contributing to brevity. In general, with the exception of Alexander and French (1946), dynamically oriented brief therapists have eschewed such techniques. By doing so, they may be neglecting an important set of intervention strategies (Wachtel, 1977), which are most certainly in keeping with the basic principles of brief therapy as outlined by Butcher and Koss (1978).

Chapter 7 by Bloom provides a description of what is probably the most "radical" form of brief therapy, that is, focused single-session therapy. After a careful review of what he calls the "extensive footnote literature" on single-session therapeutic encounters, Bloom carefully and thoughtfully applies current knowledge regarding short-term treatment in the interest of developing a therapy approach of one session duration. Bloom seems to be asking the therapist, "If you have only one session with this patient, how can you make it maximally beneficial?" His exposition of such an approach is of vast importance from a variety of viewpoints. For example, for psychotherapy researchers studying focused single-session therapy (FSST), the unit of study is substantially refined. Further, as socially committed clinicians, it is quite conceivable that we can generate interest in FSST on the part of many people who ordinarily might view mental health treatment as too time consuming, too expensive, too demanding, and so on.

The chapters by Strupp and by White, Burke, and Havens (Chapters 8 and 9, respectively), are generally more theoretically oriented than are the preceding chapters. Both contributions attempt to address the now perennial question of "what therapy, for whom, and under what circumstances?" While Strupp looks at more traditional models of ego strength and ego resources in clarifying those patients appropriate for short-term dynamic psychotherapy, White, Burke, and Havens apply a developmental perspective, which is certain to gain in significance.

The next four chapters examine the issue of short-term group psychotherapy. For a variety of reasons, dynamic group psychotherapy has been assumed to be a long-term therapy. What is the underlying reason for such an assumption? It could not be that long-term therapy has been demonstrated to be more efficacious than short-term, nor is it because individual therapy is more effective than group treatment, because neither of these has been demonstrated to be the case (Luborsky, Singer, & Luborsky, 1975). More likely, I believe, is the fact that the same biases which many therapists have regarding brief therapy (e.g., that "it doesn't go deep enough," it is "too superficial," it is "second-class therapy") are equally present as regards group therapy. Thus, for many dynamically trained therapists, short-term group therapy is an untenable marriage. At the same time, although behaviorally oriented therapists have had some interest in group treatment, they have, for the most part, basically applied individual behavioral techniques within a group setting. This is to the neglect of group processes, group dynamics, and even the social learning aspects of group therapy. Thus, there has been no real base for the evolution of short-term group therapy.

My colleagues and I have attempted in this volume to carefully describe some of the important issues in planned short-term group treatment. In my chapter with Bennett and Wisneski (Chapter 12), as well as in Chapter 13 by Daley and Koppenaal, an adult developmental perspective is applied. Clearly, such a perspective is strikingly similar to that described by White, Burke, and Havens in Chapter 9. Rather than assisting in the selection of a treatment approach, however, we use this perspective to assist us in the selection of a group focus.

The next three chapters examine the issue of marital and family therapy as a brief treatment modality. As is the case with most individual therapies, as they are practiced, marital therapy is practiced as a brief treatment (Gurman & Kniskern, 1978). Marital therapy is generally not clearly explicated as a planned brief therapy, however, nor have authors carefully and thoroughly examined the underlying elements which contribute to the brevity of such therapies. Kinston and Bentovim (Chapter 14) describe the application of Malan's model of short-term dynamic therapy to couples and families. The foci for most marital therapies are obviously the problems experienced by the couple. For Kinston and Bentovim, however, the careful, detailed establishment of the focus takes the same centrality in treatment that it does in Mann's time-limited approach to individual psychotherapy.

Weiss and Jacobson (Chapter 15) describe behavioral marital therapy (BMT) as being "brief by design and not by default." They emphasize the fact that by its short-term nature, BMT *demands* that the therapist be careful, thoughtful, active, and directive.

Finally, Gurman (Chapter 16) seeks to explicate an integrated form of marital therapy, which contains elements from the major schools of marital treatment. In his integration, he attempts to weave together these elements in a manner which maximizes treatment efficacy in the brief period that most marital therapists have with their clients.

In the last chapter, my interest is in synthesizing some of the previous contributions and then in considering where we may be heading in the field of brief therapy. It is my hope that the reader will enjoy *Forms of Brief Therapy* as much as I have enjoyed editing it.

REFERENCES

Alexander, F., & French, T. M. *Psychoanalytic therapy: Principles and applications.* New York: Ronald Press, 1946.

Butcher, J. N., & Koss, M. P. Research on brief and crisis-oriented psychotherapies. In S. L. Garfield & A. E. Bergin (Eds.), *Handbook of psychotherapy and behavior change.* New York: Wiley, 1978.

Gurman, A. S., & Kniskern, D. P. Research on marital and family therapy: Progress, perspective and prospect. In S. L. Garfield & A. E. Bergin (Eds.), *Handbook of psychotherapy and behavior change.* New York: Wiley, 1978.

Luborsky, L., Singer, B., & Luborsky, L. Comparative studies of psychotherapies. Is it true that "everyone has won and all must have prizes"? *Archives of General Psychiatry,* 1975, *32,* 995–1008.

Marmor, J. Short-term dynamic psychotherapy. *American Journal of Psychiatry,* 1979, *136,* 149–155.

Smith, M. L., Glass, G. & Miller, T. I. *The benefits of psychotherapy.* Baltimore: Johns Hopkins University Press, 1980.

Wachtel, P. *Psychoanalysis and behavior therapy: Toward an integration.* New York: Basic Books, 1977.

CHAPTER 2
BRIEF THERAPY IN THE CONTEXT OF NATIONAL MENTAL HEALTH ISSUES

Herbert Pardes
Harold Alan Pincus

It is not simply coincidental that there is so much current interest in the forms of brief psychotherapy. The development of brief treatments has been closely tied to the evolution of the overall mental health system in this country. Furthermore, the future issues and challenges that will be posed for the system as a whole are integrally linked to the future role of brief psychotherapy. Thus, this chapter examines the recent history and present context of mental health care in the United States and also comments on key factors, both scientific and political, which have had significance in the development of short-term treatments. Finally, it examines the implications of brief treatment and their link with the future of the mental health field in general.

THE HISTORICAL CONTEXT OF MENTAL HEALTH CARE IN THE UNITED STATES

In examining the evolution of mental health care over the last 40 years, one is impressed at the tremendous expansion of the treatment armamentarium during that time. In the early 1940s, there were few available treatments for mental disorders. Although there was considerable use of some organic treatments for severely ill patients, mainly electric and insulin shock as well as psychosurgical techniques, little was known about their mechanisms of action, and their use engendered much

HERBERT PARDES and HAROLD ALAN PINCUS. National Institute of Mental Health, Rockville, Maryland.

controversy. Long-term psychoanalysis was available, and for the severely disabled, there was a primary dependence on the use of long-term stays in hospitals, which were often more custodial than therapeutic. While there was the beginning of some new psychosocial efforts, no substantial cadre of mental health professionals existed. There was only modest interest in the field of mental health in society at large.

Following the beginning of World War II, a series of developments occurred that served to focus attention on mental health care. Experience with the selective service system revealed a number of startling and sobering statistics regarding the extent of mental illness. Of almost five million men turned down by the selective service system, 40% were excluded from service due to neuropsychiatric disabilities, by far the most frequent cause. Furthermore, the impressive work done in restoring people in battle to renewed active function demonstrated the value of mental health professionals and, in addition, provided for the development of new and effective techniques for treatment. Finally, wartime manpower shortages profoundly affected the already questionable care of psychiatric patients in state hospitals and assisted in bringing the situation to the attention of the media. This awakening to the extent of mental illness and the potential of psychiatric treatments, along with the efforts of various leaders in the field was an important force leading to the creation of the National Institute of Mental Health (NIMH) in 1949.

During the first 20 years of its functioning, the Institute brought promise and excitement, development of the field, and an optimism about what could be learned and what problems could be ameliorated. There was a great deal of reality in that promise. During those several decades, there occurred a revolution in concepts of mental illness and in patient care.

A wide range of psychopharmacologic agents was introduced into practice. Major and minor tranquilizers, antidepressant drugs, and therapeutic agents designed specifically for the treatment of mania were evolved. The development and use of such psychopharmacologic agents radically altered strategies of treatment and research in mental health and mental illness.

Coincident with the advent of chemotherapy was the advancement of innovative treatments in the psychosocial area. The use of group therapy became widespread, and the development of family therapy, crisis intervention, and behavioral therapies was stimulated. Mental hospitals implemented the concepts of a "therapeutic community" of increased patient participation in the therapeutic regimen and improved patient-staff relationships. In addition, there began to be greater consideration of the patient's needs in the community. There were initial attempts at aftercare, transitional living systems, and more and better activities geared toward rehabilitation. There was also an increasing emphasis on the positive strengths of the patient rather than the preexisting focus, which was predominantly on the individual's deficiencies and weaknesses.

In October 1963, the Community Mental Health Centers Act was passed by Congress and signed by President Kennedy. The act authorized NIMH to establish and fund the construction of community mental health centers in each designated catchment area throughout the country. These centers, which were to provide comprehensive services for the mental health care of each of its residents, regardless of socioeconomic status, were incorporated into President Johnson's "great society" programs, and federal funds became available for staffing them. Today there are over 750 community mental health centers around the country which are available to serve approximately 50% of the population.

Congress also authorized significant expenditures for mental health training and education, and a cadre of mental health professionals developed throughout the country. Simultaneously, there was the articulation of a team concept emphasizing the strengths of the various professionals.

These developments had the effect of making many mental patients able to function in a more integrated and appropriate manner in hospital settings. A large number of them were able to leave the institutions and return to their families and communities. In 1955, the ratio of inpatient treatment to outpatient treatment was about three to one, while in 1975, the ratio was reversed—almost one to three. The number of patients in state hospitals was dramatically reduced from close to 600,000 in the early '50s to approximately 160,000 in the mid-'70s.

All this led to a rapid expansion of facilities, personnel, information, techniques, tools, and data regarding mental health and mental illness. Toward the end of the '60s and into the early '70s, however, this phase was followed by a dramatic reversal, with the feelings of optimism and promise of the previous decades dimmed somewhat by the unrealized expectations and fluctuating sense of hopefulness and disillusionment in government and society in general and in mental health programs and professionals in particular. Confidence in the executive branch and Congress precipitously declined. An unpopular war and Watergate contributed to doubts about government, but other domestic movements for civil rights and consumer protection reflected a rebellion against traditional authorities and mores. Burgeoning health and social costs, along with the unfulfilled expectation of earlier expansive funding, led to calls for a general fiscal retrenchment.

In the mental health field, this new phase was symbolized by a sharp change in the stance of the highest levels of government toward mental health. The clinical training programs, which had developed an important cadre of mental health professionals, were identified for elimination. Impoundment suits and court fights developed between members of the mental health constituencies and the then present Administration. The research budget of NIMH was held constant and, in fact, between 1968 and 1976 was reduced in absolute dollars to a modest degree. In many ways NIMH was under seige, and the programs were dramatically influenced by this attack. It was left to Congress to annually rescue the mental health programs. In the process, however, researchers became discouraged, and a decreasing number entered the field. Clinicians, trainers, and educators felt chronically worn down by the continued threats of phase-out of support for their programs.

It is important to note, however, that the overall context of the mental health field was not quite so bleak. People in communities throughout the United States were being more supportive. Community mental health centers continued to crop up around the country, and those that were being phased out of federal funding were generally finding significant state and local support. Active programs of clinical treatment, as well as consultation and education, were having an impact on an increasing number of the nation's citizens. A larger number of people in the lower socioeconomic sectors of the community were having services made accessible to them.

At the same time, a well-intentioned effort to bring people out of custodial institutions and put them in settings where they could receive active support and treatment was having many beneficial effects on our concepts of the mental health programs. It was also sowing the seeds for a major new set of problems in the mental health field, however, given the fact that community resources were not being developed at a pace sufficient to be responsive to the people coming out of institutions.

Such was the scene when a new phase in the history of the mental health movement in this country was ushered in by the convening of the

President's Commission on Mental Health. The commission, with First Lady Rosalynn Carter as its honorary chairperson, was composed of 20 members drawn from a wide range of disciplines. It had a broad mandate to review the state of the mental health field, identify problems, set priorities, and generate recommendations for improvements. The development of the commission, the process through which it carried out its mandate, and the high visibility and support afforded it by the country and the Carter Administration all served to give a powerful "shot in the arm" to the entire mental health field.

The commission's report, delivered in 1978, became a blueprint from which major initiatives in the field of mental health could be launched by NIMH, the Alcohol, Drug Abuse and Mental Health Administration (ADAMHA), the Public Health Service, the Department of Health and Human Services (HHS), and the entire Administration. The recently developed concept of community support for deinstitutionalized patients was incorporated into the Mental Health Systems Act, designed to refine the Community Mental Health Centers Act. The act, signed by President Carter on October 7, 1980, focused more attention on the needs of underserved groups, minorities, and chronic patients and on linkages with general health and other human services. Demonstration programs were developed to identify housing for deinstitutionalized patients. Coordination was established between national agencies focusing on rehabilitation and agencies focusing on mental health. The secretary of HHS established a task force to develop a national plan for the chronically mentally ill. In addition, the institute held a research conference on the problem of stigma, in order to develop strategies to attack this pernicious and pervasive force. A task force on public understanding of the mentally ill was developed by HHS.

A new office of prevention developed at NIMH initiated a series of programs, such as those exploring the impact of the development of psychosis in parents on the children and the family and the impact of the disruption of a marriage on the children and the family.

Demonstration programs were started to establish advocacy systems for mental patients as well as to explore such improvements in the reimbursement system as exchanging two days of partial hospitalization for one of full hospitalization and extending provider status to community mental health centers.

The clinical training budget was stabilized, and the NIMH developed new programs and to develop more clinical investigators to stimulate more minority students to enter research. The entire clinical training program of NIMH was modified, so that it would more fully support the priorities identified by the Commission, including minorities, the chronically mentally ill, the aged, the young, the prevention of mental illness, and the linking of general health and mental health care.

The mental health research budget has increased substantially over the past four years. With this new support, NIMH has developed and enlarged its research programs in epidemiology, the neurosciences, the financing of mental health services, the problems of special populations, and other areas.

All this has again brought to the mental health field a feeling of zest, enthusiasm, and forward movement. At the same time, however, the nation has been developing a set of domestic problems in the areas of energy and the economy which are preeminent issues today. Given these concerns, the perception of a need for a strengthened defense effort, and the particularly dramatic rise in costs in the health care field, the renewed emphasis on mental health programs may again be in jeopardy.

THE DEVELOPMENT OF BRIEF TREATMENTS

Within this context, certain factors have played significant roles in focusing the attention of mental health providers on briefer treatment. These factors, some representing developments in the mental health field, others representing forces within society as a whole, include:

- the acceptance of more limited therapeutic goals
- the increasing development of an array of varied treatments along with a rapprochement of different therapeutic approaches
- advances in classification of emotional disorders
- the growing realization that lengthy treatments often do not meet the needs of particular populations
- an increasing concern with the costs of treatment combined with increasing access to treatment
- the growth of prepaid health plans with limited psychiatric benefits

With regard to the acceptance of more limited goals, it became apparent that in a number of instances, long-term psychological treatments did not have to be the recommended treatment for each and every person coming to a mental health practitioner. There were and are people who want relief from a specific symptom, help with a particular area of their personality functioning, improvements of their relationship with a certain person, and so forth, and there has been an increasing acceptance within the mental health provider community that such restriction of goals is consistent with a legitimate and important therapeutic enterprise.

Simultaneous with the acceptance of more limited goals has been the development of a variety of treatment modalities, as well as a change in therapist practices that demonstrates a more eclectic and pragmatic and less dogmatic approach to the field. During the 1950s, MacIver and Redlich (1959) were impressed by the division of the psychiatric profession into two camps: those using biological tools along with persuasive–directive methods, and those practicing the dynamic therapies. A subsequent study by Redlich and Kellert in 1978 showed a marked "homogenization of therapeutic approach," with practioners employing a much wider array of treatments. Family, group, behavioral, and cognitive therapies have all been used with increasing frequency. Moreover, the preexisting reluctance to combine psychological and somatic therapies has diminished substantially.

The development of such a wide array of treatment modalities has led to efforts to reconcile the various treatment approaches. On the one hand, psychodynamically oriented psychotherapists have raised the possibility of incorporating techniques from behavioral therapy into their treatment regimens (Wachtel, 1977). Concomitantly, behavioral therapists seem more ready to deal with their patients' perceptions, thoughts, and beliefs (Kazdin, 1979). The theoretical, clinical, and practical aspects of these trends have all been important in facilitating the development and use of short-term psychotherapeutic techniques.

Significant advances in the classification of mental health problems have been both a consequence of, and an encouragement to, the development of a broader therapeutic armamentarium. The delineation of specific sexual problems and the differentiation of agoraphobia into panic attacks and anticipatory anxiety, for example, have assisted in demonstrating that the use of short-term therapeutic contact is not only feasible but may, at times, be preferable.

An essential element in many of the recently developed short-term dynamic psychotherapies is their stress on the development of a clear formulation of a patient's core conflict and the notion that one can focus on that conflict and work in an active and dynamically oriented way to resolve it. In fact, Judd Marmor, in a 1979 paper on short-term dynamic psychotherapy, showed that some of the earliest psychoanalytic treatments were actually rendered in a very short time period by Freud himself. Dr. Marmor noted that Bruno Walter, the conductor, described a successful, six-session therapeutic experience with Freud in 1906. He further pointed out that Gustave Mahler's potency problem with his wife was apparently relieved in a single, four-hour session with Freud in 1908. The debate in the psychodynamic field has continued for years regarding the acceptable degree of deviation from strict psychoanalytic technique. It has been only relatively recently that a number of professionals in the field have promoted the use of short-term dynamic psychotherapy.

Underscoring these advances is the careful selection of candidates deemed appropriate for these treatments. Selection is based on specific criteria and the recognition that there are still substantial segments of those in need who require a longer term therapeutic relationship. In general, though, our ability to differentiate types of problems, sector off specific areas of functioning of individuals, and tailor our treatments to the specificity of those problems has been a catalyst in stimulating the field of brief treatment.

Related to the advances in the classification of disorders and the tailoring of particular treatments to them is the concern that long-term intensive treatments may fail to meet the needs of particular segments of the population. One of the principal findings of the President's Commission on Mental Health was the fact that there were many unserved, underserved, and inappropriately served groups. It is known that minorities are not being seen in mental health settings at rates appropriate to their need. The reasons for this certainly include problems related to the nature of the available professional personnel in the mental health field, but there have also been concerns in some segments of the minority community about the appropriateness of the typical treatments offered by the mental health providers. Some observers feel that when minorities receive appropriate preparation prior to entering longer term treatments, they are more likely to complete treatment and to ultimately benefit from treatment as much as majority populations. Still, segments of the minority community do not perceive long-term psychiatric treatment as desirable, useful, or relevant to their needs.

The elderly are known to be at high risk for a variety of mental disorders. Despite the fact that they comprise only 10% of the population, they account for 25% of the suicides in this country. They are also seen in mental health service settings in far fewer numbers than their needs would seem to require. This statement can also be made with regard to the population of children and youth. It would appear that a broad range of treatments, including brief treatments, might be far more appropriate for some of the disorders with which these populations present.

Yet another group which has been identified as underserved includes people with chronic mental disorders who require aftercare following their discharge from inpatient psychiatric settings. A focus on supportive treatments and relatively reasonably spaced, continuing treatment contacts would seem to be more appropriate for large segments of that community than intensive long-term therapy.

It is also instructive to look at the actual behavior of patients in terms of their utilization of mental health services. A large number of people come for outpatient treatment for only a relatively short period of time. Naturally, some may terminate for a variety of reasons other than a successful conclusion of the therapy. In many instances, however, it is likely that people secure their help in a limited number of treatment sessions. Data from outpatient clinics in the state of Connecticut in 1978 showed that for those patients about whom there is information, over 85% concluded their therapeutic contact within 24 sessions. A 1975 survey indicated that the median number of visits for all mental disorders treated in organized outpatient psychiatric services in the United States was 3.7, and the majority of patients concluded their treatment within 20 visits (NIMH, 1975). Generally, though, the average number of visits in private psychiatric practice is somewhat larger (26 visits for nonanalysts) (Marmor, 1975).

Thus, the behavior of patients, perhaps often in actual collaboration with their therapists, indicates that they frequently have relatively brief treatment contacts. Moreover, it is likely that there are many instances in which people leave treatment prematurely or do not come at all, because they have the impression that psychiatric treatment must be extensive and sustained. Were they to know that useful and effective treatment could be made available at an affordable cost and within a limited period of time, it is probable that larger numbers of people would be more comfortable about both coming for service and staying to its conclusion.

Increasing public attention has been drawn to the burgeoning costs of medical care. Concern about costs has also been a continually potent factor in discussions of mental health and in reimbursement of mental health services. This concern has had an impact on the use of brief treatment techniques. The worry has been repeatedly expressed that full coverage of mental health treatments would break the bank. In August 1978, hearings in the Senate Finance Committee focused on the question of Medicare and Medicaid reimbursement of psychosocial treatments. Witnesses gave dramatically contradictory testimony to a committee concerned about finding ways of economizing anywhere it could in the health field while still delivering quality health care.

In fact, when one examines the actual costs of insurance coverage, the concern that mental health coverage will break the bank does not seem justified. Lowering the obstacles of a financial nature in mental health may cause some initial increase in utilization rate for psychiatric services, but these rates level off and then remain relatively stable. Examples of such experiences are the high-option Blue Cross/Blue Shield program operating under the Federal Employee Health Benefits Program and the United Auto Workers Health Insurance Program.

In Marshfield, Wisconsin, for example, a general health plan, which at first had limited mental health services because of the fear of escalating costs, has recently been modified to eliminate the arbitrary limits and simultaneously introduce a peer review system. This change occurred as a result of the accumulation of data revealing that if the needs for care were met in an appropriate and effective way, the costs would be quite reasonable and patients would be properly served. Moreover, a recent analysis (GLS Associates, 1979) of state programs which mandate mental health benefits under private health insurance plans suggests that mental health coverage may not be viewed by state and local settings as being as uncontrollable and unpredictable as some people fear. As of December 1978, 20 states had enacted some form of private mental health insurance mandate, and 9 additional states had legislation forthcoming during 1979.

The pressure to expand access to mental health care has coexisted with pressures to control the costs of this care. Both these factors have clearly had major impact on the development and use of brief therapy techniques, which, when used appropriately, offer broader availability of scarce mental health resources in a cost-effective manner.

Not unrelated to concerns about the costs of health care have been the federal enthusiasm for health maintenance organizations and the resultant growth of various prepaid health plans around the country. This has had a significant impact on the development of the field of brief therapy. The availability of such specific, time-limited techniques, which would be cost effective and fit easily within the 20 visit outpatient limitation of most HMO plans, has been generally greeted enthusiastically by mental health providers employed by HMOs. A recent Group Health Association of America medical directors meeting in October 1979 focused specifically on the development of mental health services in these settings, and the application of brief treatments was an important focus.

It should be noted, though, that there have been questions regarding the quality of mental health care in some HMOs. They have addressed such issues as whether these systems rely too strongly on economic considerations and consequently fail to deliver an appropriate range of treatment, and whether they provide the same quality of care to all patients, for example, chronic patients. The work done at the Harvard Community Health Plan and other HMOs has been significant in demonstrating that high-quality, cost-effective care can be delivered in these settings.

This is certainly not an exclusive set of reasons for the increasing popularity of brief treatments. The combination of a broad and complex array of theoretical contributions, scientific advances, political and social forces, legislative developments, and real economic and resource constraints have all contributed to development and use of such treatments. Furthermore, the implications of the development of brief treatment are significant and are closely aligned with the development of the mental health field in general. They point toward a number of future strategies for the evolution of the mental health treatment system.

FUTURE IMPLICATIONS OF THE DEVELOPMENT OF BRIEF TREATMENTS

There is likely to be a continued expansion of the therapeutic armamentarium, along with further refinement and sophistication in the use of treatments. There is a need to develop more knowledge about which treatments work most effectively for which particular set of patients with what specific set of problems. The matching of specific short-term psychotherapeutic strategies along personality and developmental variables has already been suggested in the work of Burke, White, and Havens (1979) and in their contribution to this volume (Chapter 9).

This is important not only within the selection of psychotherapy itself, but also with regard to the combining of therapeutic modalities and techniques for the care of a single patient. For example, the work done by Klerman, DiMascio, Weissman, Prusoff, and Paykel (1974) on the complementary contributions of psychotherapy and psychopharmaco-therapy for ambulatory patients with depression is an outstanding proto-type of progress in conceptualizing and refining the use of simultaneous-ly administered therapeutic regimens.

In the pharmacotherapy area, people are working on maximizing the potency and specifity of the treatment agents while finding ways of minimizing the side effects. New treatments will be developed for those not helped by existing treatments. For example, lithium is ostensibly beneficial to some 70% of patients with manic–depressive disease; re-searchers are now focusing on the 30% of the population who do not benefit from such treatment. Such improvements in treatment techniques are likely to occur in the psychosocial area as well, with short-term tech-niques hopefully leading the way.

Policy makers have recently been raising very serious questions about the safety and efficacy, as well as the cost, quality, specificity, and appropriateness, of the various psychotherapies. While much of the pres-sure for answering such questions has been brought by forces outside the field (including some of the same factors that influenced the develop-ment of short-term therapies), these questions, in many ways, represent a series of welcome challenges to those within the field and have important implications for brief treatment techniques. The first of these challenges is to review systematically what is known about the efficacy of psycho-therapy as well as its negative side effects. Next, there is the challenge of appropriately refining the questions asked and developing plans to answer them.

A number of careful reviews of the current state of the art of assess-ing psychotherapies support the conclusion that a wide range of psy-chological therapies appear to be effective in achieving results superior to those achieved with no treatment procedures. The work of Meltzoff and Kornreich (1970), Luborsky, Singer, and Luborsky (1975), and Parloff, Wolfe, Hadley, and Waskow (1978) offer excellent reviews, which are supportive of the notion of the general effectiveness of psychotherapy.

A recent review by Smith, Glass, and Miller (1980) summarized ap-proximately 475 studies, each of which included an untreated group. It was found that in almost 90% of the studies, the psychotherapy group improved more than the control group. The median person receiving psy-chotherapy was better off than 80% of the untreated subjects. The authors concluded that their survey of research findings overwhelmingly validated the benefit of psychotherapy.

At the same time, it has also been noted that these psychotherapies are not totally benign. Inappropriately applied techniques or certain combinations of therapists' personal qualities and skills and patients' dispositions and sensitivities may result in negative side effects (Strupp, Hadley, & Gomes-Schwartz, 1977).

The work of meeting the second challenge has just begun, but simply placing these issues in a public forum has had the salutory effect of bringing psychotherapy research more firmly into the mainstream of science. Research attention is shifting away from such general questions as whether psychotherapy works and away from the search for the "best therapy." Instead, the focus is now turning toward examining which specific interventions administered by which types of therapists are most effective in reaching which specific treatment goals with which specific kinds of patients. There is also a need for research to examine the nature and importance of both specific and nonspecific factors in the process of psychotherapy. These efforts can be advanced by a continuing elaboration and refinement of brief treatment techniques. Such treatments also have the potential for use as a kind of laboratory for careful and systematic study of the process of psychotherapy.

There are also important implications for the role of brief treatments in the interface between mental health and general health. It has become increasingly apparent that a major portion of the mental health care in this country is provided by the general health care sector. Recent data by Dr. Darrel Regier and his colleagues (Regier, Goldberg, & Taube, 1978) indicated that while at least 15% of the American population suffers from a mental disorder of a temporary or long-term nature every year, only 21% receive specialty mental health services. Almost 55% of these people receive services solely through the general health care sector.

At the same time, there have been a growing recognition of the whole range of psychological, social, and behavioral concomitants of specific medical diseases and an awareness that particular patterns of behavior may predispose people to certain illnesses. Clearly, optimal treatment and a holistic approach to medical care call for a comprehensive program to address the social, behavioral, and psychological factors as well as the physiological processes.

Unfortunately, it is unclear how frequently such comprehensive formulations of, and interventions for, health care problems are actually implemented. Therapeutic compliance has been recognized as a serious problem that pervades the entire health care arena. It is estimated that as many as 50% of patients disregard advice given by health providers (Ley, Whitworth, & Skilback, 1976). Studies (Goldberg, 1979) also suggest that general health practitioners are not sufficiently sensitive to identifying people with psychiatric disorders. Moreover, even when such disorders are identified, serious questions have been raised as to general health providers' use of, knowledge about, and proficiency in various interventions, both psychopharmacologic and psychotherapeutic (Balter, 1973; Goldberg, 1978; Wheatly, 1973).

At the same time, however, the benefits of linking mental health treatments to general health care are being amply demonstrated. Schlesinger, Mumford, and Glass (1980) recently surveyed and analyzed the literature in regard to the effects of psychotherapeutic interventions on various medical problems. Their findings indicated that in each of the areas studied (asthma, alcoholism, and recovery from medical crisis), psychotherapy or psychologically informed interventions have a clearly positive effect. Their findings also indicated that there may be a substantial cost benefit as a result of the provision of these mental health services.

This has been further supported by a series of studies, known as "offset studies," which have examined the effect of the inclusion of mental health services programs on the use and cost of general health services, usually in an organized-care setting. These studies suggest that offering mental health services reduces the overall utilization of nonmental health services and also reduces their cost. In a recent supplement to *Medical Care,* Jones and Vischi (1979) reviewed 13 such studies and found a median reduction of 20% in medical care utilization. Thus, in terms of both quality and cost of care, there have been important benefits identified in linking mental health treatments to general health care.

The availability of brief treatments and the possibility of educating general health practitioners in their delivery can be an important part of a strategy to bring appropriate mental health treatment to general health settings, where the largest part of the population is actually served. Furthermore, brief treatment offers a useful tool with which both mental health practitioners and some non-mental-health practitioners in general health care settings can provide a more appropriate kind of treatment and even reduce some of the financial waste within the overall health care system.

In looking toward the future, it seems that the growth and refinement of the treatment armamentarium, the combination of different treatment components to develop tailored therapeutic regimens, the emphasis on the assessment of therapeutic modalities, and the increasing collaboration and linkage between mental health and general health, all constitute major trends within the system that are integrally linked to, and supportive of, the future growth and development of brief treatment techniques. These kinds of efforts promise benefits in ensuring that patients more regularly receive what is in their best interests to receive. They should also ensure that the patients' and the public's money is more likely to be effectively and well spent. They impress upon people outside the mental health field the value and impact of mental health treatments. Ultimately, they should make it more likely that the reimbursement of mental health services will be expanded and that greater support will be given for longer term treatments when knowledgeable clinicians indicate that such treatments are best for a specific group of patients.

The mental health field started with little before the 1940s and underwent an enormous boom and expansion in the '50s and '60s. The field overpromised, it overstated its capacity, and it tended to suggest, in a relatively indiscriminate fashion, that its interventions were helpful and appropriate for everyone. There is now a new opportunity, albeit at a time of much greater conservatism within the country. Not only is the focus on brief treatment important in terms of the technological advance it represents; it is essential to an evolving mental health system that will incorporate more in the way of specificity, differentiation of its interventions, sober assessment of its likely products, and, as a result, broader endorsement of support throughout the society. Thus, brief treatment has to be seen in this broader context and has to be recognized as offering opportunities for better care for patients of all ages and cultures throughout this country.

REFERENCES

Balter, M. B. An analysis of psychotherapeutic drug consumption in the United States. *Anglo-American Conference on Drug Abuse: Etiology of Drug Abuse*, 1973, *I*, 58–65.

Burke, J. D., White, H. S., & Havens, L. L. Which short-term therapy? Matching patient and method. *Archives of General Psychiatry*, 1979, *36*, 177–186.

GLS Associates. *Final report: Analysis of state programs which mandate mental health benefits under private health insurance*. Submitted under NIMH Contract #278-78-0040(MH), 1979.

Goldberg, D. Mental health priorities in a primary care setting. *Annals of the New York Academy of Sciences*, 1978, *310*, 65–68.

Goldberg, D. Training family physicians in mental health skills: Implications of recent research findings. In *Mental health services in general health care.* Washington, D.C.: National Academy of Sciences, Institute of Medicine, 1979.

Jones, K. R., & Vischi, T. R. Impact of alcohol, drug abuse, and mental health treatment on medical care utilization: A review of the research literature. *Medical Care,* 1979, *17* (suppl.), 1–82.

Kazdin, A. E. Fiction, factions and functions of behavior therapy. *Behavior Therapy,* 1979, *10,* 629–654.

Klerman, G. L., DiMascio, A., Weissman, M., Prusoff, B., & Paykel, E. S. Treatment of depression by drugs and psychotherapy. *American Journal of Psychiatry,* 1974, *131,* 186–191.

Ley, P., Whitworth, M. A., & Skilback, C. E. Improving doctor–patient communication in general practice. *Journal of the Royal College of General Practitioners,* 1976, *26,* 720–724.

Luborsky, L., Singer, B., & Luborsky, L. Comparative studies of psychotherapies. *Archives of General Psychiatry,* 1975, *32,* 995–1008.

MacIver, J., & Redlich, F. C. Patterns of psychiatric practice. *American Journal of Psychiatry,* 1959, *115,* 692–697.

Marmor, J. Short-term dynamic psychotherapy. *American Journal of Psychiatry,* 1979, *136,* 149–155.

Marmor, J., Scheidemandel, P. L., & Kanno, C. K. *Psychiatrists and their patients: A national study of private office practice.* Washington, D.C.: Joint Information Service of the American Psychiatric Association and the National Association for Mental Health, 1975.

Meltzoff, J., & Kornreich, M. *Research in psychotherapy.* New York: Atherton Press, 1970.

National Institute of Mental Health, Division of Biometry and Epidemiology. Unpublished data, 1975.

Parloff, M., Wolfe, B., Hadley, S., & Waskow, I. *Assessment of psychosocial treatment of mental disorders, current status and prospects.* Report to the National Academy of Sciences, Institute of Medicine, Washington, D. C., 1978.

President's Commission on Mental Health. *Report to the President.* Washington, D.C.: U. S. Government Printing Office, 1978.

Redlich, F. C., & Kellert, S. R. Trends in American mental health. *American Journal of Psychiatry,* 1978, *135,* 22–28.

Regier, D. A., Goldberg, I. D., & Taube, C. A. The de facto U. S. mental health service system. *Archives of General Psychiatry,* 1978, *35,* 685–693.

Schlesinger, H. J., Mumford, E., & Glass, G. V. *Mental health services and medical utilization.* Paper presented at the annual meeting of the American Association for the Advancement of Science, San Francisco, January 1980.

Smith, M. L., Glass, G. V., & Miller, T. I. *The benefits of psychotherapy.* Baltimore: Johns Hopkins University Press, 1980.

State of Connecticut Department of Mental Health, Statistics Section. *Outpatient psychiatric clinics in Connecticut.* Hartford: Author, 1978.

Strupp, H. H., Hadley, S. W., & Gomes-Schwartz, G. *Psychotherapy for better or worse: The problem of the negative effects in psychotherapy.* New York: Jason Aronson, 1977.

Wachtel, P. L. *Psychoanalysis and behavior therapy: Toward an integration.* New York: Basic Books, 1977.

Wheatly, D. *Psychopharmacology in medical practice.* New York: Appleton-Century-Crofts, 1973.

SECTION I
INDIVIDUAL BRIEF THERAPY:
DYNAMIC MODELS

CHAPTER 3
THE CORE OF TIME-LIMITED PSYCHOTHERAPY: TIME AND THE CENTRAL ISSUE

James Mann

Since the publication of *Time-Limited Psychotherapy* (Mann, 1973), continuing experience with this treatment method, further reflection on the process, and the stimulation resulting from the many questions raised by various audiences in the course of presentation of this treatment modality have served to refine and further define its theoretical basis, the nature of the process, and the critical principles that constitute its core. The critical principles are the conscious and unconscious meaning and influence of time and the particular method that I have devised for arriving at what I call the central issue. The central issue, in this instance, means understanding the underlying meaning of the complaints that patients bring to us and then using that understanding as a guiding principle throughout the course of treatment, from its start to the final session.

There are certain commonalities in all forms of brief psychotherapy:

1. Attention is directed to one focal issue (Small, 1971; Wolberg, 1965). Some kind of focus is established from the data provided by the patient.
2. Generally, the focal issue is apt to be one that is posed by the patient as the reason for coming for help.
3. Therapy is often directed at clarifying feelings, ideas, and behavioral manifestations in the current situation.
4. Transference may or may not be utilized. In some of the brief therapies, the use of transference is specifically ignored. In others, only those aspects of positive transference needed to

JAMES MANN. Division of Psychiatry, Boston University School of Medicine, Boston, Massachusetts.

maintain a supportive and encouraging atmosphere are used (Small, 1971).

5. The general atmosphere in the brief therapies tends to be one of crisis. It is my position, however, that except for rare instances, such as overwhelming multiple catastrophic events, all crises are exacerbations of chronic crisis states. Thus, it is important to differentiate so-called crisis intervention from any kind of more formally structured brief therapy. In crisis intervention, the aim is to restore, as far as possible, the equilibrium that preceded the acutely dysphoric state; this is done by providing for abreaction, reassuring the patient counseling with more or less direct guidance, and bringing to bear specific community resources to relieve the crisis. The intervention may include as few as one session, and perhaps up to five or six, without exerting any particular effort toward relieving the dynamic and genetic factors and forces that have induced the particular decompensation.

6. In the brief therapies, the duration of treatment may vary from as little as one session to as many as one or two sessions each week for as long as a year. The duration usually varies between 20 and 40 sessions, with the sense that when the patient feels that enough has been accomplished, treatment is over. In any case, the definition of what constitues brief therapy becomes self-defined by each therapist and relates directly either to the nature of his own training or to his particular concept of time.

The model of time-limited psychotherapy, which I have devised and refined over a period of some 12 years, is clearly differentiated from other modes of brief psychotherapy, in that it employs a specific structural framework with a precise, predetermined goal and a predetermined time limit that is the same in each case. In this chapter, I review some of the concepts of time that relate to therapy and then indicate how this manner of regarding time becomes a bridge to the formulation of the central issue, which itself also carries both implicit and explicit reference to time. Case illustrations and a variety of central issues serve to illuminate the discussion.

In a single chapter, it is possible only to detail highlights; the strategies and tactics of the actual treatment process cannot be included. A full exposition of the theory, case selection, process, and practice will be published separately (Mann, 1981).

THE IMPORTANCE OF TIME

A relatively simple way of thinking about time is to consider it as the way we integrate in our minds and in our feelings what was, what is, and what will be. At any given moment, we may consciously find ourselves thinking and feeling about a circumstance that exists at that moment. Unconsciously, we cannot restrict our thoughts or feelings to that particular moment. Events or moments that are significant to us evoke memories. We are usually not aware of this evocation of memory, because we have reasons not to remember, and whatever reasons we have for not remembering are reinforced by one or another or a number of defense mechanisms of the ego. Memories are intimately related to important people in our lives and cannot be separated from time and its meaning to us. For example, when we take a psychiatric history, or when we continue with the patient in therapeutic interviews, our efforts aim at linking time and expanding time. As we review and pick up threads of the patient's past, present, and future, we are expanding the patient's awareness of time past, present, and future. In fact, in all psychological treatment, the mutual work of patient and therapist has, as its general goal, the possibility for the patient to face up to his or her past, so as to gain some mastery over the present and be freer to determine the future. So long as we are, in a conscious state, unencumbered by the influence of any substance that alters our state of consciousness, it is impossible to escape the strictures of time. There can be no fixed moment in time, since each moment of time includes past, present, and future.

There are many ways that we employ to escape the strictures of time. We go off on holidays not only to escape responsibilities but also to escape the pressures of time. The predinner cocktail or two serve to relax us but also give us the sense that time has slowed. Whatever helps us feel relaxed also makes us feel that the pressure of time has been diminished. We take refuge from time by going to sleep; in fact, one of the common signs of depression is the escape to the bed. One of the prominent effects of marijuana is the slowing of time, sometimes to what seems to be incredible lengths. The widespread use of antianxiety drugs for the induction of relaxation, which accompanies the lessening of anxiety, makes them additionally attractive, because they, too, make us feel less pressured by time. Meditation practices provide an escape from time. The use of a steady, rhythmic, monotonous word or phrase or mantra removes us from awareness of what awaits outside of ourselves; one of the elements

we are seeking to divest is that of time. In the Benson method of relaxation (Benson, Kotch, Crassweller, & Greenwood, 1977), for example, the
meditator is advised not to use any kind of alarm to inform the scheduled
amount of time, lest he or she break and interrupt the purpose of the
method.

In mystic or ecstatic states, connections between past, present, and
future are broken, so that time is unending, an eternity. In fragmentation
states, such as depersonalization, derealization, or acute psychotic decompensation, connections between past, present, and future are also
broken, with the crucial difference that in these states, time is without
meaning and is experienced as empty. In some LSD experiences, time is
also experienced as endless, either as a state of intense pleasure or its
opposite, a state of intense pain. In our work with psychotic patients who
are in a fragmented state, we are very much aware of the pain that they
are experiencing amidst the emptiness that they feel. I have described my
experience with the analysis of so-called golden memories in a number of
patients in analysis (Mann, 1973). These memories convey a great sense
of the golden warmth of sunlight; they cannot be located in time or space
but are laden with familiarity. They have the meaning of the early
mother and of the wish to be comforted, warmed, and endlessly nurtured. I remind you of the horrible mass murder and suicide in Jonestown, where Jim Jones is said to have cried, "Mother, Mother," as he
and the hundreds of others lay dying.

If I were to choose a single element that seems to best mark the present era, I would say that it is the dizzyingly swift pace of time. The fan-
tastically swift means for communication and travel since World War II
have, in fact, shattered the more or less steady, progressive changes in
communication and travel that had been evolving over the past hundred
years. In impressive ways, we have now conquered time and space in
categorical, objective terms. These triumphs clearly carry over into the
subjective life in rather unanticipated ways. For example, this has become evident to us not only in the enormous inflation of the diagnostic
category of narcissistic personality or narcissistic character disorder, in
which the demands of the "I" for immediate gratification create great
therapeutic trials, but also in people's clear demands for instant gratification. Instant cures are demanded for emotional illness, physical disease, economic problems, and all social ills. It is as though we are, more
than ever, captives of time, which, in collaboration with the narcissistic
demands that reside in all of us—in some, more, and in some, less—

speaks to the close relationship that may exist between the objective awareness of time and the subjective or psychological awareness of time. It may well be that the current, heightened interest in brief therapies incorporates some of this narcissistic demand.

I am suggesting that man's responsiveness to explosive changes in his total environment includes a reaction that is synchronous with the very nature of the particular explosive change itself. We experience time as speeding up, so that delaying gratification appears to become increasingly difficult. Man is a remembering creature, and his memories are insolubly linked to people of importance to him in the past. Responses to people in his present are thoroughly infused with the images, memories, and affects attached to past important objects. Screen memories, amnesias, and the contraction of time in dreams and in fantasy are typically part of one's time experience. The phenomena of transference repeatedly display thoughts, feelings, and behavior which at one time speak to the past, at another to the present, then to the future, and at times to all three in the one moment. Time is unceasing, and every moment of time includes past, present, and future. This concept of time suggests that it is not a matter of succession, but rather a reciprocal relationship, in which one time mode cannot be experienced or even thought about without the other.

Time sense, its vicissitudes, and the constant relationship between time and memories point to the indissoluble connection between time and the nature of early object relations. From this we can understand that the experience of time is always accompanied by affect. The more painful and conflictual a memory is in respect to some particular personal event, the more the person will defend against and repress the affect that belongs to the memory.

This is especially evident clinically in patients diagnosed as obsessive–compulsive characters. The compulsive adherence to the demands of time (or its opposite, the compulsive need to ignore time) contributes to the excessively orderly or disorderly conduct of everyday life. In such instances, our work demands major effort in helping the patient come to know and feel the affects that have been isolated from the action taken in consonance with the felt demands of time. In both cases, there is an unusually visible unconscious imprisonment surrounding the meaning of time. Ordinarily, time is experienced as a background presence. We know that it is always there, but it does not interfere with ongoing experience. The greater the invasion of time into consciousness, the more likely the presence of some psychopathological state. In depressed patients, there is an overwhelming sense of everything being past, so that there is no present, and a future appears impossible. In the opposite state, the manic episode, time past, present, and future rush upon the patient without surcease, so that there is no day or night, no moment of rest, and there is only the unceasing barrage of the present.

Anxiety states raise concerns about future uncertainties, a fear of what may happen. The nature of the fear is unconscious, while the experience of fear is conscious and has a distinctly future orientation. The time element is present in the experience of guilt, so that it becomes necessary to distinguish between feelings of conscience, which judge the past, and guilt feelings, which warn about the future. There are guilt feelings in which the person is remorseful about some past occurrence (I should not have done or said that), and there are guilt feelings which strike pangs about the future (I should do this or I should not do that).

In contrast to other medical specialties, we are explicit about the issue of selling our time to our patients. We give patients specific appointment hours, which are usually honored rather punctually by both participants. Moreover, the patients know exactly how much time they will have for the work to be done in each visit. Therapists operate with a conscious set of conditions in regard to their time but tend to ignore the conscious and unconscious meaning and experience of time in their patients as well as in themselves. In long-term treatment, both patient and therapist cannot help but experience treatment as timeless, and neither of the two parties tends to pay much attention to the matter of time. Most often, time becomes a lively dynamic of the treatment process only when the question of termination is raised. In other instances, the importance of time may arise in connection with financial difficulties in paying for treatment, impending vacations of the therapist, the patient's consideration of a move to another city, or resistance to the treatment process.

In long-term treatment, patients' only reaction to the meaning and experience of time may be found in their unconscious fantasies in respect to the magical expectations of early, long-wished-for needs. A common fantasy is that treatment will bring patients everything they have wished for and never gotten, as well as everything they wished to be and never were. All short forms of psychotherapy implicitly propose a time limitation. Unless patients know *in advance* the duration of their treatment, however, they enter the process with the fantasy that treatment will be timeless, and the question of time will surface again only when termination, for whatever reason, is brought up. I am not proposing that all patients in psychotherapy should or even can be informed in advance. I do believe that the role of time can be most significantly revealed in any short form of psychotherapy if therapists direct their attention to it.

The greater the ambiguity as to the duration of treatment, the greater the influence of regressive, infantile, dependent wishes. The unconscious fantasy that treatment will bring with it fulfillment of certain important childhood desires is accompanied by a regression in time sense. The persistence of these wishes, enhanced by the felt timelessness of the treatment, becomes, in effect, the expectation that the therapist will *turn back time*. This is true of any therapeutic modality: of psychotherapy, psychoanalysis, psychopharmacology, and the varieties of behavior modification.

The greater the specificity in respect to the duration of treatment, the more rapidly are the infantile fantasies confronted with the realities of the adult, of real time, and of the work that must be done. To state this in another way, at the point at which a patient sufficiently overcomes his anxiety about what may happen and begins to establish a therapeutic or working alliance, he unconsciously achieves an affective return to an important early person or persons; an impressive degree of separation anxiety, always present, is temporarily relieved in the union with the therapist. Separation from the therapist rapidly becomes an important center of attention at such times as the therapist's vacation, illness, or absence for any reason. It is well documented that at such times, certain vulnerable patients become psychotic or suicidal, while less disturbed patients suffer degrees of anxiety and depression; all of these are reactions to the issue of separation and the melange of chaotic feelings it arouses, ranging from feeling deprived of vital, life-giving nurturance at one extreme to feeling punished for forbidden Oedipal wishes at the other. In effect, then, any psychotherapy, long or short, becomes for the patient an attempt at reunion and a battle against separation. The child in the adult keeps the battle alive, while we therapists depend upon our clinical assessment of the patient's functioning ego to inform us whether we will have a strong or weak ally in helping the patient eventually come to terms with rejecting union and accepting separation. This never occurs without tears, since separation is never achieved unambivalently in any instance, normal or abnormal.

In states of health, one does not *feel* the passage of time: there is no sense of one's growing older or old. In happy times, time moves ever so swiftly. People who come to us for help are in pain not unlike the pain that is felt in states of physical disease. For them, time is a felt presence and moves so very slowly and painfully.

Confining our attention to those who come to us for help, we know that in each instance, patients feel themselves to be confronted with some kind of challenging reality, outside or within themselves, to which their attention has become fixed. The challenge which they experience is not new in its unconscious and symbolic meaning to the patient, and therefore the challenge is and has been a recurrent one. How patients assess a value on their ongoing, lived time is determined by the manner in which they perceive their own state of adequacy in the face of that recurrent challenge. In such situations, the ego perceives a danger that must be met and managed in order to maintain a state of well-being as well as to keep alive one's needs and aspirations. In the face of the challenge, the question arises within the individual as to how and whether he or she can cope with it. The question will be answered on the basis of past experience, and if the answer involves fear about one's adequacy, or if the conviction is present that one *is* inadequate, then the tension that arises within the ego is experienced as anxiety, depression, or both. Which will be present will be determined by the ego's orientation in time, that is, by the assessment of one's adequacy as having a potential, a future, or by the assessment that one's adequacy is past and does not have a future. The sense of a potential leads to the mobilization of anxiety toward the end of facing the danger and mastering it. The sense of inadequacy leads to depression, with the feeling of helplessness, hopelessness, or both. In most instances, a degree of certainty and uncertainty is present, so that we see most often a mixture of anxiety and depression. From this point of view, we may understand that patients who come to us for help are saying that they are variably uncertain as to whether or not they have a future. Profoundly depressed patients, convinced that they have no future, would not be considered suitable patients for any kind of brief psychotherapy. In any case, questions about one's future are present, and affects attached to one's past, present, and future are calling for resolution.

It is this intimate connection between time and affects that becomes the bridge between time and the central issue, which we will extract from the patient's history, and to which we shall attend throughout the treatment sessions.

DEFINING THE CENTRAL ISSUE

In all varieties of brief psychotherapy, an immediate risk is to come to some determination on the work to be done in the course of treatment. While this is true in all psychotherapies, long and short, as well as in psychoanalysis, it is particularly pertinent in any therapy in which time is implicitly and explicitly limited. Most often, what seems to be the patient's most pressing complaint or symptom is likely to become the focus of the treatment. It may be the patient's depression, anxiety, anger, delayed grief, phobia, somatic complaint, or a conflict with some designated person or persons. In time-limited psychotherapy, the central issue is designed to bypass defenses, control anxiety, and, at the same time, stimulate a rapid working alliance and positive transference.

In each case, of course, evaluation interviews become the means for determining the nature of the patient's problems. Careful and thorough history taking over a period of one to three interviews should provide sufficient information for this determination. In the historical data, we look for recurrent events which have been provocative of pain in the life of the patient. The recurrent events need not be similar factually, and usually they are not, but they will be similar symbolically and in the response of the patient to them. Single, nonrecurrent painful events in the life of the patient are not apt to be significant, unless the single event itself is of overwhelming intensity, as, for example, with victims of the holocaust. *The central issue is one that is linked with time sense and with the various affects that are attached to the particular patient's time line or history.* Therefore, we extract out of the historical data what we understand to be the patient's *present and chronically endured pain,* pain which is an affective statement by the patient to him or herself about how he or she feels and has always felt about the self. It is a statement that is preconscious; that is to say, it is a chronic feeling about the self that periodically flits into consciousness but is equally quickly suppressed, denied, and warded off from full awareness by bringing into use well-established coping devices. For example, there is the person whose feelings of unacceptability to others leads to the device of being constantly pleasing to others in the hope that acceptability will follow. Sensitivity to signs of rejection is always acutely present, but when such rejection is experienced by the person, the other person is never aware of the pain inflicted, since all he perceives may be a smiling, agreeable countenance. The felt pain is rapidly extinguished by the behavioral style and the immediate denial that any injury has occurred.

This method of formulating the central issue sharply differentiates what the patient brings to us as his or her complaints and what we will determine to be the center of both the patient's and the therapist's attention in the course of treatment. Here are several clinical examples:

A 55-year-old married man presented with the complaint of dissatisfaction with his present work and career, claiming that he had achieved all that could possibly be achieved and was looking for new worlds to conquer, in terms of starting some kind of new career. His achievements in his career to date had been widely recognized, and he appeared to be caught up in the somewhat popular movement for individuals to change directions in their 40s or 50s. He wanted some help in reviewing the pros and cons of his decision.

Two evaluation interviews brought to light a very different perspective. From childhood on, this man had struggled with the pain of a chaotic and ruptured family life, out of which he had emerged with intense feelings of shame and inferiority and a sense of being different. Possessed of great energy and high intelligence, he had fought his way successfully, despite repeated instances in which he reexperienced these same feelings about himself. At the time he came to see me, a series of personal and professional events, coinciding with pressures relating to his being in his mid-50s and questions about his continuing competence, had been sufficient to raise ever more intensely the same old feelings about himself. He was looking for a way out but with no awareness that his desire for a new career was anything more than a creative solution at the right time in his life.

The central issue that was posed as the work of treatment made no reference to the urgent questions that had brought him for help. Rather, it was stated as follows: "You are a man who has been enormously successful despite many serious difficulties. What hurts you now and has always been a source of hurt to you is the difference you feel between your public image and the private feelings that you have about yourself." He was in full agreement, and treatment ended with his awareness that a new career was an attempted flight, which would have been doomed to failure, since nothing within himself would have changed. He continued in his career with satisfaction.

A 48-year-old woman was beset with problems with her teen-age daughter. She recognized areas of friction between them and tried desperately but without success to find ways of managing the relationship better. The patient's history revealed an unusual amount of control exercised over her from her earliest years both by her parents and by others. She responded passively, despite intensely frightening fantasies; to the guilt engendered by her anger, she responded with a good deal of reaction formation in the form of being understanding and helpful to others. In her own adolescence she had never rebelled, and now, confronted by an adolescent daughter who had been reared in an atmosphere of understanding and helpfulness and was now typically rebellious, she felt herself to be at her wit's end.

The central issue extracted from the patient's history, that is, her present and chronically endured pain, was stated as follows: "You are a person who has been understanding and helpful to your children and to many others. You have always had the inner feeling, however, that you are like a puppet controlled by others, and as a result, you feel and have always felt helpless.'' How she came to feel this way about herself was the work of 12 treatment sessions.

In both these cases, the central issue revealed at least three very important elements:

1. Each had always felt and was continuing to feel victimized.
2. Each was continuing to live with something about the self that once was real and, although no longer real, was being sustained as a guiding fiction about the self.
3. *The central issue included time, affects, and the image of the self.*

It is this time-bound image of the self that brings a patient to us for help, an image that is obscured by a host of complaints, symptoms, character traits, and behavioral styles. The central issue formulated in this manner does not speak to the conflict of the patient with significant others and therefore does not give rise to automatic defense mechanisms. On the contrary, the patient feels that a painfully hidden part of the self—something which the patient has never fully allowed him-or herself to know, and which has always been a source of pain—has been brought to light in a most empathic and nonthreatening manner. This occurs in a setting which informs the patient that the therapist recognizes the patient's strenuous efforts to overcome the pain (which continues despite his or her best efforts), and that it is this pain that lies hidden behind the complaints or symptoms that bring him or her for help.

It is this kind of statement of the central issue that creates a tremendous sense of optimism in the patient that he can be helped and gives rise to a rapid working alliance and positive transference. Soon enough in the course of treatment, the conflict with significant others will come to full light. This will occur, however, in a setting of trust and positive transference, with markedly diminished necessity for the automatic use of the defense mechanisms that have been the usual armamentarium of the patient.

The central statement, as we formulate it, brings the therapist to the patient's side, as opposed to the ever present sense of being victimized by others. With the sense of optimism and the feeling of unity with the therapist, the childhood expectations of the patient are rekindled and with them, the unconscious experience of reunion with the early important person(s). All these factors, along with the predetermined time limit, set the stage for the rapid development of the therapeutic process. *The goal of time-limited psychotherapy is to foster, as much as possible, the resolution of the present and chronically endured pain, that is, the persistent negative self-image.* Symptom relief is a by-product of the process and not its goal. Some illustrative central issues:

- "You have tried very hard all your life, but what hurts you and has always hurt you is the feeling that you are stupid and a phony." (A 42-year-old woman who suffered an acute, disorganizing experience in conflict with her husband, whom she feels she should divorce.)

- "You seem to be a decent sort of man and you have tried to please others, yet you feel and have always felt that you are not wanted." (A 25-year-old man depressed and given to unpredictable and impulsive fights with his wife.)

- "You have succeeded in getting yourself to be different; nevertheless, you continue to feel that you are and have always been inferior and inadequate, a loser." (A 22-year-old woman depressed and having difficulty with her job superiors.)

- "You have had a very difficult time in your life, and you have struggled to meet those difficulties. In spite of your struggles, you feel and have always felt cheated and, as a result, helpless." (A 38-year-old man in serious, self-destructive conflict with his unfaithful wife.)

- "You are a big man who has achieved very successfully, and yet, when you are alone, you feel helpless." (A 35-year-old man with an acute phobia.)

Each of these statements of the central issue communicates a distinc. message to the patient. The first message consists of an acknowledgment that the therapist is aware of the patient's very real efforts to master the present and chronically endured pain. The second message reveals that the therapist knows that despite the patient's best efforts, the latter continues to feel the pain, which is verbalized in the very terms that the patient attributes to himself. In each instance, too, the therapist adds that the work of the therapy sessions will be devoted to a mutual exploration of how the patient came to feel this way about himself.

A comment about a patient's motivation for change would be appropriate here. In the absence of severe pathology (e.g., profound depression verging on or being psychotic or acute manic or schizophrenic decompensation), I take the position that all patients who present themselves are already motivated to seek help and to change. Whether the motivation will continue in treatment depends on *(a)* the extent to which the therapist recognizes the intense anxiety present in every instance of first contact, and *(b)* the therapist's skill in managing that anxiety, so that the ever present threat of the unknown, supported by a host of frightening, unconscious fantasies, is reduced to the point where the patient comes to feel a sense of hope.

The formulation of the central issue, as noted above, comes as a summation of the therapist's recognition of the patient's deeply felt anxiety. When the patient, for his part, recognizes that the therapist knows where the patient is at, there comes a sense of relief and hope. When added to this is the therapist's statement that "we will work together to find out how you came to feel this way about yourself," there is a further increment in the relief of anxiety.

> A 38-year-old man came with the presenting complaint of mounting anxiety. His history suggested strongly that he appeared to be in the process of developing a full-blown case of agoraphobia. His anxiety included the fear that unless he was helped, he might lose his job. He had never had psychiatric treatment and was clearly agitated when he asked if I had ever seen anything like his case before, and if there was any possibility of his being helped. In the second evaluation interview, he revealed another symptom of a very embarrassing and shameful kind. In both interviews, he sat rigidly at the edge of the chair, as through about to flee. The management of his anxiety was a constant at all times in the course of the interviews.
>
> Then came the statement of the central issue: "You are a man who has always been a scrapper. You have been successful and you are aware of your competence. What troubles and hurts you and always has, however, are the feelings about yourself as being small, inferior, and bad." His response was to relax in his chair, sit back, and say with a relieved sigh, "I guess that really sums it up."

In reviewing the varieties of central issues illustrated above, it may appear that there is a certain sameness about them or, as one thinks about it, a clear limitation in the ways that this kind of central issue can be formulated. This is more apparent than real, and an explanation is in order.

If the central issue is a statement of feelings about the self, then it follows that the varieties of chronic pain are limited by the range of feelings available to every human being. It is possible to list a series of major feelings and then to show that all other feelings are only gradations or synonyms for the major feeling. Thus, one might list five major feelings:

> *Glad:* loving, happy, contented, euphoric, peaceful, wanted
> *Sad:* unhappy, discontented, depressed, unwanted
> *Mad:* irritated, annoyed, irked, angry, furious, raging
> *Frightened:* anxious, nervous
> *Guilty:* troubled, uneasy, ashamed, humiliated

The range of fantasies available to the human mind is probably limitless; the range of feelings is limited and shared by all human beings. As a result, the chronic and presently endured pain can be identified in everyone, regardless of social class, education, and cultural background. Each life story is absolutely different, one from another, in the kinds of people involved and in the events that have transpired. Each life story is absolutely similar, however, insofar as one or another of the limited number of feelings shared by all people has been experienced by all. This method of extracting and formulating the central issue in time-limited psychotherapy also opens the gate to the psychotherapeutic treatment of those patients who are often described as unavilable for so-called talking treatment.

From the foregoing, it should be evident that the central issue in time-limited psychotherapy includes time, affects, and the image of the self. The consolidation of the patient's conflict in terms of time, affects, and the image of the self inevitably and rapidly evokes memories and the objects attached to the memories. As noted earlier, however, this occurs in a setting which diminishes defensiveness and encourages constructive exposure and exploration. It may be observed that the statement of the central issue is, in fact, the paradigm of the transference that will emerge in the course of treatment. This may be understood further by summarizing briefly the manner in which the treatment proposal is offered to the patient and the general response of the patient to the various phases of the treatment process.

The evaluation process ends at the point when the central issue has been formulated and presented to the patient. In most instances, the patient recognizes the validity of the central issue and acknowledges agreement. In a small number of cases, some objection or questions may be raised; these should be understood as arising out of response to the central issue. For example, a patient struggling with anxiety about being controlled may experience the incisiveness of the central isssue as evidence of the therapist's capacity to control and may automatically seek to shy away, often by expressing uncertainty as to whether the stated issue is really the problem. In such instances, I have found it useful to ask the patient if he or she can suggest some other problem that might be more pertinent or important than the one detailed in the central issue. The invariable response is that the patient cannot think of any more important problem just now.

With acknowledgment of the central issue, the patient is then offered a series of 12 treatment sessions, usually one each week, of 45 minutes' duration, with this session being the first, and the date of the 12th and final session specifically announced. It is also explained that the work of the 12 sessions will consist of determining how the patient came to feel this way about him- or herself. The patient is then asked for an agreement to the total proposal and is encouraged to raise questions about the plan.

A CASE EXAMPLE

Let us follow a case in which the central issue is formulated as follows: ''You have had many difficult times in your life, and you have struggled quite successfully with them; however, what hurts and has always hurt is your feeling that you have been cheated, and as a result, you feel helpless.''

The first phase of the treatment process (involving the initial three or four meetings) takes place in a setting of optimistic expectation. There is an unconscious revival of childhood wishes within a framework of reunion with early important person(s); this produces positive feelings and a relatively unambivalent positive transference. In this setting, the patient tends to pour out many details of his or her victimized past and present, and the abreaction that he or she experiences further reduces anxiety and fosters feelings of closeness to the therapist. It is usual for the patient to feel much better during this phase; symptomatic relief is to be expected. In effect, it is the patient's unconscious expectation that all the episodes and incidents in his or her life in which he or she has felt cheated and helpless to do anything about it will be undone.

The activity of the therapist during this treatment phase consists primarily of encouraging continuing exploration of the feelings about the victimized self. It is a time for the therapist to raise questions, request elaborations in respect to some particular aspect of the patient's story, and exercise disciplined curiosity around any information that the patient offers which appears to have a connection, consciously or unconsciously, to the stated central issue. In some instances, the patient moves rapidly on his or her own, so that minimal interference through questioning is required. In all other instances, exchanges between patient and therapist are active and, in the mind of the therapist, always with the central issue as the guide. The usual result is the accumulation of important past and present historical data, which the therapist will ''store'' for appropriate use later in the course of treatment.

In the second phase of the treatment process, roughly the middle third of the 12 sessions, signs of disappointment and ambivalence begin to appear in the words, feelings, and behavior of the patient. In the first place, nothing magical has occurred; the optimism of the initial phase begins to fade. Most importantly, the patient may become acutely aware of having come to the midpoint of the process, although he or she more often represses this awareness and responds as noted above. The midpoint promptly foreshadows an approaching end. The therapist, now heavily endowed and invested as a transference figure, is not only failing to change the patient's life, that is, the patient's renewed negative feelings about the self, but worse than that is moving to end the relationship on a predetermined date, which clearly is approaching.

This change in the patient's feelings about the therapist becomes another guidepost for the therapist in his or her understanding of the vicissitudes of the transference already posited by the central issue. The therapist acknowledges the patient's disappointment or discouragement, thereby gaining the opportunity for further exploration of these same kinds of feelings as they have arisen in the past and are arising in the continuing present in relation to people who were and are important to the patient. In allowing the patient the right to experience his or her ambivalence toward the therapist, the stage is being set for the further clarification of the ambivalence and its effects on the image of the self. It is with this growing ambivalence about the therapist that treatment comes to the crucial termination phase, the last third of the 12 sessions, of which the final 2 are most intense.

The central issue as the paradigm of the transference now becomes transparent. All the feelings about the self, which have arisen out of the felt experiences of being cheated and left in helpless rage, have been reproduced in relation to the therapist. The central issue and the time limit have influenced the therapeutic process in this direction. The patient now experiences *in vivo*, more or less acutely, the very same feelings which have given rise throughout his or her life to the negative, painful feelings about the self, feelings which eventually brought the patient to seek help. This is not an intellectual experience; the patient *feels cheated* and *feels helpless*, because no matter how hard he or she has worked in the treatment nor how much he or she cajoles or hopes, treatment will come to its appointed end. The therapist is experienced as the victimizer. If the therapist cared, he or she would fulfill the patient's wishes or, at the least, extend the treatment to some further point of possible fulfillment. The patient does not wish to be left, as he once felt himself to have been left.

In this highly affective setting, it becomes the therapist's task to help the patient to see clearly the transference nature of these inappropriate adult responses: *that which once was no longer is.* It is in this phase of treatment that active interpretations are made regarding the nature of the patient's feelings about the therapist, past significant figures, and persons important in the patient's present life. The intensely affective is now combined with the cognitive, and together with the internalized good figure of the therapist, join to make possible changes in the patient's self-perception. Expansion of the ego takes place and, with it, the capacity to separate from the therapist with a greater sense of independence, of autonomy, and therefore of the self. Concurrently, there is a lessening of the harsh demands of the superego, so that the patient comes to regard him- or herself more charitably than before.

THE TERMINATION PHASE

Much can be said about the activity of the therapist throughout the course of treatment. I shall confine myself, however, to the particular need for such activity during the termination phase, since it is at this time that all the data previously accumulated around the central issue are brought to bear in bringing the treatment to a successful conclusion, that is, resolving the present and chronically endured pain. Of particular importance is the response of the therapist to the end phase of treatment. Psychotherapists are not accustomed to the practice of setting predetermined termination dates; to do so may precipitate anxiety in the therapist. Anxiety of this kind generally has at least two sources: the personal feelings and responses of the therapist to separations, and the need of many therapists to encourage patients' dependence upon them.

In the termination phase, the resolution of the present and chronically endured pain involves the patient not only in coming to terms with those distorted aspects of his self-image, as stated in the central issue, but also, at the same time and in intimate connection, in bearing the pain of separation and loss. The intensely affective ambience of the treatment at this point reverberates equally intensely in the feelings of the therapist in regard to his or her own experiences with separation and loss and, in particular, the extent to which he or she has mastered those feelings reasonably successfully. All terminations of treatment are difficult for patient and therapist, even more so in time-limited psychotherapy. It is at this point that countertransference reactions will press toward a reluctance to fully face the termination process or even toward actions which will serve to continue the treatment and not bring it to its agreed-upon end. The patient is the major loser if this happens.

PATIENT SELECTION

There is much to be said about the selection of patients for time-limited psychotherapy. Suffice it to say here that with time and the special kind of central issue that I have described, a thorough understanding of the functions of the unconscious mind (e.g., defenses, resistance, transference) is a prime prerequisite for accurate diagnosis and prescription. Out of accurate diagnosis, one may come to a reasonably clear understanding of the patient's capacity to engage and disengage quickly (or, stated otherwise, the patient's capacity to tolerate separation and loss). Data in this regard are obtained in the careful evaluation process. Since no diagnostician is infallible, it is a source of comfort to know that if an improper selection has been made, this discovery will be very apparent within the first two or three, or at most four, sessions, and a change in treatment can be made. It should also be known that time-limited psychotherapy is not for the beginning therapist. It is difficult, intense, and moves very rapidly. Previous experience with long-term psychotherapy is an important prerequisite as is personal therapy, preferably psychoanalysis.

CONCLUSION

I shall conclude with this statement: Time-limited psychotherapy, with its time limitation and its particular method for selection of the central issue, cannot help but bring to the forefront of the treatment process the major pain that human beings suffer, namely, the wish to be as one with another but the absolute necessity to learn how to tolerate separation and loss without undue damage to one's feelings about the self.

REFERENCES

Benson, H., Kotch, J. B., Crassweller, K. D., & Greenwood, M. M. Historical and clinical considerations of the relaxation response. *American Scientist,* 1977, July–August, p. 441.

Mann, J. *Time-limited psychotherapy*. Cambridge: Harvard University Press, 1973.
Mann, J. *A casebook of time-limited psychotherapy*. New York: McGraw-Hill, 1981.
Small, L. *The briefer psychotherapies*. New York: Brunner/Mazel, 1971.
Wolberg, L. R. (Ed.). *Short term psychotherapy*. New York: Grune & Stratton, 1965.

CHAPTER 4
SHORT-TERM ANXIETY-PROVOKING PSYCHOTHERAPY: ITS HISTORY, TECHNIQUE, OUTCOME, AND INSTRUCTION

Peter E. Sifneos

Short-term anxiety-provoking psychotherapy, or STAPP, was first used at the Psychiatric Clinic of the Massachusetts General Hospital more than 20 years ago to treat a young male patient suffering from an acute onset of phobic symptoms, which suddenly appeared after he decided to get married. The psychodynamic formulation of his difficulties pointed to unresolved Oedipal conflicts. He was treated successfully in eight interviews, over a period of three months. In the follow-up interviews, held after the end of the treatment and several years later, it was clear that he had completely recovered from his neurotic problems. He was married and free of symptoms.

At that time, long-term psychotherapy was considered to be the treatment of choice for all patients suffering from neurotic difficulties. All efforts to shorten psychotherapy were frowned upon. This attitude followed the unsuccessful efforts of Ferenczi (1926) and Rank (1929) in the 1920s to use active techniques to improve interpretations and shorten psychoanalytic therapy. Later on, despite Alexander's ability in 1946 to demonstrate that short-term psychotherapy was valuable (Alexander & French, 1946), his point of view was also generally rejected. As a result of these prevailing difficulties, the patient waiting lists in psychiatric clinics all over the United States became progressively longer.

Encouraged by the successful results obtained from the treatment of

PETER E. SIFNEOS. Department of Psychiatry, Beth Israel Hospital and Harvard Medical School, Boston, Massachusetts.

our phobic patient, we decided to try to find patients with similar problems who could be treated in the same way. This search proved to be fruitful. Over a period of four years, 50 patients were treated with STAPP, and
21 of these were seen in follow-up interviews, 1 to 1½ years later. They all
seemed to have benefited considerably from their treatment. As a consequence of this study, we were able to streamline our selection criteria and
to specify what, in our opinion, seemed to be the technical interventions
which were responsible for these favorable results.

CRITERIA FOR SELECTION OF SUITABLE PATIENTS

The criteria for selection were the following:

1. A circumscribed chief complaint. This implied that the patient was
   able to choose only one of a variety of psychological difficulties,
   assign it top priority, and concentrate on its resolution during the
   therapy.
2. A history of "meaningful" (give-and-take, altruistic-type) relationships with another person during early childhood. The discovery, as a result of systematic history taking, that the patient could
   interact with another person and was willing to make a sacrifice for
   another person signified that he or she had passed the first test for
   good interpersonal relations.
3. An ability to interact flexibly with the evaluator during the initial
   interview.
4. An above average psychological sophistication and intelligence.
5. A high motivation to change.

The latter criterion seemed to have an important prognostic value for successful outcome, so we decided to use seven additional criteria to assess the
patient's motivation. Suffice it to say that the patient's motivation did not
imply a wish for relief of symptoms, but rather an interest on the part of
the patient to alter his or her lifestyle, to understand and to be rid, once
and for all, of his or her neurotic problems.

During the 1960s, we were able to see an increasingly larger number of
patients. By 1964, when we presented our findings at the International
Congress of Psychotherapy in London, we had treated more than 500 patients with STAPP. We finished a controlled study of STAPP in 1968, and
discussed our findings at the Ciba Foundation Research Conference (Sifneos, 1968).

Because the outcome findings continued to be encouraging, the need to perfect our technique and demonstrate it explicitly, for both teaching and research purposes, became imperative. We were lucky to be aided in the early 1970s by a technical device which was to revolutionize psychotherapy research and teaching—the video tape. For the first time in its history, psychiatry had its own "microscope". On the video screen, for all to see and judge, the patients could be presented before STAPP, during the course of it, and after its termination. The whole process of the therapy, interview after interview, could be scrutinized, its techniques demonstrated, and its results studied. A marvelous technical tool for the investigation of psychotherapy had finally become available to us, and STAPP, by virtue of its brief duration, could be studied scientifically. In addition, it offered us a unique opportunity to educate those who wanted to learn to practice this form of treatment.

TECHNIQUE

What, then, are the technical requirements for this kind of dynamic therapy of short duration, which has been studied, investigated, and perfected during the last decade at the Psychiatric Clinic of the Beth Israel Hospital in Boston? They include:

1. The delineation of a psychodynamic focus underlying the patient's psychological difficulties, which both the therapist and the patient agree to investigate during STAPP, is an important requirement. This focus becomes the main theme around which the treatment is centered, and its resolution over a short period of time becomes its aim.
2. The types of problems which are thought to be amenable to such a task include unresolved Oedipal difficulties, problems relating to separation issues, and grief reactions.
3. The establishment of a working alliance, which soon becomes therapeutic, is another important, early feature of the technique of STAPP.
4. The active use of anxiety-provoking confrontation and clarifications help the therapist deal with the patient's resistances.
5. The transference is dealt with explicitly and early.
6. The therapist avoids getting entangled in pregenital characterological issues which, while of minor importance in such therapy, are

used defensively by the patient to avoid the anxiety-provoking probing of the therapist.

7. The interpretations made by the therapist are based on the systematic collection of information which has been provided by the patient. These interpretations predominantly involve connections between experiences from the past, particularly about the patient's relations with his or her parents, and attitudes which have been transferred to the therapist. These technical interventions are referred to as "parent-transference links." They play a vital role in helping the patient learn to problem solve, and they have repeatedly been shown to be responsible for the establishment of a "corrective emotional experience" and for the resolution of neurotic difficulties.

8. When the patient demonstrates an understanding of his or her conflicts and is able to offer *tangible* evidence of a change in neurotic behavior, termination of therapy should be considered. Of interest is the fact that half our patients are aware of achieving what they wanted and are the ones who initiate the talk about termination. The other half expect the therapist to talk about the end of the treatment but usually agree that it is time to stop it.

THE OUTCOME

The results from these technical STAPP interventions on a group of well-selected, neurotic patients have been investigated in our first controlled study (as mentioned above) and more extensively in two other similar studies, one of which is still ongoing.

The most striking benefits obtained from this treatment, as expressed by patients in their follow-up interviews, are:

1. a clear understanding of the dynamic conflicts underlying their difficulties
2. moderate symptomatic relief
3. general improvement in their relations with key people in their environment
4. a marked increase in self-esteem
5. a general development of new and more adaptive attitudes

6. a new learning and problem-solving capacity, which they utilize in their current lives, long after the treatment has come to an end

7. a predominantly positive feeling for their therapist, who is viewed as an educator and a friend rather than as a healer

8. a feeling of achievement, primarily accomplished by the patients themselves

From the above, it should be clear that the patients do not express a need to return for more therapy. Their ability to function as independent human beings is viewed as a major therapeutic result.

THE INSTRUCTION OF STAPP

Because the results of STAPP have been demonstrated to be effective, because of the brief duration of this treatment, and because of its economic advantages, the interest in this form of psychotherapy has soared, and the demands for its instruction have increased by leaps and bounds over the past few years.

From our experience, any young therapist who has an open mind, is well versed in psychodynamic theory, and has treated a suitable STAPP patient under intensive individual supervision can rapidly learn to practice this therapy, without a protracted period of training. What is needed is enthusiasm. Whenever it is present, it greatly facilitates the instruction of this kind of brief dynamic psychotherapy.

AN EXAMPLE OF TYPICAL INTERVIEWS

As a demonstration of the technique of STAPP, I have chosen to present an almost verbatim exchange between a therapist and a patient who was treated successfully more than eight years ago.

The problems which brought this 28-year-old male graduate student to the psychiatric clinic had to do with difficulties in his relations with both men and women. For example, he stated that he had a tendency to cover up his feelings, to wear "a mask," as he put it, so that others would not know what he truly was like. He attributed this tendency to his relations with his parents. As a result of his strong attachment to his mother, whose favorite he was, and competition with his father, he felt he had to hide his true feelings for both of them. This attitude interfered with his daily life, His two girl friends and his best friend John pointed to this problem and advised him to seek help.

The following exchange took place during the early interviews of his therapy:

THIRD STAPP INTERVIEW

DOCTOR: Well, what have you been thinking since our last meeting? Last time we covered a lot of ground.

PATIENT: Yes, you left me with a lot of heavy thoughts. I should tell you that up to last week I discussed with a friend of mine, who is in therapy, all of my actions, including last Tuesday's. I had the ability to bounce off him a lot of my feelings. Last week was an awful lot of thought about my conflict with authority figures, my conflict with feelings toward people.

DOCTOR: For example, what kinds of thought did you have?

PATIENT: They all revolve around the thought that I was talking with you last week of the mask that I put on. Of that inability to perceive it when I'm doing it. A lot of times when it becomes pretty explicit. I don't know how to explain it. I would search for a definition. But it hits me for a brief second and I realize there is a facade there. But that's only so seldom. Most of the time I am unaware of it.

DOCTOR: Yes, we know, that for instance last week during the hour there was an element of that facade.

PATIENT: There was a lot of it.

DOCTOR: Exactly. Now, were you aware of it at the time?

PATIENT: I'll tell you when I became very aware of it, at the point when I said, I don't know whether it was a slip—I think it was quite intentional—the point about threatening you. It seemed very innocuous at the time that I said it. But after thinking about that one statement, I realized what my train of thought was. I'll say this is your role. It's an antagonistic role. One, because you are an authority figure. Another one because I think I envy your role here. I envy your authority, I envy your professionalism. *[Transference is openly acknowledged.]*

DOCTOR: Now, when you say I am an authority figure, in what sense do you mean? I mean, what is my authority over you? In a sense it's nil. *[The therapist takes the opportunity to work on the transference.]*

PATIENT: Well, actually it's nil. But if I consider that . . . I was very pleased last week also. I had assumed coming in that you would be an extremely perceptive man. The point has been collaborated by a previous friend of yours.

DOCTOR: Oh, I see.

PATIENT: She highly regards your reputation. I just assume that this perceptivity grants you a certain insight into my real feelings at the time that I'm discussing them with you.

DOCTOR: Excuse me, let me ask you a question in reference to that. Is this—this so-called perceptivity of mine—because somebody else said it, or is this your own decision?

PATIENT: Both. One friend, whose name is Bob, is a very perceptive fellow also. He did make me very aware through not only knowing that I was going to come into contact with you as a professional, but also the fact that your profession in general is very perceptive. It has to be. Just through the element of time you spend looking at people. Also, realizing after you brought up the point of what I had said, it reinforced it. It wasn't an original thought at the time. I'd have to say both. I do realize that objectively that you saw through the gimmick I was pulling.

DOCTOR: Whatever this authoritative or envy of authority issue is, we can expect that the facade would come about since it's come about in situations with your father, and other men. Now, you say that sometimes you don't realize until it has happened. Sometimes you say that you are aware of it at the time.

PATIENT: Yes, sometimes I am aware of it. But most of the time, I would say a great majority, I am not aware.

DOCTOR: The one thing that is of interest here is this. That when you talked about it, both in that first hour that we had you remember at the evaluation conference, as well as last time, this attitude was particularly in reference to women. In your relationships with women. Now this has come up in terms also with men with authority. Are you talking about two different kinds of facade?

PATIENT: I don't think so. No, because I think, I feel I am defending myself against both men and women, with any person that I would really like to come close to, to be friendly or intimate, I think this facade arises. But it is most disturbing in my case in that this is where I am most interested in establishing relationships that are viable.

DOCTOR: This I understand. My question was really whether the quality of this facade . . .

PATIENT *(Interrupting)*: I don't think there's any difference. Not that I perceive right now, anyway.

DOCTOR: So are you saying then that you are hiding yourself from men, from men in authority, and from women?

PATIENT: I think I can elaborate that. It strikes me more and more that I've been looking at it, what I do, and how that I have to impress people with what I wish I were or what I assume they wish I was. You see what I mean? In other words, I anticipate expectations that I think are not real but I don't know how I can escape anticipating, as it came up in the meeting last week. I'm saying you have a certain role in mind and in quick calculation I don't know how I do it in my computer or whatever. I see your role. I assume you have certain expectations of me and try to fulfill them. Because I realize how shabby an attempt it's been. Afterwards it's been really helter-skelter and not really . . .

DOCTOR: Yes, but I'm still intrigued because there is a notion here that when you told me about the problems with your father and the facade, that was quite clear. But when you told me about your mother, and being quite close to your mother, you did not mention the facade. And this is why I was raising the question here. Whether there is a kind of difference in the nature of the facade. Certain things are to be kept out from authoritative men, including someone like me and your father, and certain other things might be kept out from women. You see what I mean? There's quite a difference. *[This is a typical aspect of the parent-transference link which the therapist makes early in the treatment.]*

PATIENT: I see very much now. I hadn't thought of it that way.

DOCTOR: Now don't think about it. Just tell me what comes to your mind.

PATIENT: I know with authority figures I tend to rebel. I tend to want to, knowing that often times I'm too submissive. You see, it's like a compensation.

DOCTOR: Well, it's a sort of rebellion.

PATIENT: It's a rebellion because I would like to be submissive and I know . . . I think I can elaborate a little more. There are many discussions with my father when I was a child, or even an adolescent. I was always brought up in the role of the authority figure as related to the Anglo-Saxon area. Now this was an implicit thing brought about by constant references to my almost 100% pure WASP nature. Very much the white supremacy type of argument led me to be an imminent leader of men. A role in which I didn't belong. I was never in a position where I could exercise it, so I was very frustrated in that role with women.

DOCTOR: Maybe you wanted to be a leader of women!

PATIENT: I might still want to be a leader of women.

DOCTOR: I see. What comes to mind in reference to women?

PATIENT: What comes to mind? Well, in general . . .

DOCTOR: Stop intellectualizing. Tell me what comes to your mind as far as your relationship with women is concerned. *[The therapist stops the patient from evading the issue and brings him back to the focus.]*

PATIENT: I don't think I could. I don't think I have an absolute possibility of leading women. I don't like women on that level. I don't want to be removed from women. I would like to be very intimate with most women.

DOCTOR: Well, it depends what it means by "leading" them.

PATIENT: O.K. There is a certain image—I would like to be that dashing character Don Juan.

DOCTOR: What associations do you have with being a Don Juan?

PATIENT: Well, I often played Don Juan.

DOCTOR: Oh, I see!

PATIENT: Because I see that role as not being a fulfilling one I could remove . . .

DOCTOR: Now don't run away from it.

PATIENT: Most of those roles are very cavalier.

DOCTOR: What does that mean to you?

PATIENT: I'm trying not to be intellectual. I'm trying to be spontaneous, but it's so hard. I've been removing myself all my life.

DOCTOR: You are just trying to run away. Now let's pursue one very simple point. This association, of "leading women." You said you couldn't. I said, well it depends on what it means. And you associated immediately to wanting to be a Don Juan. Now let's pursue that. What does that lead to?

PATIENT: It leads to Clark Gable, in my estimation he was a very handsome, very dashing fellow. Therefore, all the women he had anything to do with were very beautiful women. The fixation which I have that I know is very apparent with any of my friends at least is that I would prefer never going out with a girl that is unattractive. Not only unattractive, she has to be *very* attractive, a beautiful woman.

DOCTOR: So there is a parallel that Clark Gable equals Don Juan equals you. Right?

PATIENT: Hopefully!

DOCTOR: You are going out with beautiful women, and you *need* to. What does that mean?

PATIENT: Well, see I've intellectualized this previously.

DOCTOR: Don't intellectualize it now. I'm interested in what comes to your mind.

PATIENT: I enjoy being with beautiful women. Why do I enjoy being with beautiful women? There is a certain status associated with being with a beautiful woman. Peer group status.

DOCTOR: What was Clark Gable getting? Peer group status?

PATIENT: I think so.

DOCTOR: Are you sure?

PATIENT: I'm not sure.

DOCTOR: Maybe there was something more direct, more pleasureable, than peer group status!

PATIENT: Even on that level I do enjoy being with a beautiful woman just for the aesthetics of it, just looking at a beautiful woman. I like a fair complexion. I like the intimacy.

DOCTOR: Let me just point out something that you do. We drew a parallel between yourself and Clark Gable, and with beautiful women. An attribute which you have. You said that you would like to. I pointed out that you already have it, you like to go out with beautiful women. I ask you what is the advantage of that? And immediately you go on to something tangential, like in social status and peer groups. Now there's something much more direct. *[The therapist keeps the patient on the focus and undercuts the patient's defensive manner.]*

PATIENT: O.K. Well, if a woman goes out with me it means that I have some import to her, some value to her. You're really straining my brain.

DOCTOR: Come on! There's nothing wrong with your brain! *(Laughter.)*

PATIENT: You probably already know this, but I am trying to use your vocabulary and I'm going to try to get out of that. Because I'm not that qualified to use it. I'll try to be spontaneous. Could you rephrase the question?

DOCTOR: No. *[Again the therapist actively keeps the patient on the right track.]*

PATIENT: No you will not?

DOCTOR: You heard my question. You don't need any assistance. You can do it, perfectly well. Carry on.

PATIENT: I remember a girl named Jean that I went out with who was, I think, very, very beautiful. Facially she was extremely attractive, a beautiful complexion. A beautiful body, absolutely incredible . . . initially I started trying to date her, I'll put it at that, at about 14 or 15. At a time when I assumed that she would not like me because she was so beautiful. This is in context of the church I was going to. She was the only girl roughly my age in the church—there was a heavy pressure on dating girls in the church. And so I just assumed a rejection from her. You're talking about what affects me internally, not what I perceive externally.

DOCTOR: You're running away from my question again.

PATIENT: No, I'm trying to get towards it. I'm trying to give you all the references.

DOCTOR: That's fine. You gave me an example. I think it is fine to give an example. But what does the example say? There was a beautiful girl that you went out with. You said the assumption was—*you* made the assumption—that she would not be interested in you because she was so beautiful. Why should there be such an expectation, that a beautiful girl would reject you? Now, if so, why should that expectation be there? Now all this, however, leads us to nowhere because the question was very simple. What was it that Clark Gable, that is, *you,* was getting out of these interactions with these beautiful women?

PATIENT: I imagine sexual contact.

DOCTOR: What do you think?

PATIENT: Immediately what hit me right there was an image of very shapely breasts. I don't know why. Maybe this is what you want me to do.

DOCTOR: I don't want you to do anything.

PATIENT: I think you want me to be spontaneous. This is all I meant. I didn't mean anything else.

DOCTOR: What expectation do you have of what I want you to do?

PATIENT: I don't have elaborate expectations. You should prefer me not to intellectualize.

DOCTOR: Fine! So you had a sexual . . .

PATIENT: I see these women, all that Clark Gable has, images of beautiful women with very low-cut dresses, very shapely. This brings me into immediate contact with that.

DOCTOR: And what does that association remind you of? For example, this girl Jean?

PATIENT: How could I say it, love or something like that? It doesn't remind me of anything specific.

DOCTOR: What are you thinking about?

PATIENT: I'm thinking about . . . I'm assuming maybe I shouldn't, is what role this must play with my mother in reference to, because I also recall images of my mother nursing my youngest sister. At that time I was very attracted to my mother's nursing my sister, it was a very intimate role that I experienced at that point. My youngest sister was the only child my mother was able to nurse.

DOCTOR: And you were about 12 years old?

PATIENT: I must have been. Let's see, my sister is 18 now so I guess I was 9 or 10. Because she was quite young and she didn't nurse all the time. I recall this very intimate period.

DOCTOR: Intimate with your mother? Are you saying this because you think that's what I'm interested in? *[The therapist wants to make sure that the patient is not trying to please him.]*

PATIENT: No, I'm not. These are just images I've come across as I've been thinking spontaneously. Things that my mind refers to.

DOCTOR: What about that image?

PATIENT: I think that was the warmest period I ever had with my mother. It was not a really maternal type of love either. I'm not saying this because you want me to say it because the thought has just occurred to me. There was a tremendously warm feeling, a very warm person, showing me an intimate side of life that I had never seen. I don't know if I'd always known it was there but I had assumed that page was pretty open. I talked with my mother about nursing children before with my older brothers and sisters. She brought up the point that she would have liked to but for some physical reason she wasn't able to.

DOCTOR: Do you remember what she said?

PATIENT: I remember that she had blue milk, or something like that, so she couldn't nurse. She had attempted nursing me and wasn't able to and never tried it again until this time when the doctor said she could try it. That's about what I can recall about that. I do remember sitting beside her when she was nursing my sister and I was quite small compared to her. Of course, I was only 9 or 10. That's just what I remember as being very close. And just a tremendous feeling of warmth.

DOCTOR: Did you have any particular curiosity seeing your mother nursing your sister?

PATIENT: Well, it was strange to see my mother's bare breasts for one thing.

DOCTOR: What about that?

PATIENT: All I can remember is just mammoth breasts feeding my younger sister. Just the whole situation, as I said, was a very intimate thing with just the three of us.

DOCTOR: But you had a thought just a minute ago.

PATIENT: I was trying to refer to what my feeling toward my sister at that time was but I couldn't recall. I just liked her, I thought she was neat. Really a nice little kid. I still like very young children, children of all ages. I was trying to remember what I felt for my sister at that time and I think it was just a very warm feeling.

DOCTOR: So we really have an association which appears to be spontaneous in terms of warm feelings for your mother, probably the warmest time was when she was nursing your younger sister. You also had some curiosity about your mother's breasts. Yet, interestingly enough this association came to you from Clark Gable.

PATIENT: Yes. I think specifically it came from the woman who was standing up in the balcony in the very low-cut dress who had very apparent cleavage. I noticed it immediately. I guess you're supposed to notice.

DOCTOR: But are you saying then that the relationship that he may have had to these women was somewhat similar to your relationship with your mother? *[This is a typical anxiety-provoking confrontation.]*

PATIENT: I probably reject that feeling. I think there was a very intimate relationship and a very fulfilling one in the sense . . .

DOCTOR: What do you mean that you probably reject that?

PATIENT: Just the whole feeling of thinking about . . . again I'm complicating what I'm thinking by the concept of the Oedipal relationship.

DOCTOR: Yes, but let's forget the Oedipal relationship. Now, you didn't like this parallel of mine. *[The therapist avoids getting entangled in jargon.]*

PATIENT: Well, this has occurred to me before—what an Oedipal relationship really means.

DOCTOR: What does it mean?

PATIENT: What I think it means is this feeling of hatred for your father and sexual interest in your mother. This time that I related to my sister is the only time I can remember having sexual interest in my mother.

DOCTOR: Ah! What was the *sexual* interest? You talked about *warm* feelings.

PATIENT: Yes, I didn't think of that.

DOCTOR: Very interesting!

PATIENT: I don't know how it popped out.

DOCTOR: I don't know. It popped out from somewhere!

PATIENT: Now I'm just dealing with the feeling that I probably wanted to replace my sister. In previous references I said that my mother had said that I was the first that she tried to nurse. I think that probably I would have liked to have been in that position right then.

DOCTOR: Come now, do you view your sister's position as being sexual?

PATIENT: You mean when she was nursing? No.

DOCTOR: All right. But you used the word *sexual* in terms of . . .

PATIENT *(Interrupting)*: O.K., yeah. What I was thinking of myself is that I was allowed to feel her breasts. Also, I can remember one other time that I felt her stomach when she was pregnant. That was very intimate. I really enjoyed that intimacy at the time. I would say I would have to substitute a feeling of *warm* with sexual relationship rather than just a warm relationship or whatever I said. It wasn't so removed that there was . . .

DOCTOR: No. You don't have to substitute anything. The word *warmth* came out quite spontaneously. I think it was probably a very true feeling that you had in reference to your mother. But the word *sexual* was kept out. Then it came through this roundabout way by your associations with the Oedipus complex—and you were taken aback when you realized that your feelings were also sexual.

PATIENT: Well, it struck me almost at the same time that it struck you.

DOCTOR: I think so too. It was obviously something of interest. Now, we have to define what is the meaning of the word *sexual.* You say your mother let you touch her breasts, let you touch her abdomen when she was pregnant, and so forth. But the word *sexual* implies something which is different from the word *warm*. Right?

PATIENT: It implies quite a bit more!

DOCTOR: All right. Can you tell me what it implies to you? Not what you think I want to hear.

PATIENT: Yes, I'm trying to get away from this now. I've thought about this all week, that I must initiate responses that are honest. Your question is what is the connotation of sexual to me right now? Well, I just feel that an honest sexual relationship is the most intimate relationship I could possibly have right now with anyone. Not just the physical. In fact, I don't even think that's the most important act of the relationship. It's just very intimate and enjoyable to be with a woman that's that open. I just get the feeling that a warm relationship is one very rare in my case where I really enjoy being with someone. Should I keep elaborating?

DOCTOR: There you go again. You're asking my permission.

PATIENT: Well, I always assumed the role of the therapist would be a prodding one. I'm also looking forward to that and I also try to hide myself from that.

DOCTOR: Now, don't run away. The question now is, what are you trying to hide from? Not from me, but from what is inside you, and from what some of these associations have stirred up?

PATIENT: Sex is taboo. All through my family history that was one of the hidden parts of a relationship.

DOCTOR: Can you tell me something about that?

PATIENT: Yes, I can tell you quite a bit because I remember a lot of things that I did that were being heavily sanctioned. When I was quite young, 5 or 6 years old, there were four neighbor girls, two or three with whom I used to romp naked in the woods around my house. I was quite young then. I don't remember any particularly astounding curiosity at the fact except that they were different than I was. It was very interesting. Then in a second period of my life which came much later, I was spanked for that when my mother and my father found out about it. It was mostly my mother, though, as I recall.

DOCTOR: Wait just a minute. Are you sure? You said your mother and your father, then you said mostly by your mother. Can you remember who spanked you?

PATIENT: I just remember that most of the time I was spanked by my mother for any infraction.

DOCTOR: What was the implication here? It was that you were doing something which was bad?

PATIENT: Yes, it was wrong.

DOCTOR: You said that there was no particular curiosity that you had. Why was that so bad?

PATIENT: I don't know. I was very innocent at the time because I do recall quite vividly a couple of things. I don't know if you would say that this was very important. There were a lot of woods around the house and plenty of areas where I could be hidden from direct view of the house and my mother. Primarily the curiosity was in each one urinating. That was the extent of it. Other than that I just remember that I was caught.

DOCTOR: How were you caught?

PATIENT: That I don't recall very vividly. I just know that it was found out, maybe through the girl's parents. My parents were friendly with them. So that's the way I assume it happened. It becomes very foggy after the exact incident itself. What happened prior or after that is just very unclear. I just know that something happened that was found out by my mother. There is another incident that happened several years later.

DOCTOR: Well, before we go into the other one, what did you mother do? Do you remember specifically being spanked for this episode?

PATIENT: I remember being spanked when I was a kid.

DOCTOR: But you may not have been spanked for this specific infraction.

PATIENT: I may not have. But I assume I was. I know it was something that was serious enough so that I didn't go back to it.

DOCTOR: Now, what was this other episode?

PATIENT: I had a cousin, Martha, a girl who is about 19 or 20 now. She came to visit my family and stayed with us for a summer. I have two other cousins who are male who lived in the same general area and who used to always be around my house in the summer. The area around my house is heavily wooded. It's very removed from the urban community. We went quite deep into the woods this time, a couple of miles. There was absolutely no risk of being found out. We totally undressed. This group included myself, my two male cousins, my sister, who was the same age as Martha. This time I was much more curious in the actual genitals and what happened versus what I was doing.

DOCTOR: Now, your cousin was how old?

PATIENT: I don't recall her exact age. It just appears to me that this is about 11 or 12 years of age. So she was 9 or 10. But I'm not exactly sure.

DOCTOR: All right. What about the interest in the genital area?

PATIENT: Well, my cousins were much more informed at the time than I was about what genitals were used for. I thought that besides urinating that was the end of it. It intrigued me more than anything to find out that their concept of physical intercourse was actually collective—it could be carried off. That was the experiment at the time. Well, we did it more than once—several times—because she stayed with us all summer. In the end nothing ever really happened aside from getting in the position of physical intercourse and not knowing what to do after that. My mother did find out about it. There was a very emotional scene of crying and explaining how intimate that relationship was and that it should only be carried on by a man and wife in a very sacred relationship. That was much more vivid—both my mother's crying scene and the actual event itself—than the previous incident. That's why I kept trying to jump to it.

DOCTOR: Now, that's very interesting. In a sense both these episodes—both occurring roughly 5 or 6 years difference. Your lack of awareness or lack of knowledge is emphasized in both.

PATIENT: This is very poignant all through my life. I felt a certain lack of understanding for the male and female role, the intimate role, I don't mean the friendly role, I mean the sexual role. It was very clandestine in my parents' case. You never talked explicitly about anything having to do with sex until I was 16 or 17, with my father, and then I had a pretty good idea of what was going on.

DOCTOR: Do you think it was your mother's attitude, particularly in the second episode . . . the first one you associate more with being punished, possibly spanked. The second you associate more with an appeal to your good sense, your moral sense! Was it possible, because of that attitude in your mother that you, for example, failed to develop this interest? The interest was there in the first place. You had the interest. You were interested in looking at these girls, and you were interested in finding out what your cousins knew so much more than you did. So this points to your curiosity and interest in the second episode. You did not have, or you barely had the curiosity the first time.

PATIENT: It was just vague the first time. But the second time was a definite interest.

DOCTOR: So what happened to that interest?

PATIENT: That's a very vivid point in my memory. I remember that very clearly. I also remember a speech by my mother who said that my father's interest in girls was almost nil till he was in his 20s. Now, I don't know what this was used for because when I related it to my father in a sort of kidding way he really let out a war whoop. It seemed that that was privileged information between the two of them.

DOCTOR: So your mother was saying that your father was not interested in sex until he was 20.

PATIENT: Not only wasn't interested in it, but that it was dirty.

DOCTOR: But you were interested in sex at the age of 12, so you really had much greater interest than your father!

PATIENT: Yes, that's what struck me at the time. That I must be a pretty rotten guy because I'm interested in it so early. I enjoyed very much being with my cousins and with the girls that I recall at 5 or 6 years old. I enjoyed that communication.

DOCTOR: Was that repeated or not?

PATIENT: After my mother's sanction? Yes. I had tremendous feelings of guilt and reservation. It was like an almost uncontrollable urge. It was something that couldn't be squelched quite that fast. I had to have a lot of time to think about it.

DOCTOR: You mean it's been squelched?

PATIENT: No! I'm not a eunuch.

DOCTOR: I want to know what happened during all of this time.

PATIENT: I think that was pre-junior high school. All through junior high and most of high school the communications with any girl was basically carried on with no sexual reference. They were almost platonic relationships. I couldn't figure out why the girl I told you about was so interested in the more intimate side of the relationship. I just wanted to be with her, but I was scared.

DOCTOR: So that was, in a sense, the way to be a "nice boy" in your mother's eyes. In a way you wore a mask.

PATIENT: Primarily, I suppose.

DOCTOR: Since we know that you have an interest in sex, which still is present up to now, the point is that this interest in sex had to be submerged or to pretend that it was squelched, so that you would be a nice boy in your mother's eyes.

PATIENT: One attribute that Jean had was very early developed breasts.

That was very apparent, and still is. At the age of 14 she was developed as many 20-year-old girls. Very large breasts. She appeared much more a woman than a girl, and acted it too. And I felt quite like a boy, talking with her.

DOCTOR: I think we could recapitulate here about what we know in reference to your sexual interest in women. We went from Clark Gable and his relationships with women to your relationship with your mother, which you called warm at the time that she was nursing your sister. But then it turned out that it was warm *and* sexual. Right? The word sexual implied a great deal of interest which starts from the age of at least 5. Interest in seeing girls naked, much curiosity, but you are punished by your mother, possibly being spanked, but you're not sure about it. Interest continuing up to the age of 12 where this episode with Martha and your sister where the sexual interest is quite clear despite your being somewhat naive about it.

PATIENT: Totally naive. This was my first introduction to sex.

DOCTOR: But at that time the response of your mother is a moral appeal . . .

PATIENT *(Interrupting)*: It was very emotional!

DOCTOR: But at the same time she was telling you, not exactly maybe the same time, that your father had interests in sex that developed at the age of 20.

PATIENT: Which is 10 years later . . .

DOCTOR: And therefore you were way ahead of your father, in your mother's eyes, in this area, which was supposed to be bad. Since this interest has maintained itself up to the present time and since this interest in sex was there, the question, as I said before, was could it be that it was submerged so that your mother would not know about it. But at the same time it was being carried underground. Now, that's one possibility. Another possibility was that you and your mother had some of this intimacy between the two of you, but that your father should not know about it. In either case you wear a mask. You cover up. Isn't that what brought you to psychotherapy? This facade?

PATIENT: Yes, and the communication was intimate, much more so with her.

DOCTOR: Well, there's a lot to think about this coming week.

PATIENT: I don't like these weeks.

DOCTOR: What happens outside of this hour is just as important.

PATIENT: I dislike seeing 11:30 because I would like to carry on for another couple of hours.

DOCTOR: So I'll see you next week.

FOURTH STAPP INTERVIEW

PATIENT: I fell down from the porch and hurt myself.

DOCTOR: How do you feel about this?

PATIENT: It was a hairy experience.

DOCTOR: I can imagine!

PATIENT: It was a very brief mistake. We were on a staging that my partner and I weren't familiar with; it was called "swing staging," and one end fell and consequently the whole thing crashed down. It came down about 40 feet. We were both very lucky. We weren't injured very badly.

DOCTOR: So, have you been thinking about some of the things we talked about last time? *[The therapist, satisfied that this was an accident, brings the patient back to the focus which they had agreed to investigate.]*

PATIENT: Yes, but it's a very hard process to think about that, you know? Most of our discussion seemed to center around what I felt about my mother and myself. Primarily what I was thinking is that this area is heavily shrouded, a very taboo area, a heavy incest area; a thing like that is very negative. It was very hard to think about it. It still didn't help too much. *[The patient, an excellent STAPP candidate, is able to concentrate on the focus which has to do with the exploration of his attachment to his mother—a clear-cut Oedipal focus.]*

DOCTOR: Now tell me, what aspect of it is difficult?

PATIENT: What do you mean by that?

DOCTOR: What part is the difficult one? We talked about a lot of issues in reference to your mother, but what is it that has your thoughts stop flowing?

PATIENT: Any context whatsoever of any sexual attraction to my mother. One rejoinder you made when I indirectly made reference to the sexual feeling sort of stunned me last week. Maybe you know this.

DOCTOR: I know that. But let's just recapitulate. It wasn't my word . . .

PATIENT: No, no. I know.

DOCTOR: Remember, *you* had emphasized the word *warm,* and then later on *you* used the word *sexual.* It was not I who introduced these terms. *[The therapist is careful to undercut the patient's projection.]*

PATIENT: I know it was my word, but it was an indirect reference.

DOCTOR: All right. "Indirect" makes things a little easier, but the issues are there to be understood.

PATIENT: I was thinking about it and really not too much came to my mind.

DOCTOR: Well, let's see what comes to mind today.

PATIENT: O.K. . . .

DOCTOR: You seem to be silent.

PATIENT: I am. I'm very silent. I'm waiting for some push on your part; some jolting question, or something. Well, I was thinking last night particularly because the night before I come here I do try to gather my thoughts and think what we discussed last week. I just really can't formulate too much. I do remember when I was a little kid that I used to sleep in my parents' bed with them when I was very young.

DOCTOR: Very young, you mean . . . what age?

PATIENT: Three or four years old. I think most kids do that when they have bad dreams or nightmares. I do recall that. There were times I recall vaguely that for no other excuse, I wanted to sleep there. That's what I wanted to do.

DOCTOR: Why was that so important?

PATIENT: A lot of security. It just really felt nice to be with both of my parents.

DOCTOR: Do you remember anything specific?

PATIENT: No. Nothing really specific. That's the only reference I could make. Just that warm feeling, that contact. Other than that, not very much.

DOCTOR: Who got you in bed with them?

PATIENT: Well, my mother primarily. I think she usually came to my room if I was having a bad dream and crying.

DOCTOR: Do you remember specifically what happened?

PATIENT: No. Well, I remember a recurring dream I used to have as a kid that used to frighten me. I had that several times. It's just that I was running across a bridge. There's a bridge that crossed a road and I used to run halfway across it and start jumping over, and always wake up. That's the only thing I remember, running down what seemed like a quarter of a mile, half a mile. I just remember that distance of the dream and jumping over. I had never progressed past that point.

DOCTOR: Now, was this a dream that you had then, or is this a dream that you had subsequently?

PATIENT: That's the only thing that I can remember . . . it was the only dream I can remember as a kid—a recurrent dream—that really frightened me. It required a lot of consolation.

DOCTOR: Well now, let's get back to this situation when you had that dream, we're not sure whether it was this particular dream, or it could be another one. You had a dream, and then your mother would come to your room?

PATIENT: Yes.

DOCTOR: And then what would happen?

PATIENT: Well, I'd ask her if I could go into their bed with them and sleep with them. She usually said no. But if it was pretty bad, if it was very apparent that I was very frightened, she would take me in.

DOCTOR: So in a sense then having nightmares gave you some reward. Right?

PATIENT: Right.

DOCTOR: Now, you describe the bedroom as giving you a feeling of security. Where did you sleep, for instance? Next to your father, your mother, or in the middle?

PATIENT: Between them, or at the foot of the bed, depending on where I wanted basically to be I guess. *(Looking somewhat anxious.)*

DOCTOR: Can you tell me a little more about that? *[The therapist, sensing that the patient's uneasiness was associated with important Oedipal material, presses the patient with his anxiety-provoking question.]*

PATIENT: It's so vague right now.

DOCTOR: Yes, but let us not run away. Now, let's start from the beginning. What can you remember about all this?

PATIENT: I can remember on dark nights that if I was frightened to be by myself that I used to ask my parents if I could sleep with them. A lot of times there was no heavy evidence as to why I should and it was refused.

DOCTOR: Now wait a minute. Sometimes you were refused, and other times you were not?

PATIENT: Right.

DOCTOR: Well, what about the times you were refused? Why would you be refused?

PATIENT: Because they apparently thought I didn't need the security of that position.

DOCTOR: So one of the reasons that you would be refused had to do with the intensity of the nightmare. Were there other reasons?

PATIENT: I suppose now I can think that it would be a drag to have a little kid sleeping between you all the time. As husband and wife it wouldn't be too neat. To have a son or daughter there wouldn't be the most congenial atmosphere.

DOCTOR: Meaning what?

PATIENT: Specifically?

DOCTOR: Yes. What do you mean by congenial atmosphere?

PATIENT: I'm sure my parents enjoyed sexual relations.

DOCTOR: I would think so!

PATIENT: I would hope. There were five kids in the family. They weren't all adopted or a sea gull didn't drop them.

DOCTOR: So that would have also been a good reason why you were told "no."

PATIENT: Apparently. I would think so. *(Smiling broadly.)* *[Despite his anxiety and tendency to be vague, the patient cooperates with the therapist's questioning. This is evidence that a therapeutic alliance has already been consolidated.]*

DOCTOR: You are a bit reluctant to bring all this up.

PATIENT: Yes, well . . .

DOCTOR: Why?

PATIENT: It's a very heavy taboo area. Sex was never discussed in my family, and it just is a very hard thing to relate.

DOCTOR: So it's time for us to sit around and discuss it. *[Again the therapist pursues relentlessly the Oedipal focus.]*

PATIENT: That's why I'm here.

DOCTOR: Yes. That's what we have to understand.

PATIENT: I read something that got me onto this track of thought. I read an old psychology textbook. So that initiated a lot of thought which seemed to relate to what we have been discussing. Still it doesn't make it any easier to be that frank. The only reference I can ever remember in my family that had anything to do with sex is very negative. The whole church doctrine was incorporated in my parents' philosophy. The church was used to reinforce their philosophy or they reinforced the church's, I don't remember which. It doesn't seem that important right now.

DOCTOR: In a sense it is of some importance because, on the one hand, as you say, and you smiled when you thought about your parents obviously enjoying their sex life because they had five children. At the same time you got the message that all talk about sex was supposed to be taboo. Yet when your mother was nursing your sister you saw that it wasn't as taboo as that.

PATIENT: No, it wasn't entirely taboo. Premarital sex was taboo. Anything concerning sexual activity, heavy petting, anything premarital like that was taboo. This came very explicitly in a lecture from my mother once. I was telling you last week that my cousin Martha and my sister were intimate with my other two cousins. Well, my mother found out about this somehow, I'm not sure how. I think my sister told her or something. She asked me to see her. I knew it was something heavy because just the tonal quality of her voice and of the attitude that she had when she wanted to talk with me alone, I knew there was something special. She made a roundabout reference to sexual activity and broke down crying—it was a very emotional scene—about how this was an act reserved only for the postmarital relationship. It was something not even to be considered. I think I told you last week about what she told me about my father's attitude toward women. That was all a very reinforcing, very emotional conversation that "do not think about it till after you're married." That's where the taboo lies, you know, premarital relations. Even contact was prohibited. It seemed very hard for me to separate being with a woman and touching her in some way, desiring to extend that to sexual intercourse. Even at 18 or 19 I couldn't . . . which may seem funny. At any age that late most kids are very aware of what's happening. It was very hard to segregate the thought of just being with a woman that I liked, being a friend with her. Not wanting to go to the stage of total intimacy.

DOCTOR: But obviously this was then due to a wish at least, to please your mother because you knew that your mother would have disapproved if this were to take place.

PATIENT: Oh, yeah. It was a heavy thought all the time. That conversation impressed me so much that it's one of the memories that was so outstanding that I never could repress it, I never could lose it. It was always there.

DOCTOR: Yes, you mentioned it already last time and I can see that this was of great importance. But this does not mean, as we said last time that your curiosity disappeared.

PATIENT: No, it seemed to wane pretty much though and through my junior high school years . . .

DOCTOR: All right then, let's leave that just for a minute here. We'll get back to the junior high school years. We know that your curiosity was at its height when you were 5 years old, from that first episode at the forest, remember? And then when you were 10 this episode with Martha and your sister. You were about 10, weren't you?

PATIENT: Ten or twelve.

DOCTOR: Anyway, around that time. It was also in between that time that you had seen your mother nursing your sister. That was when you were about 7 or 8?

PATIENT: Yes. I think it was Doris that I saw her nursing.

DOCTOR: I see.

PATIENT: No, I'm pretty sure it was Jane because Jane is the only child my mother nursed after myself. You see, I think I brought out that point also. I figure Jane is 20 and I'm 28, so I was 7 or 8; yes, it had to be Jane.

DOCTOR: So it was? All right. Now the episode in the forest with the two girls. Was that Jane also?

PATIENT: It was my sister Doris and my cousin Martha.

DOCTOR: O.K. And two of your male cousins? The episode with your mother nursing Jane that you described to some length was difficult for you. And the first time that you went into the forest with that other little girl, who was your neighbor, was when you were 5. Now, your curiosity was quite impressive. We have an additional aspect here which might be of some interest. That is, that you used to go to your parents' bedroom. That was around the age of 4 which even precedes the episode with the neighborhood girl. You used to go to sleep in your parents' bedroom associated with these nightmares.

PATIENT: It didn't always have to be a nightmare.

DOCTOR: But you associate it with some need for security. At times you were successful—your mother would get you to sleep with them—and other times you were not, and we thought that maybe this had something to do with your interfering with your parents' sexual life.

PATIENT: Yes, that is one possibility.

DOCTOR: What other possibility?

PATIENT: They might have wanted to sleep and I might have been a disturbance also.

DOCTOR: All right. Now, sometimes you said you slept in the bed, between the two of them, sometimes you slept—where was it? . . .

PATIENT: . . . at the foot of the bed.

DOCTOR: At the foot of the bed. Now, you slept closer to your father or to your mother? What was the arrangement, and what do you remember of it?

PATIENT: Well, the only thing, that's very strange. If I ever slept at the foot of the bed it seems that my head was on the other side of the bed and my feet towards my mother. Also, another thing that just popped into my mind that may be of significance or not—and you can tell me as you have whether it is or not.

DOCTOR: You are the one who decides whether it is significant or not, what I tell you makes no difference. *[The therapist again undercuts the patient's attempt to depend on him. This is obviously a regressive maneuver so as to avoid anxiety.]*

PATIENT: Actually it does because I go off in tangents. Every time that I wanted to take a nap or go to sleep when my parents weren't sleeping I slept in my parents' bed. It always seemed more comfortable than my bed. I always assumed my father's position in the bed. But for some reason his pillow or his side of the bed was more comfortable. Now, I don't know what significance that has. But that just struck me as another time that I did . . . *(Looking anxious.)*

DOCTOR: What significance does it have?

PATIENT: Well, assuming my father's role apparently! That's what I think the significance is. It's a dangerous assumption. *[Despite his anxiety, the patient cooperates beautifully, bringing additional pertinent information around the Oedipal focus.]*

DOCTOR: What about assuming your father's role?

PATIENT: Well, I suppose I wanted to be the dominant force. As I told you, a lot of things my father talked about was being a leader and all this business. I think I would have liked to be the *main man* in my family. I wouldn't have liked to totally knock my father out of the position, but I would have liked to be the *head* influence in the family. It was very frustrating. In fact, when my parents went out at night I was often the baby sitter—most often. And I exercised quite an authority role then. I was very brutal, in fact, as a kid.

DOCTOR: Brutal?

PATIENT: Yes, very physical.

DOCTOR: Was your father physical?

PATIENT: Not very. Every once in a while he did spank me but it wasn't a role that he seemed to get into. He's a relatively gentle man.

DOCTOR: Now, when would be the times that you remember that he spanked you?

PATIENT: I don't really remember specific incidents of his spanking me, but I do recall incidents when I was supposed to do things for him that I didn't do that he was quite angry at me for.

DOCTOR: Now, is there one episode that stands out? Times when he really spanked you physically?

PATIENT: No. I know that he did, I know that I've stored that away somewhere, that he actually did spank me at times, but I don't recall any incident. Isn't that interesting?

DOCTOR: Why?

PATIENT: Well, that just wasn't my father's role.

DOCTOR: You just told me that you wanted to take over your father's role. You even slept in his side of the bed. You told me that you took a kind of authoritative role when you were a baby sitter for your brothers and sisters. Now, you couldn't remember when your father spanked you, although he did occasionally.

PATIENT: Well, he used to correct me verbally which was a much stronger . . .

DOCTOR: But I meant physically. Because this is the role that you emphasized to your brothers and sisters.

PATIENT: Well, that's the only authority I had over them.

DOCTOR: Yes, I don't question that. My interest is in what was the authority your father had over you when he spanked you.

PATIENT: I don't know. He didn't even have to spank me. It was much more painful for him to reprimand me than to spank me.

DOCTOR: Did he ever spank you, for instance, because you slept in his bed?

PATIENT: I don't think so. No, that was too much of a taboo.

DOCTOR: Probably at face value, but what about your having to take over his role in bed?

PATIENT: I don't think he was too threatened by my taking over his role.

DOCTOR: I've no interest in what your father thought. I've more interest in what's inside your head.

PATIENT: I don't think that thought ever occurred to me. I just can't recall it now. I'm straining to think of things like that but I don't think that it ever occurred to me.

DOCTOR: All right, maybe if your father didn't spank you because of that, what other situation might have come up for which he would spank you?

PATIENT: You leave the field so wide open to speculate.

DOCTOR: What comes to your mind? Let's worry about my speculations afterwards. *[Again the therapist persists in obtaining information which the patient is resisting.]*

PATIENT: Nothing in particular.

DOCTOR: Is this your way of running away from your anxiety right now?

PATIENT: It could be.

DOCTOR: I wonder.

PATIENT: As I told you I didn't recognize it all. I'm thinking of one incident. I don't know if it's related so I blank it out a little bit. But I'll tell you anyway and then you can determine if it isn't.

DOCTOR: *You* are going to determine whether it is or not.

PATIENT: O.K. Well, I'll just tell you. As a kid, being the oldest, I had to assume a lot of responsibility. I was physically the biggest—the oldest male—I was not too diminutive as a kid. I was bigger than my brothers and sisters. So my father built the house we lived in and as the time came that we needed more room, we built. One task I can remember, I was supposed to be working on the porch of the house and height frightened me quite a bit. Well, it didn't frighten me when he was up there because I could always rely on him to zip down and help me if I was ever in a scary situation. I was supposed to be working on the porch. It wasn't a very rough job. I just remember I was pretty severely reprimanded for it when he got home with my mother. I remember he had been out shopping or something and had been gone two or three hours and I could have done quite a bit, but I . . .

DOCTOR: O.K. You were reprimanded because you didn't do the work on the porch?

PATIENT: No, I did not.

DOCTOR: I see.

PATIENT: I fooled around. I sat up on the porch and didn't do anything.

DOCTOR: It's an interesting association to happen at the time when you fell off the porch and hurt yourself. Can you tell me just for a minute the details of what happened? *[The therapist belatedly returns to the subject which he should have explored more earlier. That was a mistake on his part.]*

PATIENT: Every summer for the last few years I've painted. Usually it's been on one- or two-story houses at maximum. My partner works quite independent of me. He takes whatever he thinks we can handle. He took tenement dwellings. He took a couple of contracts which are three-story dwellings, three apartments, one on each level. We were up on the floor, there was a porch, working on what they call "swing staging." Swing staging works on two eyebolts. There were eyebolts about every 24 feet on these houses. There was a block on the top and a block on the staging that the ropes went through. You haul yourself up on the ropes and you tie them off. Now, I had untied mine and was holding it to lower ourselves down. My partner couldn't untie his and yanked it and pulled his block out of the end of the staging, and his end just zipped down. He grabbed his rope and luckily I grabbed mine. I burnt my hands pretty bad. I burnt some of my fingers and I had several bruises on my side. We hit the ground and I knew I hurt my knee, I didn't know it was this bad. It wasn't as painful then as it is now. That's how that occurred. But I do remember incidents like being on the porch of my house and looking over, just constantly looking over the edge to see how far down it was, and being frightened of it and backing off.

DOCTOR: So we had one interesting association here above and beyond the present of what happened, when your father wanted you to be exposed to something that you were clearly frightened about, that is, working on the porch, and you were reprimanded for not doing it. What was the fear of height all about?

PATIENT: Falling off, primarily I would think.

DOCTOR: The dream about the bridge?

PATIENT: Yeah, that was a high bridge, that was falling into the road below or something.

DOCTOR: All right. Any thoughts about the nightmare?

PATIENT: Well, I just remember that I was straddling the side of the railing on the bridge. This bridge has a railing about 4 feet high which would be very easy to get over if you wanted to get over it. I just remember, straddling it. It was this compulsion to jump off of it and not wanting to, fearing to jump off of it. For some reason I woke up.

DOCTOR: Is there any connection?

PATIENT: I don't know.

DOCTOR: Tell me what comes to mind because I think there might be something here.

PATIENT: I think there was a feeling of imminent death in both situations. If I did fall off the porch I would be really badly injured. And it wasn't that high because my brother John used to keep jumping off the porch. It was only about 8 or 10 feet high, and he used to jump off into a sand pile. You do remember my brother John. I think that was significant.

DOCTOR: I haven't forgotten your brother John, but let us stick to the issues.

PATIENT: John did these feats of jumping off the porch. He used to love to be up on it and jump off. We had this sand pile at one end of the house and he used to just leap off the side of it into the sand pile.

DOCTOR: But this is fear of death, which in this situation comes through the reality of your recent hurt. In your dream jumping off the bridge is somewhere associated with your father who is not a brutal person, who is a very gentle person.

PATIENT: I hadn't made these connections before.

DOCTOR: Of course, that's why you're here. What about these connections?

PATIENT: Well, I don't know. I suppose I could be thinking that my father was forcing me into a situation that would imperil me.

DOCTOR: Yes. So why?

PATIENT: The connection that actually comes to mind is that I assume through the role . . . now I'm very hesitant to say this because I do think there is a certain line of questions, but the train of thought would be that of course because I wanted to be the boss, but I'm not sure that it is a valid consideration.

DOCTOR: You made the point clearly before. You did not want to "knock your father out of his position." These were your words. You see, it may have nothing to do with your father at all. These are the thoughts going on in your head.

PATIENT: You see I don't feel that connection, even now. I don't feel that my father was in that position. *[The patient is obviously very resistant, but the therapist persists because he is aware of the importance of this subject. This is typical STAPP technique.]*

DOCTOR: That's what I'm saying. It is very possible that it was never anything that your father thought of, but that you created this particular situation to protect yourself from some feelings that you had about your own competition with your father. After all, we have seen your competition with your father clearly in all kinds of situations. This we know, we've known all along since the first time I saw you. But the question was what does one do with feelings of competition with someone whom one loves?

PATIENT: Suppress them, I imagine.

DOCTOR: Or, another way?

PATIENT: Vent them, I don't know.

DOCTOR: Vent them how? Towards one's brothers and sisters, or on oneself, or by feeling guilty?

PATIENT: Yes, I suppose. Guilt would be a tremendous outlet on that, just feeling that I should do something, but how dare I do something, it's wrong.

DOCTOR: Is there another way?

PATIENT: Yes, vent them in a clandestine manner.

DOCTOR: Yes, how?

PATIENT: Doing things that I know he'd envy but never letting him know about it.

DOCTOR: Any other way? What was your chief problem?

PATIENT: My chief problem? You mean assuming his role?

DOCTOR: We delved into that. But that isn't what you said. Your chief problem you said was covering up your feelings and getting into trouble with your father as well as people in authority. Does that clandestine way of yours take care of it? Your facade . . .

PATIENT: Yes.

DOCTOR: Yes, I agree. So you see how many interesting maneuvers one could use in a situation which was a competitive one.

PATIENT: Yes, that's very strange.

DOCTOR: What's so strange?

PATIENT: I had just never thought of that. But I suppose you could do hidden things, do things physically, and then become more and more sophisticated in this and not even have to do this physically. Just hide what you think or what your feel and still have the very conscious or just slightly subconscious feelings and never reveal them. I suppose that's just as effective a way of hiding what you feel and what you do, as physically hiding them. That's still a very shaky feeling; it still isn't very crystal clear, but I can see the direct line of logic there anyway. *[Despite his resistance, the patient shows insight with his defensive maneuvers.]*

DOCTOR: Now what are your thoughts right this minute?

PATIENT: Well, what I was referring to, or what I was hinting to exactly then was why in the hell do I get up to three stories if I really don't like it too much. Why don't I just refuse to? I know directly. I don't want to frustrate my partner too much, make him too anxious about the situation. And also, initially between my partner and I, no matter what job we had, I always assumed the role of high man, the highest ladder, stuff like that. He doesn't like to go up there. I was less reluctant to go up than he was. But I always assumed I was the peak man, doing the peak work and stuff like that.

DOCTOR: Can you tell me something about your partner?

PATIENT: He's my boss. An authoritative figure.

DOCTOR: He's older than you?

PATIENT: Yes, he's 45. In some ways he's older. Physically older. *(Smiling.)*

DOCTOR: Why are you smiling?

PATIENT: He's just a funny guy. He has a tremendous sense of humor. I really enjoy working with the guy. Our train of thought is very much the same way. He's very overt in his sexual references to his exploits of women. He was the first guy I think that it ever became clear to me that this wasn't dirty if someone could talk about it that way. It wasn't that long ago. I must have been 17 or 18 when I started talking with him.

DOCTOR: Can you give me an example?

PATIENT: He's in a very topsy-turvy marriage. He assumes a very rigid code of what marriage should be. It's a one-time relationship. But he has left his wife several times, but always comes back feeling pity for her or something, I don't know exactly what. During these bouts he has had several different relationships that seem very glamorous to me. For example, he moved out to Texas for a little over a year—that was about 3 years ago—and then came back in the summer and we worked together and discussed about what he'd done. His exploits were just really crazy!

DOCTOR: Such as, for instance?

PATIENT: I'm getting into some very private things. He moved out to Texas and he had an affair with a woman who was also married, but made it very explicit that he was going out with other women. His wife knew about it. His cousin introduced him to this one woman . . . it's very funny all these things that pop into my head. The woman was very active sexually. He would just make reference to that sometimes. She fulfilled a lot of the demands that he made, like being a good wife—fixing breakfast and being very congenial. He asked her why she had left her husband. She said that the only things he had on his mind was sex. In fact, I discussed this yesterday with him. It really was funny because she was very active sexually. Another instance is that he is . . .

DOCTOR: But why do you view that this sexual activity of hers is funny?

PATIENT: Oh, also she made reference to the church. The Assembly of God, the A of G, that's what I refer to it as, as a thing that would mess up your head. The thing that she came back with is that she doesn't go to church because it'll mess up your head. I thought that was very funny because I agree with her. I think just that for anyone else to refer to it is . . . sorry if I make your job so difficult.

DOCTOR: I'm very amused. I'm amused by the ways you are slowly and steadily trying to hide yourself from having to reveal some things that might be of some importance. Is this your way of hiding your feelings? You do it here with me. *[The therapist brings up the transference here.]*

PATIENT: Well, I think the things that are of importance are of course very hard to reveal. I don't like to reveal them.

DOCTOR: I understand. But I think what is of importance is to try—it isn't a question of revealing them to me, but it is really bringing them into the open so that we can understand them together. *[Here reference is made to the therapeutic alliance.]*

PATIENT: There are other heavy significant things that I suppose that I should talk about. I am going to break off from this and refer to something that I had told you very early in this conversation. The conversation that I had with my mother about my sister. I thought about this and it's very hard to reveal. But there was a very apparent incestual relationship between my sister and I at a very early age, and it really bothered me, and it still does. It's a weird feeling.

DOCTOR: Can you tell me something about it? What did it involve?

PATIENT: Well, the incident that I told you in the forest, in the woods there with my cousin, we were all naked. I did attempt, as did my cousins— all five of us experimenting back and forth with physical intercourse— I don't think we ever accomplished anything, it physically hurt my sister and my cousin to try it, so we stopped it there, but there were several incidents after that where I just physically touched my sister's vagina and her genital area.

DOCTOR: What were your feelings about that? On the one hand obviously this talk with your mother . . .

PATIENT *(Interrupting)*: What I felt even before that was the feeling that that was a *no-no*. But that there was no possible way of venting it anywhere else. My sister knew about my feelings like that.

DOCTOR: So what you have just told me in response to the question that I asked you earlier in this interview was that your curiosity did not disappear even after your mother's lecture.

PATIENT: No it did not.

DOCTOR: So it had to go underground. It had to go through this more clandestine type of relationship with your sister. It may have gone on in other areas. But what is important is that it would have been much worse if it disappeared. Don't you think?

PATIENT: Well, I think so.

DOCTOR: The fact that you have a healthy sexual interest is a perfectly normal thing to have. Now, obviously there were problems that were associated with it, and obviously the attitude of the church also was important. But the fact that you continue to have a perfectly healthy, normal sexual interest is understandable, so let's not forget the reality.

PATIENT: That's very funny. That it wasn't as hard as I thought it would be. It wasn't as uneasy. *[In response to the therapist's clarification, the patient reacts very positively.]*

DOCTOR: Maybe our work is working.

PATIENT: Maybe. I don't feel quite as abnormal as I thought I would. That's the only feeling.

DOCTOR: As long as you don't feel, as I said before, that you are confessing to me like you did in church—expecting that I am going to absolve you by saying that this is all good or this is all bad, a sin and so on.

PATIENT: No. It's the opposite feeling—you're not going to absolve me. You are working with me. *[The therapeutic alliance has been solidified. Both therapist and patient are ready to proceed with the therapy.]*

DOCTOR: All right. See you next week.

These two interviews show clearly some of the technical interventions used by the therapist in STAPP. It should be apparent that so early in this therapy (the third and fourth) interviews, patient and therapist have established a strong therapeutic alliance. Despite his anxiety and his attempts to evade it when pressed by the therapist, the patient brings up valuable associations from the past, which reinforce the problem-solving task so vital for this kind of therapy. All this work is done within the Oedipal focus, which is constantly clarified in the patient's relations with both men and women.

The therapy with this patient lasted four months (13 interviews in all), and it was successful. In terms of outcome, the patient gave up his tendency to hide his feelings. When seen in follow-up, he was having a meaningful relationship with a young woman who was "unattached." (He had a tendency to be attracted to women who were "attached," such as his mother and a great number of others.) He had no symptoms and had a good insight into his relations with his mother and father, which were the focus of his therapy.

CONCLUSION

"Where is short-term dynamic psychotherapy going? What is its future?" The answer is simple. It is here to stay. Why? This answer is also simple. Short-term dynamic psychotherapy has eliminated, once and for all, several of the cliches or myths about psychotherapy in general. These myths emphasized that long-term dynamic psychotherapy was the treatment of choice for all forms of neurotic difficulties, that research in psychotherapy was almost impossible to do, that no controlled studies could be developed, that the transference should not be touched unless it appeared as a resistance, and that the principle of "minimal activity" on the part of the therapist was the only proper way to relate to the patient. This latter attitude, which is a caricature of what is supposed to be "true psychoanalytic technique," has tended to frustrate many a healthier patient and lengthen the therapeutic process.

By emphasizing the importance of proper selection of patients based on clear-cut criteria, by introducing revolutionary, active, technical interventions, by studying the outcome over a long-term period with adequate scientific follow-up methods, and by using video tapes to illustrate its process, short-term dynamic psychotherapy was able to demonstrate its effectiveness conclusively and convincingly, not only for patients suffering from mild neurotic difficulties but also for those with much more severe problems (Davanloo, 1978; Malan, 1976a, 1976b; Mann, 1973; Sifneos, 1979). Systematic investigation of this kind using similar techniques must be tried with sicker patients.

Generally speaking, I do not foresee any dramatic change taking place in the next decade as far as the technique of short-term dynamic psychotherapy is concerned, since what is being done at present has been shown to be highly effective. Nevertheless, it is possible that more systematic investigation of the interventions which appear to be most useful, such as is the case at present with the parent-transference link, will demonstrate the efficacy of other such technical requirements.

I do foresee, however, the expansion of short-term psychotherapeutic techniques in child psychiatry, in work with couples, in family and group therapies, and, with major modifications, in psychosomatic medicine.

The future of short-term dynamic psychotherapy is bright. Its horizons are unlimited.

REFERENCES

Alexander, F., & French, T. *Psychoanalytic therapy: Principles and applications.* New York: Ronald Press, 1946.

Davanloo, H. *Principles and techniques of short-term dynamic psychotherapy.* New York: Spectrum Press, 1978.

Ferenczi, S. *Further contributions to the theory and technique of psychoanalysis.* London: Hogarth Press, 1926.

Malan, D. H. *The frontier of brief psychotherapy.* New York: Plenum Press, 1976.(a)

Malan, D. H. *Toward the validation of dynamic psychotherapy.* New York: Plenum Press, 1976.(b)

Mann, J. *Time-limited psychotherapy.* Cambridge: Harvard University Press, 1973.

Rank, O. *The trauma of birth.* New York: Harcourt Brace, 1929.

Sifneos, P. E. Learning to solve emotional problems: A controlled study of short-term anxiety-provoking psychotherapy. In R. Porter (Ed.), *Ciba Foundation symposium on the role of learning in psychotherapy.* London: J. & A. Churchill, 1968.

Sifneos, P. E. *Short-term dynamic psychotherapy: Evaluation and technique.* New York: Plenum Press, 1979.

CHAPTER 5
THE COMPLEX SECRET OF BRIEF PSYCHOTHERAPY IN THE WORKS OF MALAN AND BALINT

James P. Gustafson

FROM INTUITIVE TO CONCEPTUAL MASTERY

"Why is it that the secret of brief psychotherapy keeps getting lost?" Malan (1963) asked at the start of *A Study of Brief Psychotherapy*. Freud (Breuer & Freud, 1895/1955; Freud, 1905/1953, 1909/1953), Ferenczi and Rank (1925), Alexander and French (1946), all had a period of dramatic short cases, only for this therapeutic secret to disappear as mysteriously as it had come. I suspect that this history is repeated in a minor way by most of us who practice psychotherapy. It is one thing to have some successful brief treatments, and quite another to have a systematic method of brief therapy that is consistently reliable. Because the practice has so many necessary elements in complex relation to one another, we are unlikely to hold them together for long. As we identify one critical element in our technique and take delight in learning more about it, such as interpreting the transference, we lose elements which we practiced intuitively, such as staying close enough to the patient to help him bear his pain. Thus, intuitive mastery is essential to early success, while integration of the relevant concepts of brief therapy is essential to retaining this mastery.

Balint provided the intuitive brilliance for this school of brief psychotherapy at the Tavistock Clinic in London, as Freud, Ferenczi and Rank, and Alexander and French did before him in other centers. The necessary elements are shown in his book *The Doctor, His Patient and the Illness* (Balint, 1957), where we shall begin. Malan then provided the passion and capability for scientific clarity by pinning down some of these necessary

JAMES P. GUSTAFSON. Department of Psychiatry, University of Wisconsin, Madison, Wisconsin.

elements. In a series of books, he has defined early, middle, and current acquisitions of "focal psychotherapy," as this body of work has come to be known.[1] At each stage, we will identify these conceptual gains, which have been essential to retaining the complex art of this method over the past 25 years of their clinical research.[2]

This school of brief psychotherapy is vital not only for its intuitive clinical capability and integration of concepts. It has continually posed the most fundamental questions about psychotherapy itself and has proposed bold hypotheses in reply. What repertoire of relationships offered by the doctor bring about the intense contact necessary to the start of brief therapy (Balint, 1957)? Is it inevitable that psychoanalysis has changed from being a brief psychotherapy to a long-term method; or can this be reversed (Malan, 1963)? Can psychotherapy be planned for each patient in advance, as a thought experiment (Malan, 1976a)? Is it possible to show the continuum from a simpler "psychotherapy of everyday life" to more complex psychotherapy (Malan, 1979)? Is interpretation a sufficient method for bringing about change (Balint, Ornstein, & Balint, 1972)? When a new theory makes predictions opposite to the current theory of psychotherapy practice, we have a scientific clash. These situations are of the greatest interest when the clash is over fundamental questions in psychotherapy, since evidence may be introduced to decide which theory makes the reliable predictions, and we may choose between the rival theories.

Yet every kind of scientific project, in its delimiting and defining aspects of reality, has to ignore some aspects and take others for granted. Something is aways lost; some fixed assumptions are made, which facilitate the research, even though they may later be shown to be rough approximations. At every stage of this project, Malan chose to hold onto the classical psychoanalytic theory of technique of Glover (1955), Strachey (1934), and Karl Menninger (1958), despite an immediate loss of many of the interpersonal and existential elements in the technique of Balint, and despite a continuing series of complex cases which Malan describes beautifully but which do not fit his classical model. Thus, the intuitive elements remain together in the case descriptions, although they are excluded from the theory of technique.[3]

I shall propose alternative models to account for these complex case descriptions. To anticipate this argument in one sentence, I may say that the actual technique that has been successful in their hands is more difficult than Malan's theory of technique contends. Often, is is a technique in three steps that is described by a two-step theory. Furthermore, this technique, as it is practiced, cannot be reduced to verbal interpretations, as argued by Michael Balint and demonstrated by him in the only full-length description of brief psychotherapy we have from this school, the book *Focal Psychotherapy* (Balint *et al.*, 1972), which I will fully present. Finally, I shall close with a review of the remarkable contributions we have received from Balint and Malan, both intuitive and conceptual.

THE COUNTEROFFER: *THE DOCTOR,*
HIS PATIENT AND THE ILLNESS (BALINT, 1957)

We are not surprised by Freud's startling offer to his patients, because we have heard it over and over: say whatever comes to mind. We have been assured already that he will not be the forbidding and didactic man that we fear. Hence, we can scarcely imagine what it must have meant to be invited to lie down in a room of classical wealth and wander as freely in one's associations as possible—a romantic contrast to Victorian parents, which is lost on us.[4] As Alexander and French (1946) would later argue, this difference between the transference expectations and the actual doctor brings on the intense contact that is essential to brief therapy. We can get a little feeling for this in our own terms when we consider how psychotherapy has come to mean seeing the accepting doctor and talking endlessly. What a contrast when James Mann (1973) tells his patient that 12 sessions will be all that he will need! This is the kind of surprise that Balint was interested in.

While Freud never organized his account of his activities in interpersonal terms, Balint decidedly did. Prior to the first focal therapy workshop, Balint experimented with brief therapy in the general practitioner (GP) workshops. All the elements necessary for brief therapy by the analysts of the focal therapy workshops were present in the earlier work with GPs, who were relatively untrained in psychological matters.

Balint and his colleagues offered a new kind of relationship to medical patients, as Freud had. Unlike Freud, the account in *The Doctor, His Patient and the Illness* (Balint, 1957) is directly interpersonal. Even the "illness" is conceived of as an interpersonal construct. It is the result of offers by the patient (e.g., symptoms, complaints) being met by counteroffers by the doctor. Together they "organize" an illness. Balint argued that the usual way for an illness to become organized is for the patient to offer bodily symptoms, whereupon the counteroffer of the doctor is to work them up, to some extent, by clinical investigation. Gradually, perhaps even irrevocably, a state of bodily distress, often occasioned by painful life events, is organized into a physical illness.

Balint now proposed that the initial offers of patients, although in the form of physical sensations, could be met by deeper counteroffers by the doctor, often in the form of a "long talk." Balint's colleagues would later offer intense but brief contact through very spontaneous emotional reactions on the part of the doctor—the so-called "flash" method (Balint & Norell, 1973).[5] Either a long and deep talk or a sudden, deep connection would provide a dramatic contrast to patient and doctor slowly working up a physical illness together. If the patient met this new counteroffer with a deeper response of his or her own, they might together "organize" an illness which offered a better hope of treatment than would a chronic, physical illness.

Not only was the viewpoint more directly interpersonal than that of Freud—Balint spoke of two-body psychology being more relevant than one-body psychology—but the doctor was given much more flexibility, more room to be active. The doctor, especially if untrained, could be none other than himself, with his "apostolic" notions of how his patients should behave when ill. The aim would be not to stop this, but to make it less automatic and bring it to conscious awareness, so the dose of "the drug doctor" could be controlled. Freud's counteroffer had been to remove himself and allow the patient to organize a new illness within him- or herself, namely, an intrapsychic conflict, that had a better chance of being cured. This, of course, put great restriction on the doctor's movements. Balint's doctors might also make the specific counteroffer Freud made—to listen deeply—but they, from the start, might make many offers other than that of being the psychoanalytic doctor. The kind of offer often depended on the practitioner's own personal bent, which was given great latitude to emerge.

One counteroffer, then, might be psychoanalytic. The doctor might listen deeply and comment on the conflict, hovering evenly between the impulses and the prohibitions (see especially Case 19 in Balint, 1957).

Another counteroffer might be for the doctor to simply listen deeply while putting him- or herself "with" the patient as much as possible, "being" and "staying" with the patient through thick and thin. Havens (1976) argued that this is the essence of the existential therapeutic relationship. Balint emphasized this alternative a great deal as having specific potential for the GP (see especially Case 16 in Balint, 1957), who could always be at hand. He referred to this never-ending partnership as the "mutual investment company," putting an existential idea in terms a doctor could appreciate.

Another counteroffer might be more in the tradition of interpersonal psychiatry (Havens, 1976), inasmuch as it would involve removing from the doctor the projections that interfered with care. This might require great skill, as the doctor would have to be taught to accept some projections (e.g., that giving tonics is a sign of a caring doctor) while gradually approximating to more emotional topics.

Finally, Balint did not shrink from explicitly behavioral conceptualizations or treatment relationships. If the patients of England had been "trained" to expect pills and physical diagnoses, they could be "untrained." The doctors would often simply reinforce the different kind of working relationship that they wanted, whether it was about when night calls would be made or when pills might be gotten. Balint was also shrewd enough to couch *his* offer to GPs in behavioral terms or, more exactly, in the objective–descriptive terms of medicine (Havens, 1976). His opening paragraphs considered that the most important drug in the pharmacopoeia—the "drug doctor"—has no pharmacology. Balint shows here the kind of bold offer of relationship that takes into account the specific relationship needed by the client.

It is amazing to consider that Balint intuitively offered at least the four kinds of relationships prominent in modern psychiatry and psychotherapy (Havens, 1973): the psychoanalytic, the existential, the interpersonal, and the objective–descriptive. He also knew how to offer the right kind of relationship to the right client. In the case of GPs, he knew well enough that they respected an objective–descriptive endeavor like pharmacology, so he offered them, first, an opportunity to take on the most critical drug of all, with careful attention to specifying the action, the dose, and the follow-up results. He knew they felt lowly and disrespected and bossed by specialists, so he offered them the chance to be themselves and make "independent discoveries." (See Balint, 1954, for the strategy of his seminar method.) One would have to look to the cases of Alexander and French (1946) for an equally deft assessment of the kind of relationship that would be different enough from the old, painful relationship to allow intense, new contact and to provide new endings to old experiences and for an appreciation of the full range of relationships available to modern psychiatry. These are the necessary tools for a complete technique of brief psychotherapy, which Balint carried over from his enormously varied and deep clinical experience, especially the recent experience with the GP workshops.

Perhaps Balint decided that his psychoanalyst colleagues in the first focal therapy workshop had to be themselves, that is, to be strictly psychoanalytic in their offers to patients and in their thinking. In any case, with the first book on focal therapy itself (Malan, 1963), the interpersonal and existential elements brought out by Balint disappeared into the background, only reappearing 12 years later in the complicated case reports of later books on focal therapy. The reader of the first series of cases in *A Study of Brief Psychotherapy* (Malan, 1963) will be struck by how every case is met with a counteroffer of Oedipal interpretations, sometimes augmented by Kleinian interpretations (of the bad feelings spoiling the good breast). Certainly, these doctors were offering deep relationships.

Indeed, Malan argued that they "discovered" that deep transference interpretations were often the only way to keep open a contact that was bogged down immediately by transference. It is difficult to say, from the outside, how much of the narrowing down of the therapeutic offers and thinking to the psychoanalytic and the objective–descriptive comes from the other therapists in the workshop and how much from Malan who took over the clinical research leadership. I suspect, from Balint's ironic conclusion to his chapter on the "history of the focal therapy workshop" (Balint *et al.*, 1972), that it is Malan as well as many of the others. Regarding the second workshop (1956–1961), Balint wrote:

> Although the reasons for its termination were many and complicated, one that is perhaps worth mentioning was that most of its members, being fairly new qualified analysts, were perhaps too absorbed with traditional analytic thinking to be able to proceed with the tasks that lay ahead. It was very difficult indeed to realize that the new techniques and way of thinking did not endanger psychoanalytic theory and practice: that they were supplementary and not antagonistic to each other. (Balint *et al.*, 1972, p. 13)

Although this is said in criticism of Malan, that he narrows down considerably from Balint's wide range of therapeutic relationships, it must be equally stressed that he increased the power and precision of the psychoanalytic and objective–descriptive frames of reference for brief therapy. Indeed, in his later books, he makes it entirely clear that he finds himself in a historic battle to vindicate Freud's discoveries, which have been denied their proper recognition by historical forces. He brings a passion for both a radical, "penetrating" psychoanalysis and a scientific rigor and objectivity that corrects many of Freud's failings (e.g., not sorting observations carefully from theories). He even writes with some of the style of Freud, with a novelist's power of description and storytelling combined with both elegant and trenchant thinking. He does not simply draw from a single case at a time, but from an entire ensemble of cases with memorable names. The Neurasthenic's Husband, the Pesticide Chemist, the Gibson Girl, the Indian Scientist, the Stationery Manufacturer, and the Falling Social Worker return again and again in different combinations.

He also draws upon the whole maternal side of English analysis that has been so fertile in clinical and conceptual achievements—from Anna Freud on the defenses, from Melanie Klein in the conception of depressive and paranoid positions, from Winnicott on "good enough" mothering and the need for ruthlessness. Malan's capacity to integrate opposites is very impressive. Qualities which, for others, are merely dichotomies become, for him, possible in the same man and the same breath, very much like Freud again: boldness and cautionary tales, ruthlessness and sympathy, high drama and science, Holmesian shrewdness and wonder.

While all of this, I think, is his due, I must conclude that the change from Balint's leadership to that of Malan results both in narrowing and in very high powered development in the focused areas. The model of technique becomes heavily and classically interpretive. The model of selection is a very powerful combination of psychoanalytic and objective–descriptive psychiatry. The Balint emphasis on interpersonal flexibility and existential staying-with-the-patient recedes into the background. This is especially true of Balint's understanding of nonverbal and preverbal archaic relationships, "basic faults" that cannot be healed by words but must be handled by ways of relating. Interpretation becomes the central device. We shall see, however, that these Balint elements do remain in the cases, although they are less prominent in Malan's models to account for the cases.

Perhaps this is inevitable with complex secrets like brief therapy. A man has only so much attention, so that concentration of interest on one side cannot but lead to neglect of other matters. Perhaps we should simply be grateful to Malan for the increase in power that he has given in his selective interest. Having sketched the main line of our story of 25 years of brief therapy at the Tavistock Clinic, we now turn specifically to the early, middle, and recent stages of this remarkable development, in order to see what has been the context at each stage, what has been attempted, and what has been grasped scientifically so that this complex secret might be retained.

BREAKING THE TRADITIONAL BONDS OF PSYCHOANALYSIS:
A STUDY OF BRIEF PSYCHOTHERAPY (MALAN, 1963)

CONTEXT

Why had psychoanalysis become a longer and longer method of treatment, so that few could have its benefits? How had it continued to stay disconnected from science, so that its discoveries remained unaccepted? In most quarters, this context has been not altered from 17 years ago, since few understand how Malan and his colleagues boldly set themselves against the two major problems of psychoanalysis and, I think, solved them both. I can only recommend to the reader who finds himself blocked by these questions to turn at once to Chapters 2 and 3 of *A Study of Brief Psychotherapy,* only the bare outline of which I can provide here.

WHAT WAS ATTEMPTED

What have been the "lengthening factors," Malan asks, which changed psychoanalysis from a brief therapy to a long-term therapy? Psychoanalysis seemed to "discover" more and more inevitable, lengthening factors in the patient: "1. Resistance, 2. Overdetermination, 3. Necessity for working through, 4. Roots of neurosis in early childhood, 5. Transference, 6. Dependence, 7. Negative transference, connected with termination, 8. The transference neurosis." Some lengthening factors could directly be located in the change in analysts, however: "9. A tendency towards passivity and the willingness to follow where the patient leads, 10. The 'sense of timelessness' conveyed to the patient, 11. Therapeutic perfectionism, 12. The increasing preoccupation with ever deeper and earlier experiences" (Malan, 1963, pp. 8–9). If these were the lengthening factors, were they inevitable? Or could the focal therapy workshop deliberately set itself against *all* these lengthening factors, either by interpretation or setting limits? This was the therapeutic project.

What were the antiscientific factors separating psychoanalysis from the main body of scientific inquiry? "1. The failure to publish sufficient details of individual cases, with the result that an independent observer is rarely able to draw his own conclusions; 2. The tendency to select only the most successful cases for publication, so that no lessons are learnt from failure; 3. The utter neglect of the vital necessity for developing psychodynamic methods, based on published evidence, for assessing therapeutic results; 4. The partial neglect of the equal necessity for long follow-up" (Malan, 1963, pp. 35–36). The scientific project was to correct all these failures at once, with detailed case reports, psychodynamic outcome criteria with published evidence (including the failures as well as the successes), and strict and long follow-up.

This was a pilot study of 21 patients, with 7 therapists who were supervised by their colleagues in the workshop (including Balint), all of whom either were analysts or had had several years of training in psychoanalytic psychotherapy. Between January 1955 and Easter 1956, patients were seen from 4 to 40 times; all but 3 received less than 20 sessions. Follow-up for assessment of psychodynamic change continued for 3 months to 5 years beyond treatment. The criteria for success were defined as follows: 0 meaning no change, 1 meaning only symptomatic change but no new methods for handling the stressful conflict, 2 meaning symptomatic change *and* evidence of facing comparable stress without new symptoms and with new coping strategies, 3 meaning ability to handle these stressful conflicts in both major spheres of life (both at work and at home), with both men and women. The interest was in whether or not brief psychotherapy could produce clinical results that would compare favorably with long-term psychoanalysis, that is, scores of 2 or better, indicating stable psychodynamic change, rather than a change that was symptomatic or temporary or obtained by withdrawing or avoiding the central conflicts. The critical test (scores below 2 or above 2) bears repeating, because it is central to the claim that brief therapy can compare favorably with long-term analysis. The idea is that a central conflict in a patient can be considered improved only when the patient shows evidence of tolerating the full force of the conflict, with appropriate coping strategies and without symptoms. For example, if the patient has a central conflict about rivalry with other men, which causes anxiety, lengthy obsessive preparations, and withdrawal from competition, he can be considered "psychodynamically improved" only when he faces new situations of rivalry with men without these symptoms and with full capacity to do his best. This concept is essential to the scientific status of psychoanalysis, for it makes possible objective measurement of what psychoanalysis seeks to change at the heart of the neurosis.

The intended clinical experiment was based on the conservative anticipations of the therapists in the workshop. They believed that only mild cases of recent onset would do well, and that the transference should be avoided, deflected, or ignored because of fear of the "transference neurosis,'' that is, that the clock should be turned back to the primitive psycho-analytic technique, before transference was made central to the technique.

The actual clinical experiment, as Malan noted, brought together two populations which would do what was most natural to them: the analysts, who would use their interest and skill in transference interpretation, and the Tavistock patients, who would demonstrate their long-standing and severe character disorder problems. As Malan suggested, it was an experiment in nature, an ''ecological'' event.

OUTCOME

From the methodologic point of view, the clarity about dynamic criteria for change is superb, but the histories of ''all known disturbances in the patient's life'' are very weak (e.g., strictly oriented to Oedipal phenomena, the ignoring of separation–individuation events), as are the accounts of the therapies (e.g., listing therapist interpretations but very little about the responses of the patients).

Despite Malan's heralding, the clinical results read as a succession of failures, with an occasional dramatic success. Only 6 of the 21 patients scored either 2 or 3 on outcome, 3 scored 1, and 10 scored 0 (2 were unscored). On the three- to four-year follow-up, however, 3 of the 6 star cases had scores which improved from 3 to 4.[6] Certainly, this powerful and stable psychodynamic change in brief therapy is not consistent with the conservative psychoanalytic position.

THE EARLY MODEL OF SELECTION

The conservative Hypothesis A in the literature had suggested that only mild neurotic problems of recent onset would be suitable for brief therapy. Hypothesis A was refuted, to the surprise of the workshop members themselves. In fact, mild problems of recent onset were not among the successes at all. Instead, all but one of the cases in which dynamic change (score of 2 or better) occurred were chronic character disorders with disabling anxieties, phobias, hysterical symptoms, and deficient interpersonal capacities of at least several years duration. The only exception was the Lighterman, with severe panic attacks two to three months prior to treatment. The most severe disturbances, of paranoid and psychopathic characters, indeed failed as predicted. Hypothesis B was confirmed: ''The prognosis is best in those patients who show evidence from the beginning of a willingness and an ability to *work in interpretive therapy"* (Malan, 1963, p. 178).

THE EARLY MODEL OF TECHNIQUE

The conservative hypothesis of technique was that the transference had to be avoided. Malan argues that this Series 1 showed that *(a)* radical interpretation of the transference did not bring on the feared effects, *(b)* it often was "inevitable" to resolve an early deadlock of communication, and *(c)* the more radical the technique, the better the results. Radical or complete transference interpretation included the parent-transference link, early genetic material, negative transference, and termination experiences. With the thinly reported cases, it is very difficult for this reader to judge whether propositions *(a), (b),* and *(c)* hold up as consistently as claimed by Malan. I will return to these claims again, where the evidence is more complete in the replication of Series 2. In any case, the early model of technique offered nearly complete freedom from the constricting belief that interpreting the transference should be avoided. It was *either* not harmful, inevitable for continuing, or essential to success, depending on how one judges the evidence.

THE FIRST OVERALL CONCEPTION OF BRIEF THERAPY

Malan (1963) summarizes as follows:

> Prognosis seems to be most favorable when the following conditions apply: The patient has a high motivation; the therapist has a high enthusiasm; transference arises early and becomes a major feature of therapy; and grief and anger at termination are important issues. (p. 274)

The most important result of this pilot study was that the two major obstacles to brief therapy from classical analysis had been effectively challenged—the inevitability of the lengthening factors, and the inevitability of subjective judgments. Even if the star cases were a small minority, Malan and his colleagues had demonstrated that powerful and stable psychodynamic change could be brought about in brief therapy, and that the subjective events of psychoanalysis could be handled objectively. The deadening assumptions had been broken, and the second study could be planned.

THE POTENTIAL FOR PLANNING BRIEF PSYCHOTHERAPY IN ADVANCE OF TREATMENT: *THE FRONTIER OF BRIEF PSYCHOTHERAPY* (MALAN, 1976a), *TOWARD THE VALIDATION OF DYNAMIC PSYCHOTHERAPY* (MALAN, 1976b)

CONTEXT

Despite the radical evidence from *A Study of Brief Psychotherapy* (Malan, 1963) and from Sifneos (1972) and Mann (1973), the same spectrum of opinion about brief therapy continued as before, and psychoanalysis and science continued their separate ways. Apparently, the argument for the clinical paradigm of focal psychotherapy and the scientific argument for the validity of the evidence would have to be strengthened. Malan elected to write *The Frontier of Brief Psychotherapy* (1976a) for clinicians, and *Toward the Validation of Dynamic Psychotherapy* (1976b) for psychotherapy researchers, dividing what had been the double labor of *A Study of Brief Psychotherapy* (1963), in recognition of the reality that these audiences remained quite separate.

WHAT WAS ATTEMPTED

Series 1 had been a pilot study. Series 2 would be a replication, with the clinical acumen gained from the first series and stricter scientific standards. The second focal therapy workshop (1956–1961), consisting of 10 therapists, treated 39 patients and followed up 30 of them successfully, with a median follow-up of five to six years after treatment. Of the 30 cases, 22 were actually brief therapy cases of less than 30 sessions; the other 8 went on to long-term therapy.

The selection criteria were much stricter than in Series 1. At the referral stage, before the patient was seen, those with grave pathology were excluded, following Hildebrand's exclusion criteria: serious suicidal attempts, drug addiction, convinced homosexuality, long-term hospitalization, more than one course of electroconvulsive therapy (ECT), chronic alcoholism, incapacitating chronic obsessional symptoms, incapacitating chronic phobic symptoms, gross destructive or self-destructive acting out. At the second stage, that of interview and psychological testing, a prima facie case for brief therapy would be necessary. The patient had responded to interpretation, a focus was conceivable, and the dangers were not inevitable; that is, the patient was not likely to break down into serious depression or psychosis along the way or be unable to terminate. (See Malan, 1976a, p. 69, Table 3, for an excellent summary.)[7]

OUTCOME

The median outcome score rose dramatically, from 1 in the first series to 2.11 in the second. The reader will recall that the 2 score represents symptomatic relief plus evidence of having managed the stressful conflict in appropriate new ways. Taking a score of 2 or higher as a favorable outcome, and less than 2 as unfavorable, the 30 patients divided into several distinct groups. There were 9 short favorable cases (9 SF), of which 7 had moderately severe neurotic problems and 2 were drastic cases, to which we shall return. There were 6 long favorable cases (6 LF), making a total of 15 out of 30 clear successes, in which psychotherapy brought about significant dynamic change. There were 9 short unfavorable cases (9 SU), 4 false-positive cases (4 F) which were short in duration and brought about by spontaneous remission long after a negative result from therapy, and 2 long unfavorable cases (2 LU).[8]

In regard to predicting outcome from content analysis of the technique (therapist notes), the higher percentage of parent-transference links made by the therapist gave the only successful correlation with higher outcome. In addition, the patients who ranked highest in receiving parent-transference interpretations had the best outcome. Malan argues that this is the first validation of a psychoanalytic principle with empirical evidence.

THE EMERGENT MODEL OF SELECTION

The trouble with the emphasis on motivation as the central indicator for selection (Malan, 1963) is that motivation varies a great deal, depending on what difficulties have to be faced. What we want to know is whether motivation will remain high as patient and therapist go through each stage of brief therapy and as they link separate areas of the patient's experience. How can one anticipate the effect of these difficulties?

The reply is that the therapist can conduct the therapy in advance as a thought experiment. This is possible because Malan has clearly defined the typical dynamic events of brief therapy and the kinds of experiences in the patient's life which will help or hinder these events in brief therapy.

What, then, is the logic of the interaction in brief therapy? It is very

straightforward. The patient must be capable of beginning effective therapeutic work within the first four sessions. This will not happen if the therapist cannot make emotional contact with the patient, or if he must work
for a long while either to generate motivation or to penetrate the defenses.
The patient must be capable of terminating therapeutic work after the
focal issue has been worked through. This will not happen if the issues are
too complex, or if the dependency aroused cannot be given up. Finally, the
patient must be capable of carrying on his life without breakdown as the
focal conflict is being faced. This will not happen if the depressive or psychotic potential is considerable, and if there is little or no support in the patient's outside life. (See Malan, 1976a, p. 69, Table 3.)

In effect, brief therapy has a beginning, a middle, and an end, for
which the patient must be capable. Malan defines six different arenas
where we may test this hypothesis in advance of therapy:

1. the psychiatric history
2. the psychodynamic history
3. the history of interpersonal relations
4. the present outside relationships
5. the relationship made with the interviewing therapist, especially in
   response to trial interpretations
6. the projective tests

The material in all six sectors should integrate into a recurrent, un-
solved conflict (what Mann, 1973, would describe in existential terms as
"the present and chronically recurring pain"). If the same focal conflict
keeps reappearing in all six sectors of the inquiry, there is likelihood that
these areas may be linked by the therapist in the course of the brief therapy
itself. It is foolhardy, Malan suggests, to miss any one of these sectors of
inquiry by imagining one has a plausible case from one or two. This was
learned by some very painful errors, which comprise the "Cautionary
Tales" in the closing of *The Frontier of Brief Psychotherapy* (Malan,
1976a).

In the ideal assessment, the therapist predicts in advance, from his
survey of the six sectors described, the current conflict, the nuclear conflict and its relation to the current one; the patient responds to initial interpretation of this conflict, with a rise in motivation; this conflict is about
to emerge in the transference; and the termination version of the conflict
can be imagined clearly. For example, the patient is conflicted about becoming a painter against her parent's wishes. She has always felt that her

parents were easily injured by her independence, and she experiences a surge of determination when the therapist tells her that it is not easy to feel your strength is so overpowering. It is evident that the patient will become concerned about hurting the therapist's feelings with her intensity (the transference), especially in the termination, when she is likely to direct the ending on her own terms. (See Malan, 1976a, pp. 92–100, for a case such as this, i.e., the Almoner.)

The stages in the selection can be clearly demarcated:

1. The therapist eliminates the absolute contraindications (Hildebrand's exclusion criteria) at the point of referral.
2. The therapist declines brief therapy in the first interview, if the dangers of beginning, surviving, and ending the therapy are inevitable for the patient.
3. The therapist attempts to define the focus from the interview and the projective test, which will integrate the dynamic events in all six areas of the inquiry.
4. The therapist offers the focus to the patient.
5. If the patient responds to this offer with deeper material and increased motivation, the therapist will set up an agreement to see the patient for brief therapy, ending on a definite date—after 20 sessions if the therapist is experienced, or 30 if the therapist is a trainee or the therapy has some other special complication. For example, a long-standing, outside, dyadic relationship in difficulty may take longer. The patient is told that if and when he needs to talk further, he may return after the termination on an ad hoc basis.

THE EMERGENT MODEL OF TECHNIQUE

Havens (1973) wrote of Freud:

> He possessed to the highest degree what Napoleon called the supreme desiderata of generalship: complete patience and utter decisiveness. We can consider whether he had the same emotional flexibility but we need to understand at the start this striking power: both to act and not to act. (p. 94)

Malan's general scheme of technique for brief therapy appeals to the military general in us all. The plan for battle is to stick completely to interpretation, the one and only necessary weapon. The "strategic aim" is that of psychoanalysis itself: to bring into consciousness the emotional conflicts. The only difference from classical psychoanalysis is that the brief therapist usually limits him- or herself to analysis of a single conflict. This "focal conflict" is often the very same "nuclear conflict" which would be at the center of a lengthy analysis. In exceptional cases, the "focal conflict" chosen would be more superficial than the nuclear problem. In any case, the "strategic aim" is the same as that of psychoanalysis itself, except that it takes a single conflict as its object rather than a series of different conflicts that are handled in a full-scale analysis. The "tactical aims" are taken in two steps:

1. Analysis of the defense and anxiety allows analysis of the repressed impulse in one sector of the patient's life, ordinarily his present outside (O) situation being taken first.
2. This battle having been won, it is linked to the other two major sectors, the transference (T) and the genetic past situation with the parents (P)—in Malan's favorite schematic terms, the O/T and O/P links and, most essentially, the T/P link.

The theory of therapy, always assumed but rarely discussed by Malan, is that unconscious conflicts from childhood govern adult life, unless they are made conscious (Glover, 1955). Interpretation mobilizes this material into contact with the adult ego, which assimilates what has been repressed and arranges more appropriate solutions.[9]

THE EMERGENT UNIFIED CONCEPTION OF BRIEF THERAPY

I hope it is apparent to the reader by now that Malan plans the attack in brief therapy with a schematic clarity and thoroughness of preparation that is not likely to be surpassed. The optimal result is what he calls "dynamic interaction," which may be thought of and even measured as a summation of motivation, focus, and the percentage of parent-transference interpretations. A graph (Malan, 1976b, p. 265) of motivation + T/P% plotted against outcome shows that all but a few cases, which are "exceptional" on clinical grounds, fall along the slope showing that outcome is proportional to the degree of "dynamic interaction" measured in this way.[10] The scheme for focal therapy has become highly organized.

UNEXPLAINED COMPLEXITY

I do not believe, however, that it actually works this way. There are three different sets of clinical observations provided by Malan himself. Correct as he has been to give the independent observer a chance to come to his own conclusions on the strength of the published evidence, these observations are not explained by his model of technique.

1. The model does not explain the difference in outcome between the short favorable (SF) and the short unfavorable (SU) cases.
2. The very cases that are described at length show much more complicated mechanisms of improvement than the theory can allow for.
3. The model does not explain anything about the other mechanisms of improvement (besides interpretation) that Malan (1976b) admits in the conclusion of *Toward the Validation of Dynamic Psychotherapy* are significant.

Let us take these three sets of clinical observations one at a time. A minimum requirement for a theory of brief therapy is that it explain the difference between successful and failed cases. Now, if we compare the seven short favorable neurotic cases with the seven unfavorable neurotic cases,[11] what kind of explanation for the difference can Malan's theory provide us?

On the basis of initial motivation, three of the seven SF cases are negative, while only two of the seven SU cases are negative. Motivation itself is no explanation. The reply must be that the therapist's selection of the correct focus and his vigorous interpretation of the parent-transference connections explain the favorable outcome as opposed to the unfavorable.

But if we inspect the case reports of the unfavorable cases, we find no lack of vigorous interpretation. Rather, we find that the four "false" cases were put in touch with powerful affective experiences that they could not control, leading to flights from therapy. The three other SU cases are obviously patients with very uncertain identities, which will remind readers of Kohut's (1971) "disorders of the self." It is not surprising to such readers that these patients would be put in touch with powerful Oedipal feelings without being able to manage them. All seven of these patients were engaged in "dynamic interaction" but could not contain it. It is no wonder they broke off from "dynamic interaction" and consequently scored low on focus and T/P%. Of course, Malan surely might give counterexplanations for these failures to the ones I have offered. The point is not that I am correct in my interpretation, when indeed I am much farther from the realities of these cases than he was. Rather, I argue that "dynamic interaction" is no explanation at all for the difference between the successful and failed neurotic brief cases. As Malan himself admits

(1963, p. 36), an adequate model of brief therapy must face the failures and explain them.

The second set of unexplained clinical observations are the cases of successful brief therapy cited at length in *The Frontier of Brief Psychotherapy* (Malan, 1976a). They are admirable pieces of clinical work, vividly described. It is even possible for Malan to link together all the associations of the patient with his minimum set of concepts: defense, anxiety, and impulse, and current outside, transference, and parental problems. But the decisive interventions of the therapist are not explained within this scheme.

Consider the frustrated young man, the Zoologist. The current problem is that he has given up his love for biology, in deference to his father's ideas about a career, but then has angrily spoiled his success in college. He is very intense about his love and his anger but has to defend against both. Already Malan is obliged to construct (correctly, I think) two triangles of defense, anxiety, and impulse, for the love and for the anger. But the therapist's first decision is what to take up with the patient, given these two possibilities. The frustration is so prominent that he is tempted to go after the anger, interpreting the defense, anxiety, and impulse, but the patient does not respond. Then he simply tells the patient there is a "choked" quality in his voice when he speaks of what matters to him, that "he seemed to have a lot of intense feelings that couldn't come out." The patient suddenly opens up, telling of how a young girl had once put her hand in his and said, "I like you," one of the proudest moments of his life.

The Zoologist tempts the therapist to see only his frustration and hate. When the therapist, like the little girl, appreciates his loving side, he opens up. Several interviews later, the therapist must pass the same test, this time over why the patient feels like "wandering off" from therapy. The therapist is tempted to emphasize the anger, true as it may be, but instead tells the patient that the latter wishes the therapist would "actively show him that I loved him." In summary, the patient has to have his love appreciated before he is willing to engage about his hatred. I could argue that this is a *necessary sequence* for this patient. When the therapist shows that he appreciates the loving side of the patient, the patient is reassured he can show his hatefulness without losing love. If the therapist persisted in pushing for the anger, however sophisticated he might be about taking the defense and anxiety ahead of the impulse and choosing the current outside sector or past relationship ahead of the transference, little could be expected.

In fact, this therapist intuitively follows the first plan, understanding the patient's initial need for love, then vigorously facing his hatefulness, alternating back to the need for love when reassurance was needed. He handles being tempted to the wrong issue by not being tempted—the critical *test*—and he keeps to the right order or *sequence* of issues. The two critical decisions described cannot, however, be directed by the theory or concepts Malan has available. The best he can do is acknowledge that there are *two* defense-anxiety-impulse triangles, and that the therapist shows great intuitive "skill."

All the other cases described at length in *The Frontier of Brief Psychotherapy* (Malan, 1976a) have a similar set of tests, in which the therapist must do more than "interpret" the defense-anxiety-impulse relations and the connections between current outside, past, and transference problems. In all of them, he is tempted to be like the transference expectations and, as Alexander and French (1946) have argued, must show that he is different. By tempting the therapist to repeat the traumatic activities of the parents, the patient tests him to be sure he is different, to be sure it is safe to bring out the deeper feelings (Sampson, 1976; Weiss, 1978; Weiss, Sampson, Caston, Silberschatz, & Gassner, 1977). The Magistrate's Daughter has literally been seduced by her brother and continually flirted with by her father. She arranges an increasingly steep set of tests for this therapist, to be doubly sure he will not repeat the trauma. She gives him a fascinating set of sexual details, tempting him to go deeply and fast. She becomes indecisive and confused about where she wants to go, inviting him to take over. She tempts him to keep her in therapy "even though she might run out of things to say." Miss Persistence is another remarkable case, in which the therapist puts a stop to all the "great expectations" held out to this patient through years in the clinic and years with her parents and boyfriend. This patient is now able to be angry, knowing her therapist is strong enough to resist and calm her.

In the case of the Falling Social Worker, Malan admits a complex set of themes, that the "use of complex foci requires a great deal of further exploration." But what he calls the exception to his classical model of technique is shown by his own full examples to be the rule. By my reanalysis of all nine short favorable (SF) cases in Series 2, all but the Indian Scientist show this same evidence of either a complex *sequence* of issues or a series of difficult *tests* in which the therapist must show him- or herself to be different from the transference expectations, or usually both.[12] The intuitive mastery of this method shows through, despite the conceptual model of pure interpretation.

The third set of unexplained clinical observations is tucked away in the research book that most clinicians will not read, *Toward the Valida-tion of Dynamic Psychotherapy* (Malan, 1976b). There they are least apt to contradict the classical paradigm of technique which Malan wants to em-phasize. There he acknowledges that maturing, finding a satisfactory mar-ital partner, taking responsibility for one's life, and gaining insight from sit-uations which involve little dependence or transference interpretation can bring about lasting dynamic change. This is evident from the follow-up study conducted by Malan on patients seen for one interview at the Tavi-stock (Malan, Heath, Bacal, & Balfour, 1975) and from the "spontaneous remissions" of the false cases in Series 2 of the focal therapy workshop. What does Malan do with these contradictions to his clinical paradigm? He admits that both "nonspecific" mechanisms and "specific" interpre-tive mechanisms can bring about dynamic change, as if interpretation were the only way to give the patient assistance that is specific to his psy-chodynamics! Alexander and French (1946), Balint *et al.* (1972), and Kohut (1971) surely would not agree. The therapist can be quite specific about what kind of interaction a particular patient needs to solve his or her problems or what specific emotional experience must be shared by another. The interpersonal and existential methods can be quite as specific as the in-terpretations of psychoanalysis without telling the patient about it.

In summary, *The Frontier of Brief Psychotherapy* (Malan, 1976a) and *Toward the Validation of Dynamic Psychotherapy* (Malan 1976b) demonstrate a powerful new capacity for organizing brief therapy, both in the logic of selection (conducting the therapy as a thought experiment) and in tight battle plans for the therapy itself. The unifying conception of "dy-namic interaction" also allows the outcomes to be roughly encompassed.

THE CURRENT METHODS OF SELECTION AND TECHNIQUE: *INDIVIDUAL PSYCHOTHERAPY AND THE SCIENCE OF PSYCHODYNAMICS* (MALAN, 1979)

CONTEXT

Malan's double project remains the same: to bring psychoanalysis to its rightful honors, and to bring out its abstract core of scientific truth. Now he brings these aims back together in a new form, a textbook on psycho-therapy. Traditional psychoanalysis is held to be an immutable set of truths, but its order is reversed. No longer is long-term therapy the central paradigm of psychoanalysis, with brief therapy a special variation. Now brief psychotherapy is the central paradigm, because it shows the basic principles of psychodynamic knowledge clearly and succinctly, and long-term analysis is a special variation for patients with more complex issues and deeper deprivation. At once, Malan upholds the principles of orthodox psychoanalysis, while reversing the relative priority of long-term and short-term treatment! It is a very quiet and clever revolution. The scientific failures of psychoanalysis are attacked more directly and simply. Psychoanalysis has kept apart from science and biology, maintained an esoteric language, and turned to ideology.

THE ATTEMPT

The generative idea of this book is to separate the reliable clinical observations of psychoanalysis from its ideology. Malan starts with the most elementary and familiar and proceeds in language as plain as possible toward the strange and more difficult problems, keeping a continual eye on man's biological past and future. As he moves toward the more strange and difficult problems in patients, Malan emphasizes the uncontrolled problem of aggression in man himself. He ends with five powerful chapters on assessment for psychotherapy, which emphasize that we must be sympathetic but ruthlessly honest about what we can do about all this. This is not a textbook in any conventional way, but rather an extended position paper on where we stand with our psychodynamic knowledge.

THE CURRENT MODEL OF SELECTION

The planning methods of *The Frontier of Brief Psychotherapy* (Malan, 1976a) remain as stated there, but Malan is able to render them even more concisely by facing two strategic problems:

1. How can one have the benefits of deep contact with the patient—to see the patient's ability to work with interpretation, his motivation, and the suitability of the therapist's focus—without the risks of arousing hopes, disturbance, and attachment that may be dashed?
2. How does one balance psychodynamic contact with traditional

psychiatric inquiry? the essential subjective events with the history of objective events?

The "fundamental law of psychotherapeutic forecasting" says that the extremes of psychopathology discovered by psychiatric history are likely to return in an intense period of psychotherapy but are apt to tell little of how the patient may take advantage of psychotherapy. In plain English, the essence of the two questions may be stated as follows: How does one care for the patient and ruthlessly face facts? By dealing with these potential contradictions, Malan reaches a new integration of psychoanalysis and objective–descriptive psychiatry.

At the risk of becoming overly schematic myself, I will outline the logic of Malan's proposal (1979, Chapter 17) for the steps in selection:

1. If there are known disturbing facts, or if the patient hints at severe deprivation or psychotic experiences, the interviewer proceeds directly to the psychiatric inquiry before making much contact. For example, a social worker sought a "training brief therapy" in order to "come to life in my work." Rather than follow this emotional lead, the interview shifted directly to asking about when she had ever "come to life" and discovered her coming to life in the last therapy had been way out of control, with her smearing carbolic acid on her face. Better to find this out, certainly, before setting contact in motion again (1979, p. 213)!

2. If psychotherapy openings are not available, one also restrains contact for the same reason.

3. One may risk interpretive comments to make some contact, but no more than necessary.

4. If the disturbance seems containable, therapy is available, and contact has been made, the interviewer should proceed vigorously with trial interpretations.

5. The interviewer should gently halt when he or she has sufficient information.

6. The interviewer must be prepared to take responsibility for situations created by the interview.

In summary, Malan solves the two strategic problems of selection interviews: (1) the interviewer controls for the dangers of contact prior to making it; and (2) the interviewer uses psychiatric history to face the worst, and psychodynamic contact and history to find out what the patient can do to change.

THE MODEL OF TECHNIQUE IN BRIEF THERAPY, FROM ELEMENTARY TO COMPLEX

The technique of psychotherapy will no longer be vague when we can describe what the psychotherapist actually does. Malan's reply is that he lends to the patient definite capabilities that the patient lacks. In "the psychotherapy of everyday life," other people provide what the patient lacks, but if these talents are not available, the psychotherapist can supply them.

In Chapters 1 and 2, he tells us simply that the complexities of psychopathology arise from "unexpressed painful feeling." The Economics Student, enjoying herself with a young man in Spain, becomes jealous when her girlfriend joins them and takes over the interest, but she cannot express this painful jealousy because of shame and fear of losing control of her anger. She hints to them of her distress, and they read between the lines to her pain. Were her friends unable to read this, she might turn to a psychotherapist to appreciate the source of her pain. This is the simplest version of what we therapists do. We take a history, reading back to where the pain began. We face the unbearable feelings that the person cannot tolerate alone, so that he or she can find a more direct way of relieving them. In Chapter 3, Malan adds the ability to translate unconscious communications, and in Chapter 4, the ability to face conflict fearlessly and evenhandedly, both of which patients may not be able to do for themselves. In Chapter 5, Malan reminds us that taking an accurate history may be all that is necessary. The patient may have the remaining talents to face the situation and take a new course, making one interview psychotherapy quite common! (See Malan, 1979, Chapter 4, the Geologist.)

Now he takes the reader beyond "the psychotherapy of everyday life" to consider, in Chapters 7, 8, and 9, the "sexual problems in women," the "problems of masculinity in men," and "transference." Here it is also possible to be economical with theory, paring down psychoanalytic theory on Oedipal issues to its recurrent clinical observation that adult conflicts become intelligible when linked to the sexual dilemmas of children. He demonstrates the variations on the theme when this light is cast.

Finally, in Chapter 10, Malan explains the overall strategy in which the described actions of the therapist are employed: "The aim of every moment of every session is to put the patient in touch with as much of his true feelings as he can bear" (1979, p. 74). The therapist can decide if he or she is proceeding in this true direction by judging whether rapport is increasing or decreasing, this being the "universal indicator."

In Chapter 11, Malan demonstrates that the most successful area for applying this strategy is in the problems of assertion. He believes these are workable in two basic steps: (1) identify the defense against aggression and the anxiety about losing control, which will allow the patient to experience his true angry feelings in one sector (transference, outside, or past), and (2) link this experience to the other areas, where the patient will repeat his advance.

BEYOND THE BASIC MODEL OF TECHNIQUE: THE CORRECTIVE EMOTIONAL EXPERIENCE AND TERMINATION

I was startled to discover a break from this orthodoxy hidden away in Malan's Chapter 13 on "regression and long-term therapy." Here, in three pages (140–142), is a clear exposition of what Alexander and French (1946) had argued, and how it had been misconstrued on the way to throwing it out. The "corrective emotional experience" is not the attempt to provide the nurturance missed from the depriving parents. Indeed, one cannot make up this failure. But one can help the patient to experience the longings, giving up those that are impossible and seeking what satisfactions life can offer. The good therapist fails to nurture the patient as much as the latter would like to be nurtured. The therapist is "corrective" in that, unlike the parents, he or she is willing to face this failure and help the patient bear it. This is the "new ending" that Alexander and French said was possible.

But how should the therapist *behave* in order to bring about the "new ending," if, indeed, he or she is not going to make up the failure? Malan here stops short of explaining Alexander and French. Perhaps that would be going too far from the classical model. But he shows a perfect working understanding of their principles in Chapter 16 (regarding termination) without ever making them explicit.

What "the new ending" means, specifically, is that every termination is somewhat different. This is by far the most flexible model of termination current in brief therapy. In the Geologist, the therapist accepts the gratitude of the patient without trying to hold him beyond the single interview. Yet, in the Factory Inspector and the Neurasthenic's Husband, the therapist opposes the flight of the patient. In the Factory Inspector, he compromises, suggesting the patient try out his new-found potency for three weeks and then come back to discuss it. Why the differences? How would one know which way to go, since one would certainly be tempted to either let go or confront in nearly every case? The governing principle, which Malan illustrates beautifully but never states, is that the therapist *behaves differently* from the patient's parents, specifically avoiding the kind of trauma they would inflict about ending. Hence, a "new ending" becomes possible. That is, the Geologist was trying to free himself from a possessive mother, which required the therapist not hold on to the patient at the end,[13] whereas the Neurasthenic's Husband had a weak father, who could not handle the strength of his child, which required his therapist to be boldly confronting, so that the patient would know the therapist was ready and capable of tolerating his anger at the end. In the case of the Factory Inspector, it is even more subtle, since the therapist ends up showing that he is glad for the patient's new-found potency, yet does not need him to leave. Confronting him could have been an attack on his new, marvelous claim, while letting him go could have signaled unwillingness to get closer. The final two termination cases, the Swiss Receptionist and the Man with the School Phobia, are powerful and extremely bold versions of the principle of being different from the parents. In the first, the therapist bears with a woman who lost her mother at 14 years of age, not relenting from the time limit, while in the second, the therapist bears with an extreme problem of rage, using a series of emergency adjustments.

REINTERPRETATION OF THE INTUITIVE MASTERY IN MALAN'S CASE EXAMPLES

AN ALTERNATIVE HYPOTHESIS OF TECHNIQUE FOR THE COMPLEX NEUROSES

In the background of my exposition on *The Frontier of Brief Psychotherapy* (Malan, 1976a) and *Individual Psychotherapy and the Science of Psychodynamics* (Malan, 1979), I have been sketching the lines of an alternative explanation of Malan's technique, which I will now bring out as clearly and directly as I can. Let us take, as a starting point, the case that Malan (1979) has made up to exemplify his conception of technique, the Imaginary Case (pp. 81–89).

Here we have a young man who, when he was a teenager, lost his mother from a terrible cancer. This was so shocking to the boy's father that he withdrew, and both father and son retreated into numb silence and work. This loss was worsened for the boy by his having had a quarrelsome relationship with his mother for years before her death. Now, as a young man, he comes for psychotherapy because of his relationships with young women, where he loses feeling for them after a promising start, and finds they become angry and disappointed in him.

The classical theory, of course, finds no difficulty in linking the past and the present outside problem to predict the two problems in the transference. The patient will have difficulty getting close to the therapist, and he will have difficulty with anger at the therapist, as he had with his mother and girlfriends. Malan has his imaginary therapist-in-training make two major mistakes in this Imaginary Case, one with each of the transference problems. After initial closeness, the patient backs away, as he has with young women he starts to care about. The therapist is tempted to confront the patient about this defense against his true feelings, pointing out the defense and the anxiety. This confrontation leads to a breakdown in communication. In the termination phase, as the patient is getting angry about being left by the therapist and is worried about letting go with the anger, the therapist again is tempted to confront the patient about these true feelings, his defense against them, and the anxiety about loss of control. Again, the communication is disrupted.

In both instances, Malan (1979) has the imaginary, experienced supervisor caution the therapist-in-training against confronting the transference resistance too deeply and too fast (pp. 83, 89). These are two instances of his precept that the "skill" of the therapist is in knowing "how deeply to interpret, at any given moment, with any particular patient" (Malan, 1976a, p. 262). Yet, both errors are consistent with the model of technique: to interpret the defense, anxiety, and impulse or true feeling, and to connect the present, outside version with the past and with the transference. Malan has to go outside the theory for practical help to an ill-defined something called "skill."

An alternative psychoanalytic theory of technique, whereby we may predict the temptations and errors of the therapist, takes us beyond these limitations of the original theory of the defenses, which Malan adopted from Anna Freud, Glover, and Strachey. This new "control-mastery" theory of Weiss and colleagues (Sampson, 1976; Weiss, 1978; Weiss *et al.*, 1977) builds upon the early ego psychology of the defenses, as well as more recent advances. Sandler and Joffe (1969) suggested that defenses are not lifted until the patient is reassured that it is safe to do so and is sure he will not be traumatized again ("the conditions of safety"). Patients then have to protect themselves against the repeat of the old trauma by being defensive.

Weiss (1978; Weiss *et al.*, 1977) and Sampson (1976) take this further.

They argue that the patient unconsciously tempts the therapist to repeat the earlier trauma, to test whether the therapist is actually different from the traumatic parents—whether, in the terms of Alexander and French (1946), the therapist is capable of providing or allowing a "new ending" to the "old problem." In Malan's (1979) Imaginary Case, control–mastery theory predicts that the therapist will be provoked by the patient (1) to either reject him or withdraw from him, as his mother did by dying and his father by becoming suddenly unavailable, and (2) to get into fights with him, which would make him feel very guilty. If the therapist does not fall to these specific temptations, the patient will be reassured that he can become close, without the danger of being left suddenly again, and get mad, without fear of protracted quarrels.

The fascination of Malan's Imaginary Case is that Malan intuitively shows his appreciation that therapists-in-training will fall to these very temptations which the classical theory cannot define for the trainee in advance, but which are predicted specifically by control–mastery theory as the critical tests of the therapist. As we have seen, Malan frequently refers to the idea of Alexander and French (1946) that the new ending comes about because the therapist is different from the transference expectations. Malan, the workshop therapists, and the therapists of his brief therapy unit continually show that they intuitively appreciate this critical idea, but when pressed to provide a conceptual model, they revert to the orthodox concept.

Of course, Malan is right that monitoring of "rapport" is essential and will help the therapist correct a divergence away from what is useful to the patient. He also has two methods for slowing down the confrontation with what is most difficult for the patient to bear: (1) by facing the defense and anxiety ahead of the impulse, and (2) by choosing the sector in which to face it, that is, transference, outside present relationship or past relationship. Why, then, do therapies get into trouble, even when the therapist is most tactful about showing the defense and anxiety first and in the most tolerable sector?

There are two reasons. First, even if interpretation makes the patient aware of the defense and anxiety, he or she may not be able to control the impulse when it is reexperienced. Hence, several kinds of preliminary steps are often necessary before interpretation. Second, interpretation of the transference may help to distinguish therapist from parent, or it may not. If the therapist makes a demanding interpretation, for example, he or she may become the essential, demanding parent.

Patients acquire the necessary "control and mastery" of the defenses either by finding a new control in themselves or by borrowing control temporarily from the therapist. Of the first type, patients may be stubborn because they are afraid of passivity that will endanger them. As they practice being stubborn with the therapist (and the therapist accepts their willfulness), they become reassured that they can always revert to being stubborn, should they lift their defense and be passive. The defense comes under conscious control, allowing it to be used selectively and reliably. Of the second type, patients may invite the therapist to do what is traumatic, to be sure in advance that the therapist is capable of withstanding the temptation and providing the control that is protective. Given the same problem of stubbornness and fearful passivity, patients might tempt the therapist to take over and run a session by forceful interpretation that is frightening. When the therapist does not take over, patients are reassured that they may show the passive longings, because the therapist will not assault them. Thus, the same danger may be controlled in advance of its full appearance either by a new capability of control in the patient (especially by more skillful use of the defense) or by proof of capable control in the therapist (Weiss, 1971). When these steps are omitted by the therapist who moves directly to pure interpretation, retreat by the patient is predictable.

When the dynamics are very similar according to the classical theory (e.g., in problems of assertion), the routes of control may be opposite, as may be the tests of the therapist. For example, the Interior Decorator (Malan, 1979, pp. 75-79) fears his temper because of being able to threaten his weak father. After a bold start, he becomes tentative and submissive, tempting the therapist to explore the latter topic. But the therapist does not fall to this temptation, which the patient's father would have preferred, and challenges the patient about the contrast between his start and his backing off. The patient now is reassured that the therapist can handle his forcefulness and brings out his propensity for finding fault in bigger men and bringing them down. He relies on the therapist to control these attacks without being hurt by them.

The Pesticide Chemist (Malan, 1979, pp. 101-107) has a similar problem with rage, but the route of control is opposite. The patient's approach is to learn to reduce the demands on him by others, so that his rage will not be so stimulated and too terrific to contain. He refuses to accept the therapist's challenges to go deeper, getting the therapist to stop being so demanding! Now it is possible to bring out the anger, knowing in advance that he can keep the amount down by not letting others push him around.

The patient relies on his own new capacity of control. In the Interior Decorator case, the therapist's challenging of the patient proves the therapist different from the weak father and capable of providing the control, whereas in the Pesticide Chemist, the therapist's backing off from challenging the patient allows the patient to control the amount of anger induced in himself.[14] Thus, similar dynamics may require opposite responses before interpretation.[15]

Hence, most neurotic problems cannot be reduced to Malan's two-step model of pure interpretation, that is, to interpret the defense, anxiety, and impulse and to interpret the link to other sectors. Only the Indian Scientist appears to work this way. All the other short favorable (SF) cases in Series 1 and 2 and all the extended case reports in *The Frontier of Brief Psychotherapy* (Malan, 1976a) and *Individual Psychotherapy and the Science of Psychodynamics* (Malan, 1979) are three-step cases:

1. The patient acquires the capacity to control the danger of the impulse, either by testing to be sure the therapist is different from the parent and is able to supply the control or by the therapist permitting the patient to practice a new control of his or her own.
2. The patient then exposes the dangerous impulse, and practices and masters it in one sector of his or her life.
3. The patient finally links this to the other sectors (transference, present outside relationship, past relationship), where the mastery is completed.

CROSS-VALIDATION OF THE CLASSICAL THEORY

Popper (1962) emphasized that a scientific hypothesis is no better than the tests to which it has been subjected. Correlations are always made to back up new theories and will continue to hold up, even if statistical calculations show they are significantly far from random distribution, as long as no serious attempts are made to disrupt the correlations with challenging experiments. After all, one could show that good health correlates with drinking milk in a dairy state (e.g., Wisconsin), because the healthy would tend to drink the favorite drink of the state, while the unhealthy would turn to other tonics. As long as one stayed in the dairy state, one would have powerful correlations to back up the theory, since no serious attempt would have been made to get outside the state, where the correlations could be disrupted.

Therefore, the importance of interpretive linking to dynamic change

cannot be considered corroborated until experiments are done in which
therapists try to avoid making interpretations. If the experiments fail, then
we may be more sure that parent-transference links are as necessary as
Malan would have us believe. In fact, in the two therapies in his series in
which the therapists designed the therapy in advance to avoid interpretation, namely, Mrs. Morley and the Stationery Manufacturer, the outcomes were outstanding. Thus, a minor experiment by Malan's colleagues
suggests the correlation is easily disrupted.

Indeed, this kind of testing of one psychodynamic hypothesis against
another is exactly what is needed to judge to what extent interpretive measures are necessary. One current set of such experiments are those by Weiss,
Sampson, and colleagues (Weiss *et al.*, 1977). They use a tape-recorded
analysis of a patient by an analyst in another city, who is unfamiliar with
their theory of change. Independent judges predict the course of the
therapy from the first ten sessions, one team using the classical theory,
another team the control–mastery theory. The relative adequacy of the
theories can be tested over the predictions which are opposite.

Not until more of these experiments are conducted can we judge the
validity of one theory against another. Even on the basis of the clinical evidence Malan provides, I hope I have shown that the interpretive two-step
model does not explain the clinical events. I am not claiming that my
counteranalysis is more correct (a preposterous idea, since I am much farther from the actual case histories than Malan), but rather that an alternative explanation is, at least, plausible. Brief therapy could provide the evidence in manageable complexity to decide between these rival theories.
Not until these decisive experiments are carried out can Malan consider his
theory of technique to be corroborated.

THE NEGLECTED STUDY OF TECHNIQUE:
FOCAL PSYCHOTHERAPY (BALINT *ET AL.*, 1972)

CONTEXT

Balint (Balint *et al.*, 1972) realized that the scientific project led by Malan
was strongest in specifying the dynamic criteria for outcome and following
up the cases and was weakest in the study of the technique used by the
members of the workshop (p. 5). He believed that the close study of an
outstanding case might begin to remedy this weakness. He did not say that

many of the intuitive elements in his technique were being lost because of Malan's narrower construction of psychoanalysis. Rather than lecture against this trend, he gave a remarkable clinical demonstration to show his technique at work, bringing back all the necessary elements we began with in *The Doctor, His Patient and the Illness* (Balint, 1957).

Nowhere are they missed more than in the brief psychotherapy of more disturbed depressive and paranoid patients. A moment's reflection will show why. A successful brief psychotherapy must arouse the very disturbance it seeks to remedy, but it must do so within the limits of control that the patient and therapist can muster. In more deprived patients, the impulses are huge, and the fears of renewed trauma are terrifying. Yet, Malan proposes only to interpret in the Kleinian tradition. These patients are told about their primitive defenses, fears, and impulses, and the parallels between present outside, past, and transference are clarified. Should we be surprised that the impulse, although well described, still feels wildly out of control to the patient? or that the therapist, interpreted as different from the parent, still seems very much like that parent? No wonder that the preliminary steps of control necessary to neurotic patients are even more essential here. The desires, rage, and retaliatory fears are enormous. Without preliminary phases of control, the dosage of intensity is usually neither tolerable nor safe. The treatments are erratic and often stopped by the patient without warning.[16]

But the problem is not only quantitative. When the child has been failed by his parents long before words were available to him, interpretations are not likely to come close enough to the disturbance.[17] The nonverbal climate or atmosphere matters more. Actions speak louder than words, how the patient and doctor fit together, "hit it off." These are the very elements left out by Malan's emphasis on interpretation but brought back into the center of treatment in *Focal Psychotherapy* (Balint *et al.,* 1972).[18] We shall see that these qualities allow the therapist to contain and control the primitive experience, which has to be aroused in the course of the treatment.

THE CASE

The patient, Mr. Baker, was apparently a very able and successful man. At the age of 43, he was a joint director of a stationery manufacturing firm, deeply in love with a loving and admirable wife, and the father of three children. His chief complaint, however, ran very deep. He had become increasingly preoccupied with his wife having had another suitor before they were married. On psychological testing, it was apparent that he was overwhelmed by fear of a powerful, phallic woman and was desperately defending himself by ruthless, jealous attacks. In other words, here was an extreme, jealousy paranoia in a man with considerable strengths. He was treated by Michael Balint from November 1960 to February 1962 in 27 sessions. The long follow-up was in two interviews, the latter in November 1966, and in letters until Balint's death in 1970.

THE NEW METHOD FOR OUTLINING CLINICAL EVENTS

Balint and his two coauthors, Enid Balint and Paul Ornstein (Balint *et al.,* 1972), attempt to make intelligible the interaction between this patient and this doctor, as reconstructed from Balint's notes after each session. Two-thirds of the text consists of the session reports (with commentary), in a very interesting form, which draws upon Balint's concepts of the doctor–patient interaction:

A. initial expectations
B. atmosphere in interview, with changes, if any
    1. patient's contribution
    2. therapist's contribution
C. and D. main trends and therapeutic interventions given
E. therapeutic interventions thought of but not given
F. therapist's focal aims in interview
G. outcome of the interview
H. afterthoughts

Perhaps at first glance, this session report form is not remarkable. In using it in experiments with my own psychotherapy cases, however, I have found that it redirects my attention very effectively away from interpretation and toward the nonverbal and interactive events. You begin with your own feelings and hopes in advance (A), which set the stage for the atmosphere (B) (e.g., where the contact is strained or boisterous or alters over the course of the interview). The main trends and interventions given are itemized (C and D) as a set of offers by the patient and counteroffers by yourself. In the next category (E), you write down all the interpretations you were tempted to make but refrained from making, aiding your self-restraint in the session itself. You can locate your brilliance afterwards on the form, rather than having to dazzle the patient. Your intelligence goes into bringing about a certain kind of interaction, specified by the focal aims (F), rather than into explaining matters to the patient. In other words, "focal therapy" need not mean "interpretation of focal conflict" but, rather, "focal aims" for a specific kind of interaction.

THE GENERAL OUTLINE OF THE TREATMENT

Balint discovered in the first two sessions that two breakdowns had occurred previously, one in the mid-1950s when the patient had moved himself and his wife into a new house and his father-in-law had died, the other in the spring of 1960, a half year prior to seeing Balint, when the patient became a director of the firm, replacing his father. Oversimplified, his formulation was that the patient could not tolerate these Oedipal victories, because they threw him back upon relations with women that were extremely primitive. His calm was destroyed when he succeeded, because the fathers (men) were no longer available to protect him.

Balint does not propose to explain this to the patient. He does not formulate a "focal conflict," which would construe the situation in verbal, intrapsychic terms, for a man in danger of falling into the black depths of his early deprivation, which is the "basic fault." Instead, Balint sets up "focal aims" to bring about a specific kind of interaction which will protect him. They are, first, to help him accept his triumph over his male rivals and, if that is too ambitious, to help him share his wife (symbolically) with the therapist (another man).

In general, the treatment divides into two distinct phases. In the first 13 sessions, Balint and the patient become very close, with great relief to the patient, but the attempt to "tail off" treatment brings back the disturbance. In the last 14 sessions, the patient pushes Balint to the limit with his jealous rage, finally calming himself down and making most of the interpretations himself. The result on follow-up is spectacular. What could easily have become a chronic paranoid psychosis, like the Schreber case, instead showed complete symptomatic relief and an ability to weather the kinds of stress that had brought about previous decompensations (i.e., the retirement of his father, competitive athletics with his son, the factory badly damaged by fire, and his son wishing to become independent of him and to take over the business). This outcome was scored 3.75 (the mean of four independent judges) at the follow-up of three years and four months.

MALAN'S ACCOUNT OF THE TREATMENT

In *The Frontier of Brief Psychotherapy* (1976a), Malan gives a lengthy account of this treatment in an attempt to fit it into his classical psychoanalytic conception. According to Malan, the first half is about all the interpretations given and not given, requiring many pages to explain but defying summary. This view is completely at odds with that taken by Balint and his coauthors. They believe that nonverbal or noninterpretive moves by the therapist are, in fact, equivalent to verbal ones and should be scored as such. When the total number of these interventions were divided into those based on previous psychoanalytic knowledge (PPsaK), those made strictly from current observations with the patient (CO), those which were mixed (M), and those that were independent discoveries of the patient (ID), only 2 out of 120 interventions were rated (PPsaK). According to Malan, the second half of the therapy has only two interpretations, consisting of "working through" and confronting the patient with reality. Balint and his coauthors emphasize that the final six sessions contained an equal number of interventions by the therapist and independent discoveries (IDs) by the patient, namely, 13 of each.

Malan ends up with an account of the first half, which is so dense with interpretive content that it cannot be followed, and an account of the second half, which is virtually empty. He writes, in summary, "Balint stuck to very limited interpretation and confrontation with reality," leaving us with what analysts like to call "supportive psychotherapy," which is completely lacking in specificity. We meet again the usual dichotomy present in Malan's thought between specific interpretive treatment (truly psychoanalytic) and nonspecific treatment (not very psychoanalytic). This misses the whole point of Balint's attempted treatment and attempt to explain what he did; that is, that it is possible to be very specific about one's interaction with the patient without interpreting all of this to the patient. But this takes one out of the classical psychoanalytic model and toward interpersonal and existential methods, which Malan continually eschews.

THE NEGLECTED POWER AND INTELLIGIBILITY
OF BALINT'S TECHNIQUE

Because this treatment is simply intelligible in interpersonal terms, as Balint claimed, because the neglected power of this point of view has been obscured in Malan's hands, and because this was such a brilliant therapy, I have decided to present it here.

Session No. 1. After Balint listened to "this dreary and very painful story" in the minutest detail about the patient's wife, the other man, the various alternative suspicions, and so on, Balint "brushed it aside," "not brusquely but in a friendly manner," telling the patient that the details were not important but that his feelings were, and that he needed someone to act as a "sounding board." The patient returned to this idea several times, very moved and grateful.

Session No. 2. In this session, Balint made a different counteroffer, to "look into things more deeply that had gone wrong," and the patient broke off treatment for 15 weeks.

Session No. 3. Here Balint had learned from his success in the first session and his failure in the second. He brushed aside everything but the fact that the patient was subjecting his wife to cruel harassment, but the truth was that he had won, he was the powerful man, and why couldn't he accept that! This brilliant maneuver set up the success of the treatment. It reassured the patient that *he* was the powerful man, respected rather than overrun by Balint. It actively countered the projection, so easily aroused in Session No. 2, that Balint would "look into him" as the intruding parent. At the same time (with the other hand, as it were), he was confronted with the malignant activity that he must stop. This is the kind of balancing maneuver practiced by Sullivan and recently described by Havens (1976).

Sessions No. 4–8. The patient now brought out spontaneously that his feeling of inferiority must have come out of childhood, when he was frightened by his father. His need for love made him accept homosexual advances at the expense of his self-respect. Malan goes into enormous detail about this. The essential point, however, is that Balint displaced away from himself any idea the patient had that Balint would ridicule or assault him for this need and for what he had allowed.

Session No. 9. After yet another counterprojective move by Balint, to the effect that "no wonder you were so vulnerable to homosexual advances," the patient revealed he had had a dream of a big snake curled up with him, and he entered a period of marvelous symptomatic improvement.

Very specific to his "focal aim," Balint made being close to the powerful father (i.e., the big snake) safe by differentiating himself from the assaulting father. Although he was continually tempted by the patient to ridicule, criticize, or make pronouncements that would belittle the patient, Balint refused to be tempted, passing the tests which differentiated him from the father, displacing these negative projections away from himself.

Session No. 10. Now the patient could use Balint to help him cope with women. He literally brought his wife to this session to share her with Balint. The patient calmly enjoyed his victory, having the powerful father close to him to ward off any dangers from the primitive mother.

Sessions No. 11-13. The attempt to "tail off" the treatment did not work, since the patient could not manage separation from Balint without losing the power Balint had loaned him.

Sessions No. 14-17. There was now an enormous build-up of rage directed against Balint.

Sessions No. 17-24. The patient began to treat Balint as if Balint were the child assaulted by the father, as if the patient had become the father. This route is not an uncommon one in psychotherapy, according to Weiss *et al.* (1977), when the therapist will permit the patient to use it. It is a reversal of the transference, what they call turning "passive into active." The patient subjects the analyst to what the child received from the parents in order to learn from the analyst how to handle it. Balint was now called upon to use all his resources.

Session No. 17. Baint took a firm stand against the patient's attempt to "mangle" his wife and "trip them (his wife and Balint) up" in complications; yet, in the same sweep, he showed the patient he was "tormenting himself" as well. Here Balint was placing himself over against the father-like assaults on others or himself, with that part of the patient which was helpless to do much about this. This is what Havens (1980) has called counterintrojection, namely, helping the patient to not be overrun by his powerful introjects.

Session No. 18. Here Balint empathized with the patient's requirement of a completely harmonious, archaic relation (Balint, 1959, 1968). No wonder the patient was so ruthless!

Session No. 19. Balint carefully avoided getting ahead of the patient, not offering interpretations which would carry the danger of making Balint the phallic mother or father. Instead, he let the patient make the independent discovery that he had been conditioned by his parents to see himself as inferior.

Sessions 20-23. Balint finally just had to stay with the patient, wondering if this assault would go on forever. In brief, Balint was subjected to a severe series of tests, tests of whether he could stay with the patient and still show him how to ward off these assaults.

Session No. 22. Just as Balint had begun to despair, the patient revealed that he felt calm, because he felt completely understood by Balint.

Sessions No. 23-27. The patient now emerged spontaneously with a series of "independent discoveries," starting with fear of abandonment, how he came to feel inferior, empathy for the position in which he had put his wife, and so forth. He now was carrying away Balint with him, inside.

Reviewing this interaction in very broad strokes, I would emphasize the following points. In the first half, Balint had to make it possible for the patient to take him close for protection; he did this by separating himself from previous assaults by "fathers" (counterprojection). In the second half, Balint had to weather all the assaults of the introjects with the patient, staying with him by understanding his archaic needs, standing with him against the introjects (counterintrojection), and letting the patient make independent discoveries.

I have been suggesting all along that the clinical capability of this school of brief therapy is greater than its concepts would allow, and I have used various alternative concepts at different points. This technique of Balint in the case of Mr. Baker shows all of them together. The overall idea is this: The patient is invited to run a major risk in the course of a few months, namely, to lift a defense (ruthless attacking) that is giving a lot of trouble. How does the patient decide to run this risk? The general answer is that the patient will go ahead if it is safe enough to do so, if he believes the big dangers will be avoided en route. The specific technique for the specific patient, however, must be in the hands of the therapist. The specific concepts of technique are demonstrated by Balint's handling.

First, Balint recovers from an early mistake, in which he suggests he "will look into" the patient's problems with him. He backs off a purely interpretive attitude, which is too terrifying to the patient, grasping that a "prior step of control" (Weiss et al., 1977) is necessary before much can be said to him. Most of the therapy deals with securing this control rather than clarifying it for the patient with interpretation. Indeed, the patient does the interpretation for himself.

Second, Balint has to take the issues in the right order or sequence (Weiss et al., 1977). The patient cannot borrow Balint's friendly power until Balint is distinguished clearly from seductive, powerful people who have assaulted him. Balint takes this first.

Third, as Alexander and French (1946) argued, it is necessary for Balint's *role* to be sufficiently different from that of the frightening parent. Since the father was bossy and demeaning, Balint had to be the opposite, giving the patient all the credit as a man and letting him make all the discoveries independently (very similar to the role taken by Alexander in his Case A).

Fourth, he must not succumb to temptations offered by the patient to revert to the father's traumatizing behavior, thus passing tests that he is indeed different and the new situation safe (Sampson, 1976; Weiss *et al.*, 1977).

Fifth, neither the neutral analytic attitude nor the role taking suggested by Alexander and French is enough to reassure some patients, such as this, about the difference between the dangerous past and the new present ending.

Balint not only had to be different in his behavior from the feared projections, but he also had to actively counter the role forced upon him, displacing it into others who had assaulted the patient, where the danger could be clearly focused (Havens, 1976). Certain people did seduce the patient; no wonder he must be careful about getting close. In other words, in order for a patient to feel adequately protected in the risk to be run, he or she may need methods and relationships specific to schools of psychiatry *other than psychoanalysis* (Havens, 1973), such as this use of counter-projection. This is the full technique of Balint, which we have previously seen, in part, through the many complex, successful cases described by Malan.

THE REMARKABLE CONTRIBUTIONS REVIEWED

We have followed the development of 25 years of experimentation with brief therapy at the Tavistock Clinic, led by Balint and Malan.

- They have attempted to retain the complex secret of the art by defining a science of brief therapy. At each stage, we have kept track of the intuitive clinical capabilities and the progress in conceptual clarity.
- Balint provided the generative idea that patients could be offered new kinds of relationships, allowing doctor and patient to organize new forms of brief treatment relationships corresponding to the four modern schools of psychiatry. Thus, in *The Doctor, His Patient and the Illness* (1957), he supplied the necessary equipment with a minimum of theory to secure this intuitive knowledge.
- In *A Study of Brief Psychotherapy* (1963), Malan broke the long-standing bonds of traditional psychoanalysis, which held that the lengthening factors were inevitable, and that subjective judgments inevitably separated psychoanalysis from the objective traditions of science.

- In *The Frontier of Brief Psychotherapy* (1976a) and *Toward the Validation of Dynamic Psychotherapy* (1976b), Malan became so clear about the dynamic events of brief psychotherapy that he could demonstrate how to plan the selection and technique in advance. At the same time, he introduced the complex clinical observations distorted by this conception.
- Malan's current thinking in *Individual Psychotherapy and the Science of Psychodynamics* (1979) allows him to provide a clear line of procedure through the complexities of selection and termination and through definition of the specific clinical capabilities of psychoanalysis, from the elementary skills to the complex.
- This clarity about the tools of psychoanalysis succeeds until Malan reaches the complex neuroses, where the conduct of the actual cases cannot be explained by his ideas of pure interpretation. An alternative hypothesis is offered by this author.
- The neglected power of Balint's technique, lost in Malan's narrowing conception of brief therapy as the essence of psychoanalysis, is represented by Balint, Ornstein, and Balint in *Focal Psychotherapy* (1972). The "focal aims" need not be to "interpret focal conflict," but rather may be to bring about a specific kind of interaction that the patient needs.

This tradition gives us, then, the complex secret of brief psychotherapy both in intuitive clinical brilliance and in increasingly sharpened concepts. The clinical acumen in Balint's *The Doctor, His Patient and the Illness* (1957) and *Focal Psychotherapy* (1972) and in the complex cases of Malan's *The Frontier of Brief Psychotherapy* (1976a) and *Individual Psychotherapy and the Science of Psychodynamics* (1979) is exemplary. The specific conceptual tools could not be clearer:

1. the methods for providing complex clinical observations in short form to allow independent assessment
2. the objective criteria of dynamic change
3. the powerful model of selection that integrates psychoanalysis and objective–descriptive psychiatry
4. the capacity for planning technique in advance of brief therapy
5. the most flexible of termination strategies, based on the logic of the "new ending"
6. clarification of the specific capabilities that an analytic psychotherapist loans to his patient

Balint provided the intuitive mastery of relationships that made possible the beginning of this tradition, while Malan provided the militant, integrative, organizing power of psychoanalysis and science to retain it. True to objective science, Malan has kept before us both his hypotheses and the clinical observations in all their complexity in order to allow continued building of the complete science of brief psychotherapy.

ACKNOWLEDGMENTS

I am indebted to Brooks Brenneis, Simon Budman, Joseph Kepecs, David Malan, Karin Ringler, Steven Stern, William Swift, Mark Trewartha, and Michael Wood for critical suggestions on the manuscript and its concepts and for their encouragement. I am particularly grateful to Dr. Malan for his generous, scientific spirit about our points of difference.

NOTES

[1]For those readers who prefer early definition, I may add that the idea of "focal psychotherapy" has been used by this school of brief therapy in several ways. Malan chiefly uses it to mean a brief psychotherapy in which the therapist limits himself to interpretation of a single "focal conflict." Balint, however, uses "focal psychotherapy" to refer to a therapy which has "focal aims." A focal aim may be to interpret a focal conflict, but it may also be to bring about a *specific* kind of interpersonal interaction with the therapist, which will represent a new kind of mastery for the patient. A focal aim may also be to help the patient bear certain feelings which have been unbearable to the patient alone, such as grief (cf. Malan, 1979, "The Nurse in Mourning"). In other words, the focal aim of a focal psychotherapy may be psychoanalytic, interpersonal, or existential. Whatever the focal aim, the brief therapist has to accept the reality that he cannot make up to the patient the ways in which the environment has failed him. This "basic fault" is a given. He must consider whether a small but well-chosen additional supply to the patient's life will have a multiplier effect that will produce a big difference. What will do this? In general, if the patient can safely lift one of his major defenses, there can be major ramifications. The focal aim is then to supply the right kind of relationship in which the patient can lift a single but major defense, with full control of the consequences (control against the recurrent trauma and control of the unrepressed capability that is allowed to emerge). For the most fully described and analyzed case from this entire school of brief therapy, see Balint *et al.* (1972) and the section of this chapter entitled "The Neglected Study of Technique": The patient, Mr. Baker, achieves control and mastery of the defense of ruthless persecution.

[2]In other words, the aim of this chapter is to be helpful to the clinician. Research findings have been discussed where they directly influence clinical method. I have made no systematic attempt to present or evaluate the research methodology or content of these works. That would be another large project.

[3]A recent article reviewing the different schools of brief psychotherapy (Burke, White, & Havens, 1979) gives a distorted account of the work of Malan and Balint, primarily because it

takes the model of technique offered by Malan at face value. From this, the authors argue that the entire school uses heavy interpretation, didactically weaving together present and past. They have not read the successful cases carefully. Balint is said to have offered a heavily interpretive technique in *Focal Psychotherapy* (1972), when, in fact, his whole aim was to avoid interpretation. The errors continue: Malan is said to have emphasized exclusion criteria, when, in fact, the ability to work in interpretive therapy (Hypothesis B) has been of equal or greater importance all along. Patients with deep-seated characterological problems are said to have been handled through the use of a more superficial focus, when, in fact, most of the star cases have had deep-seated characterological difficulties and have had their central problems taken on. Termination is said to have been downplayed by Malan, when, in fact, it was considered to be very important. A flexible strategy of termination does not deny its importance. The summary table used by these authors for comparison then collects these errors in one place (p. 184). Of course, it is not easy to carry out sweeping comparisons because of the sheer amount of study required. Minor errors should be forgiven when broad strokes are intended. These distortions, however, are large. The present chapter may allow more accurate comparisons to be made in the future between this and other schools of brief therapy.

[4]For a vivid introduction to the Victorian world, see the novel of Fowles (1969). Given this context, it is easier to appreciate the surprise of Freud's approach. This is also captured by the recent film, *The Seven Per Cent Solution,* in which Alan Arkin plays Freud in a manner which contrasts with our sober expectations. Malan (1979) has also written a similar paragraph about Freud (pp. 141–142).

[5]Strictly speaking, this school of brief psychotherapy divides into two main streams: brief psychotherapy by GPs, and brief psychotherapy by specialists (analytic psychotherapists). I will be considering only the latter, but we should not forget the continuing development of the GP line of work. For further reading, compare Balint and Balint (1961) and Balint and Norell (1973).

[6]Between the first scoring for *A Study of Brief Psychotherapy* (Malan, 1963) and the second scoring of Series 1 (Malan, 1976b), Malan and his colleagues added the possible score of 4 to the scale. The score of 3 now meant "substantial resolution" but with "some important reservations," whereas the score of 4 meant hardly any reservations (Malan, 1976a, p. 61).

[7]The ideal research arrangement, Malan suggested, would be to have two separate judges for judging the patient factors in the selection phase, two for analyzing the content of the technique, and two to judge the outcome, all making totally independent judgments, in order to correlate factors in the patient (selection criteria) and in the therapy (technique), on the one hand, with outcome on the other. Because Malan and Eric Rayner were contaminated by the knowledge of selection and the conduct of the therapies due to being two of the workshop therapists themselves and participating in the discussion of the cases of their colleagues, Malan decided to separate himself and Rayner, as the contaminated judges of outcome, from two other, totally uncontaminated judges of outcome. Since reliable assessment of psychodynamic outcome was the most important objective, this would provide two teams (of two judges each) for outcome, one team contaminated, one not, thereby allowing measures of interrater reliability between the two teams. After outcome judgments were made, Malan and Rayner went back to content analysis (from therapist notes) and finally back to evidence on patient factors in the selection phase. Two new uncontaminated judges of selection factors were added later. In general, interrater reliability was superb.

[8]In regard to predicting outcome in the selection phase, recent onset and mild pathology (Hypothesis A) again did not predict good outcome. Motivation for insight gave the best correlation but was not statistically significant. What was powerful and interesting was that high motivation in the patient and a consistent therapeutic focus from the therapist between the fifth and eighth sessions were reliable predictors of outcome. In other words, therapies "going well" ended up with the high outcome scores, whereas therapies "going badly" after the introductory phase ended up with low outcome. Either the patient and therapist "hit it off"

in a powerful way soon after the first four sessions or they never did. If this result were replicated, patients and therapists would have a powerful argument for stopping therapy after the first ten sessions if nothing had seemed to come of it by then. The situation is somewhat more complicated than this, however. Whereas the short favorable (SF) cases had become high in focus and motivation by the fifth to eighth session, the long favorable (LF) cases tended to be high in motivation only, the focus coming clear only later. The high motivation allows patient and therapist a long but successful search for a more complex focus, since the motivation will carry them through the periods of frustration and confusion.

[9]As a theory of psychotherapy, the classical model emphasizes the dynamic and economic points of view. The psyche is represented as a dynamic equilibrium between instinctual forces and superego forces, mediated by the ego. Strachey (1934) offered one of the clearest and most subtle versions of this theory of technique. In the first stage of interpretation, the analyst, by taking a position which is less harsh than the constraining superego, releases some of the impulse energy from repression. The dosage of the impulse released is kept in moderation so as to keep the patient's anxiety within tolerable limits, because the original anxiety in relation to the phantasy objects is aroused by this first stage of interpretation. In the second stage of interpretation, the patient grasps the difference between the phantasy object and the analyst as object, allowing relief from the original anxiety. Thus, in these two stages, the single weapon for arousing and then resolving the danger is interpretation.

[10]Here Malan treats psychoanalytic technique as if it were a simple, quantifiable entity, as if patients received varying doses of a completely purified medicine called "dynamic interaction." Those who received bigger doses got better, with occasional exceptions. Those who did not tolerate this "dynamic interaction" medicine were selection errors, that is, patients unsuitable for this drug. This is the baldest statement of the proposition that the drug "psychoanalytic doctor" can be given in some pure, standardized form. This is the simplest version of Malan's attempt to put his therapeutic concepts into a form which can be subjected to empirical tests (i.e., scientific methods). I believe he is correct in stating that psychoanalysis must be translated into propositions which can be corroborated or refuted. I disagree, however, that he has succeeded (cf. the section of this chapter entitled "Cross Validation of the Classical Theory"). Malan admits that clinical practice itself should not necessarily follow this logic of "dynamic interaction", that is, the more, the better, but it serves as a rough approximation of his recommendations. I am completely in sympathy with Malan's attempt to pare down psychoanalytic concepts to a consistent set of propositions. The ad hoc theorists will attack him for this, unfairly, I believe. My argument is rather for another consistent set of propositions whose predictions can be tested.

[11]To compare with the seven short favorable (SF) cases of neurotic type (leaving aside the Stationery Manufacturer and Mrs. Morley as instances of psychotic or near psychotic proportions), I have attempted to make a similar division of the short unfavorable (SU) cases. By admittedly crude reckoning, it appears from the clinical evidence presented that the three short unfavorable (SU) cases plus the four false (F) cases included in *Toward the Validation of Dynamic Psychotherapy* (Malan, 1976b) are all neurotic or narcissistic personality disorder cases. All the short unfavorable (SU) cases in *The Frontier of Brief Psychotherapy* (Malan, 1976a) are of psychotic proportions. Therefore, I have excluded the latter six (SU) cases from the comparison. It is interesting that Malan grouped the short failures (SU, F) between the two books in this way. It has the effect of obscuring the technical problems which the workshop therapists had with the neurotic cases. In any event, I am comparing the following: (SF)—Almoner, Buyer, Gibson Girl, Indian Scientist, Pesticide Chemist, Zoologist, Maintenance Man; (SU, F)—Company Secretary, Factory Inspector, Mrs. Hopkins, Au Pair Girl, Gunner's Wife, Mrs. Lewis, Representative.

[12]In terms of control–mastery theory (Sampson, 1976; Weiss *et al.*, 1977), all nine of the cases (indeed all psychotherapy cases) involve control against repetition of the old trauma prior to the patient lifting the defense. Some patients, like the Indian Scientist, who are simply han-

dled with analytic neutrality and interpretation, will find in the neutral and matter-of-fact analyst an object sufficiently different from the frightening parent (e.g., different from the overpowering father of the Indian Scientist) that the patient is reassured enough to bring out his forbidden impulses. As Weiss and Sampson would say, these cases have easy tests for the therapist to pass. The other cases in this series involve either steeper tests (to separate analyst from traumatizing parent) or prior steps of control by the patient over his own impulses. See the section of this chapter entitled "Reinterpretation of the Intuitive Mastery in Malan's Case Examples" for a full discussion of Malan's successful cases in terms of control-mastery theory.

[13]In the Gibson Girl, there is also a history of a nervous mother and a boyfriend pestering the girl for intercourse. In the course of brief therapy, she frees herself from giving in to these things and wants to stop. The therapist is probably in error to pester her to continue, but she has the good sense to leave anyway (Malan, 1979, p. 195).

[14]The case of the Pesticide Chemist is complicated by the therapist's interventions, which are highly erratic. The responses of the patient, however, show the problems of the traditional theory and the advantages of the control-mastery theory very clearly. There is no doubt that this man's desperate defense of trying to please everyone is, as Malan (1979) points out, "a desperate wish to prevent himself from unwittingly expressing his angry feelings against the firm, and thus causing a disaster to them—and, of course, to himself as well" (p. 102). But putting him in touch with his anger, his anxiety about it, and his defense against it is no reassurance to this man that the anger is controllable—just because he has this full interpretation of it! Indeed, in Session No. 2, the patient tempts the therapist to go directly after the anger by suggesting that the boss had criticized him unjustly. The therapist tries to go "to the heart of the matter" at once, saying that it was impossible to be angry with father, too. The patient retreats immediately, saying that the boss had now stopped being critical, and in next session, he wants to quit treatment. In Session No. 3, the therapist "completes the triangle of conflict over and over again," pointing out "the anxiety about his outburst, and the clamping down as a defense and the hidden part of himself that wanted to let go and make a mess." Although Malan emphasizes that the man is now willing to continue treatment, the next session, Session No. 4, is a blank. The turning point is in Session No. 5: "The patient now said that, if he understood the therapist correctly, he had made a conscious attempt at putting aside childish feelings and growing up, and that this was the cause of his trouble. He *didn't agree* [italics added]—everybody has to grow up and learn to be responsible and rational" (p. 105). In essence, the patient tells the therapist to reduce *his* demands to get at the anger, and then the therapist appreciates the point that the immediate task of the patient is to keep his anger under control. This becomes the route for his improvement. As he gets the therapist to reduce his demands and stop angering the patient, so he gets others to stop their excessive demands and stop making him so angry. This is the step of control, first practiced by the patient with the therapist and then accepted by the therapist, which makes it safe to acknowledge the anger, because its stimulation can be kept down within safe limits. The patient then practices this method of control with others and continues the excellent advance. Although the therapist intuitively follows this method of the patient, he cannot restrain himself from more "brilliant" interpretations, which are contrary to this method. In one instance, the patient dismisses the interpretation, and in the other, he nearly produces a disaster with his wife again. This is the danger of a theory of pure interpretation. Sometimes, the therapist intuitively gets the idea of the method of control, and the therapy goes well, but sometimes he does not, and the treatment is highly erratic. The traditional theory does not point to the essential matter, so only the intuition of the therapist keeps the therapy on track. Indeed, the traditional theory tempts the therapist away from the route of advance by the patient into "deep" and "true" interpretations.

[15]In their extremely detailed study of the case of Mrs. C., who was treated by an analyst who held traditional theories, Weiss *et al.* (1977) have shown that the testing of the analyst and the

emergence of the repressed impulse preceded, by many sessions, the interpretation of the impulse by the analyst. This finding is inconsistent with the traditional theory, which says that the impulse is released by interpretation. It *is* consistent with control–mastery theory, which says that patients lift defenses when they test that is safe to do so (Step 1). Weiss *et al.* (1977) take a position very similar to that of Balint *et al.* (1972), which claims that patients read therapists for "conditions of safety," utilizing either their actions or their words (interpretations) as evidence. Perhaps actions speak even louder than words (according to the unconscious). In any case, Weiss *et al.* (1977) argue that interpretations and actions of the therapist are roughly equivalent, that what is essential is whether they are consistent with the patient's unconscious plans to solve his problems, whether they pass the tests of the patient to differentiate the therapist from the traumatizing parent.

[16]In Series 2, these unsuccessful, disturbed cases include the Bird Lady, the Cellist, the Military Policeman, the Receptionist, the Sociologist, and Mr. Upton. Their erratic, uncontrolled course can be compared to that of the Stationery Manufacturer and Mrs. Morley (Malan, 1976a), in which the therapist deliberately planned a method of control, which was extremely successful. A case which falls between the two extremes is the Playwright (1976b), who was first handled with maximum direct interpretation, which produced only more extreme feelings and defenses, and was later handled successfully with warmth and respect for his intelligent ideas. There are some successes. They strike me as heroic ventures for both patient and therapist. In the depressive cases, the therapist translates the problems of the patient (i.e., hating the very person that he loves) directly into the relationship with the therapist. In the paranoid cases, the therapist directly interprets the patient's projection of his own murderous and sadistic impulses onto others, including the therapist. These interpretations are based on Melanie Klein's ideas (1975) about the depressive and paranoid positions. As Malan (1979, p. 162) himself points out, these direct transference interpretations are tolerated by certain patients who have an unusual capacity to bear the extreme feelings which are evoked. This direct method may even be necessary to such patients. This is impossible to know without comparative clinical studies. It is also difficult to know how rare such patients are and thus how rare are the indications for this heroic technique. In any event, the case reports are extremely dramatic. Compare, especially, the Personnel Manager (Malan, 1979, pp. 153–162) for a depressive problem and the Cricketer, the Refugee Musician, and the Foster Son (Malan, 1979, pp. 163–192) for a series of extreme paranoid problems. They make the most compelling text.

The danger is that these extremely unusual cases may be taken as a major paradigm for psychotherapy of major depressive and paranoid disorders, forgetting that most disturbed patients require more modulated control, and that there are methods for conducting psychotherapy with them that provide much more control of the dosage of extreme feelings (Balint *et al.,* 1972). The failure to heed this principle yields the kind of erratic therapies of disturbed patients referred to in Series 2 (as well as in Series 1). The Kleinian therapist had better have very demanding criteria of selection, very strict agreements with the patients about responsibility in crises, frequent visits, and reliable emergency and hospital back-up. Indeed, this is what therapists like Kernberg (1975) require.

[17]Some of the most interesting consideration of preverbal object relations and technique is in Balint's earlier books (1959, 1968).

[18]Every rule has its exception. A small conceptual movement back toward the interpersonal and existential ideas is made by Malan in *Individual Psychotherapy and the Science of Psychodynamics* (1979). Compare, especially, "The Nurse in Mourning" (pp. 116–124), where the emphasis is on being and staying with the grief of the patient, who has had "too many deaths." This, rather than interpretation, is the "greatest service" here. As I have emphasized repeatedly, the case reports have implied these concepts all along, but here we have Malan espousing them directly.

REFERENCES

Alexander, F., & French, T. M. *Psychoanalytic therapy*. New York: Ronald Press, 1946.

Balint, E., & Norell, J. S. *Six minutes for the patient*. London: Tavistock Publications, 1973.

Balint, M. Method and technique in the teaching of medical psychology, II. *British Journal of Medical Psychology*, 1954, *27*, 37–41.

Balint, M. *The doctor, his patient and the illness*. New York: International Universities Press, 1957.

Balint, M. *Thrills and regressions*. London: Hogarth Press, 1959.

Balint, M. *The basic fault: Therapeutic aspects of regression*. London: Tavistock Publications, 1968.

Balint, M., & Balint, E. *Psychotherapeutic techniques in medicine*. London: Tavistock Publications, 1961.

Balint, M., Ornstein, P. H., & Balint, E. *Focal psychotherapy*. London: Tavistock Publications, 1972.

Breuer, J., & Freud, S. *Studies on hysteria*. In *The complete psychological works of Sigmund Freud* (Vol. II). London: Hogarth Press, 1955. (Originally published, 1895.)

Burke, J. D., White, H. S., & Havens, L. L. Which short-term therapy? *Archives of General Psychiatry*, 1979, *36*, 177–186.

Ferenczi, S., & Rank, O. [*The development of psychoanalysis*] (C. Newton, Trans.). New York: Nervous and Mental Diseases Monograph, No. 40, 1925.

Fowles, J. *The French lieutenant's woman*. Boston: Little, Brown, 1969.

Freud, S. Fragment of an analysis of a case of hysteria. In *The complete psychological works of Sigmund Freud* (Vol. VII). London: Hogarth Press, 1953. (Originally published, 1905.)

Freud, S. Notes upon a case of obsessional neurosis. In *The complete psychological works of Sigmund Freud* (Vol. X). London: Hogarth Press, 1953. (Originally published, 1909.)

Glover, E. *The technique of psychoanalysis*. London: Balliere, Tindall & Cox, 1955.

Havens, L. L. *Approaches to the mind: Movement of the psychiatric schools from sects toward science*. Boston: Little, Brown, 1973.

Havens, L. L. *Participant observation*. New York: Jason Aronson, 1976.

Havens, L. L. *Explorations in the uses of language in psychotherapy: Counterintrojective statements*. Unpublished manuscript, 1980.

Kernberg, O. *Borderline conditions and pathological narcissism*. New York: Jason Aronson, 1975.

Klein, M. *Love, guilt and reparation*. London: Hogarth Press, 1975.

Kohut, H. *Analysis of the self*. New York: International Universities Press, 1971.

Malan, D. H. *A study of brief psychotherapy*. New York: Plenum Press, 1963.

Malan, D. H. *The frontier of brief psychotherapy*. New York: Plenum Press, 1976.(a)

Malan, D. H. *Toward the validation of dynamic psychotherapy*. New York: Plenum Press, 1976.(b)

Malan, D. H. *Individual psychotherapy and the science of psychodynamics*. London: Butterworth, 1979.

Malan, D. H., Heath, E. S., Bacal, H. A., & Balfour, F. H. G. Psychodynamic changes in untreated neurotic patients, II: Apparently genuine improvements. *Archives of General Psychiatry*, 1975, *32*, 110.

Mann, J. *Time-limited psychotherapy*. Cambridge: Harvard University Press, 1973.

Menninger, K. *Theory of psychoanalytic technique*. New York: Basic Books, 1958.

Popper, K. *Conjectures and refutations: The growth of scientific knowledge*. New York: Basic Books, 1962.

Sandler, J., & Joffe, W. G. Towards a basic psychoanalytic model. *International Journal of Psychoanalysis*, 1969, *50*, 79–90.

Sampson, H. A critique of certain traditional concepts in the psychoanalytic theory of therapy. *Bulletin of the Menninger Clinic*, 1976, *40*, 255–262.

Sifneos, P. E. *Short-term psychotherapy and emotional crisis.* Cambridge: Harvard University Press, 1972.

Strachey, J. The nature of the therapeutic action of psychoanalysis. *International Journal of Psychoanalysis*, 1934, *15*, 127–159.

Weiss, J. The emergence of new themes in psychoanalysis. *International Journal of Psychoanalysis*, 1971, *52*, 459–467.

Weiss, J. *A new psychoanalytic theory of therapy and technique.* Unpublished manuscript, 1978.

Weiss, J., Sampson, H., Caston, J., Silberschatz, G., & Gassner, S. *Research on the psychoanalytic process, I and II.* Psychotherapy Research Group, Department of Psychiatry, Mount Zion Hospital & Medical Center, San Francisco, Bulletin No. 3, December 1977. (Available from Ms. Janet Bergman, San Francisco Psychoanalytic Institute, 2420 Sutter Street, San Francisco, California 94115.)

SECTION II
INDIVIDUAL BRIEF THERAPY: ALTERNATIVE MODELS

CHAPTER 6
BEHAVIOR THERAPY AS A SHORT-TERM THERAPEUTIC APPROACH

G. Terence Wilson

INTRODUCTION

In order to discuss behavior therapy as a short-term treatment approach, I needed a definition of what is commonly accepted as short-term therapy. Accordingly, I turned to Butcher and Koss's (1978) recent review of brief and crisis-oriented therapies. They have the following to say about the length of short-term therapy: "Today, most practitioners agree that 25 sessions is the upper limit of 'brief' therapy, with as many clinicians recommending courses of treatment lasting from one to six sessions as the longer 10 to 25 session treatment" (p. 730). Given this time frame, behavior therapy unquestionably qualifies as one of the many forms of short-term therapy. This conclusion will hardly surprise anyone familiar with the development and nature of behavior therapy. From the first, starting with Wolpe's (1958) initial series of clinical cases, for which he claimed a 90% success rate, the brevity of behavior therapy has virtually always been identified as one of its distinguishing characteristics vis-à-vis psychoanalysis and its various derivative psychodynamic methods. Indeed, the speed with which Wolpe and other early behavior therapists claimed to have achieved treatment success provoked almost as much controversy and skepticism as the apparently unprecedented success rates themselves. By and large, contemporary behavioral treatment methods for a wide range of diverse clinical disorders continue to be relatively short term in nature, although this once controversial aspect of these methods is now regarded as commonplace.

G. TERENCE WILSON. Graduate School of Applied and Professional Psychology, Rutgers University, Piscataway, New Jersey.

Before turning to an analysis of the technical and theoretical niceties of behavior therapy as a form of short-term treatment, I would like to review some summary examples of different behavioral treatment strategies for commonly encountered clinical problems. I should also make clear my conception of the nature of behavior therapy. By this less than clearly defined but nonetheless still useful term (Wilson, 1978), I do not mean the radical behaviorist approach of Skinner (1953), a nonmediational model of human behavior that eschews the serious analysis of private events or symbolic processes and proclaims that, aside from genetic influence (and these are usually given short shrift in operant conditioning analyses of behavior), all behavior is under the control of external environmental factors. Nor am I restricting myself to what I have called the neobehavioristic S-R approach of Wolpe's (1958) and Eysenck's (1960) pioneering contributions to the development of behavior therapy. Rather, I view behavior therapy from the perspective of social learning theory, with its emphasis not only on classical and operant conditioning procedures that characterized the early behavior therapy methods, but also, most importantly, on cognitive mediational processes and self-regulatory capacities (Bandura, 1977a, 1977b; Wilson & O'Leary, 1980). Consistent with this broader theoretical framework is the relatively recent emphasis in clinical behavior therapy on cognitive principles and procedures—or what is often referred to as "cognitive behavior therapy" (Foreyt & Rathjen, 1978; Meichenbaum & Cameron, in press).

According to social learning theory, the influence of environmental events on the development and regulation of behavior is largely determined by cognitive processes. These cognitive processes are based on prior experience and determine what environmental influences are attended to, how they are perceived, whether or not they will be remembered, and how they might affect future functioning. In contrast to the essentially unidirectional, causal model of behavior posited by radical behaviorism, with its reliance on environmental control of behavior, social learning theory is predicated on a reciprocal determinism model of behavior, in which psychological functioning is a product of interlocking sets of personal and environmental influences. As Bandura (1977a) put it:

> Personal and environmental factors do not function as independent determinants; rather they determine each other. Nor can persons be considered causes independent of their behavior. It is largely through their actions that people produce the environmental conditions that affect their behavior in a reciprocal fashion. The experiences generated by behavior also partly determine what

individuals think, expect, and can do, which in turn, affect their subsequent behavior. (p. 345)

In its clinical application, this social learning approach bears a marked similarity to Lazarus's (1971, 1976) broad-spectrum or multimodal behavior therapy approach to assessment and treatment. The details of how this social learning approach overlaps and differs with other conceptual views within the broadly defined compass of behavior therapy and its implications for clinical practice are discussed elsewhere (Bandura, 1969; Rosenthal, in press; Wilson & O'Leary, 1980).

CLINICAL ILLUSTRATIONS OF SHORT-TERM BEHAVIOR THERAPY

PHOBIC DISORDERS

Specific phobias, such as fears of snakes, heights, enclosed spaces, darkness, elevators, and so on, seem to yield readily to no more than roughly a half-dozen sessions of participant modeling or graduated, *in vivo* exposure, a performance-based technique that has been shown to be the most effective form of behavior therapy for most phobic disorders (e.g., Bandura, 1977a; Marks, 1978). More significantly, clinical research shows that complex phobic disorders, such as agoraphobia, are typically treated on a short-term basis with significant success (Marks, 1978; Rachman & Wilson, 1980).

Fairly typical of the treatment programs and their effects in this connection is the comparative investigation of Gelder, Bancroft, Gath, Johnston, Mathews, and Shaw (1973) in England, which meets the requirements of both methodological rigor and clinical relevance. Briefly, flooding was compared to both systematic desensitization and an attention-placebo control condition in the treatment of phobic clients. Treatments were carried out by experienced therapists explicitly trained in the administration of the different methods. An attempt was made to induce a high expectancy of success in half the subjects by describing the treatment and the therapist in very favorable terms and showing them a video tape of a patient who had benefited from the treatment they were to receive. Of the 36 patients, half were agoraphobics; the other half, a mixed group of specific social or animal phobics. Patients were assigned to treatments and therapists in an experimental design that permitted an analysis of the possible interactions among treatment effects, therapist differences, types of phobia, and levels of expectancy. Therapy consisted of 15 weekly sessions that included both imaginal and real-life exposure. Sessions lasted from one to two hours. Treatment effects were evaluated in terms of multiple measures of behavioral avoidance, blind psychiatric ratings, client self-ratings, physiological responsiveness, and standardized psychological tests. The subjects were evaluated at the end of treatment and at a six-month follow-up. The adequacy of the control group in eliciting expectations of success comparable to those evoked by the two behavioral methods was assessed directly. The expectations of improvement were comparable across all three treatment conditions.

Both of the behavioral treatments, particularly flooding, produced greater improvement than the control condition on the behavioral avoidance tests, physiological arousal measures, and psychiatric ratings of the main phobia and the patient's self-rating of improvement, although only the flooding, as opposed to the control condition comparison, reached acceptable levels of statistical significance. These treatment gains were maintained successfully at follow-up. Simply put, flooding was roughly twice as effective as the powerful attention-placebo treatment. An important finding in this study was that the placebo control treatment was markedly less effective than either flooding or systematic desensitization with agoraphobics than with the other subjects. This result provides evidence that the success of behavioral methods, such as flooding and systematic desensitization, cannot be attributed solely to the role of placebo factors or expectations of favorable therapeutic outcome.

Successful treatment of agoraphobics using *in vivo* exposure methods, such as flooding and participant modeling, has been reported by different groups of clinical investigators working in different countries (Marks, 1978). Particularly encouraging is the fact that uncontrolled clinical trials have shown that group treatment (Hand, Lamontagne, & Marks, 1974), home-based treatment, in which husbands of agoraphobic women followed a treatment manual in acting as cotherapists (Mathews, Teasdale, Munby, Johnston, & Shaw, 1977), and hospital-based treatment, in which nurses acted as the primary therapists (Marks, Hallam, Connolly, & Philpott, 1977), have all produced comparable treatment success, despite a considerable reduction in the time spent by the professional therapists in direct contact with the patients.

OBSESSIVE-COMPULSIVE DISORDERS

Another excellent example of the broad applicability and clinical relevance of behavior therapy is the treatment of obsessive–compulsive disorders. There is wide agreement among clinicians of different theoretical orientations that obsessive–compulsive disorders are among the most severe and disabling psychiatric problems. They have remained notoriously resistant to successful treatment of any kind, and they provide a searching and decisive testing ground for potentially effective therapies. As in other areas, the behavioral treatment literature shows a definite progression toward the development of increasingly refined and more effective therapeutic techniques. After methods like imaginal systematic desensitization proved to be largely ineffective, more effective alternative techniques, such as *in vivo* exposure and response prevention, were developed (Rachman & Hodgson, 1980).

The evidence of behavioral treatment of obsessive–compulsive disorders may be illustrated by reference to a clinical outcome study by Hodgson, Rachman, and Marks (1972). They compared the efficacy of three treatments: *(a)* flooding *in vivo, (b)* modeling *in vivo,* and *(c)* flooding combined with modeling *in vivo.* The severity of the subjects' compulsions is indicated by the fact that six were unable to work, while the others were severely hampered in their work. Family relationships were often completely imperiled, as in the case of an affectionate mother who was unable to touch her three children for fear of contamination. The clients were hospitalized for a seven-week period. After an initial week's evaluation, all subjects received 15 one-hour sessions of relaxation training over the next three weeks. This extended period of relaxation therapy was designed to serve as an attention-placebo control. Thereafter, the subjects were randomly assigned to the three treatment conditions for an additional 15 sessions of therapy during the final three weeks.

Flooding consisted of encouraging subjects to engage in their most feared activities. The *in vivo* modeling treatment was similar to participant modeling. The therapist modeled a series of increasingly threatening behaviors, which the patient then imitated under the therapist's supportive supervision. All the subjects were asked to refrain from carrying out their rituals between treatment sessions, but there was no nursing supervision to ensure that this instruction was followed. Subjects were assessed before treatment, after the three weeks of relaxation therapy, at the end of flooding or modeling, and at a six-month follow-up. The measurements taken included self- and psychiatric rating scales, attitudinal responses, behavioral avoidance tests, which were tailor-made to the individuals' specific problems, and direct measures of compulsive acts.

Both flooding and modeling were significantly more effective than the relaxation control treatment on all measures, but they did not differ from each other. The combined treatment did not increase the success of either method alone. A subsequent two-year follow-up (Marks, Hodgson, & Rachman, 1975) revealed that of the 20 patients who had been treated, 14 were judged to be much improved, 1 improved, and 5 unchanged. Notice, however, that many patients received booster treatments after discharge from the hospital: 9 needed antidepressant drugs, 2 required marital therapy, and 1 received assertion training. Marks et al. (1975) commented on both the importance of the therapist–patient relationship in prompting patients to comply with instructions to desist from their rituals and the value of the active involvement of family members. Indeed, 11 patients in all had a mean of three home visits following discharge, and of the patients who failed to improve, all but 1 refused to cooperate in following instructions once they returned home.

Rachman and Wilson (1980) have summarized the clinical and experimental evidence as follows:

> It is reasonable to conclude that behavioral treatment is capable of producing significant changes in obsessional problems, and rapidly at that. Clinically valuable reductions in the frequency and intensity of compulsive behaviour have been observed directly and indirectly. Significant reductions in distress and discomfort are usual, and the work of Boulougouris and his colleagues . . . suggests that psychophysiological changes of a kind observed during the successful treatment of phobias take place. The admittedly insufficient evidence on the durability of the induced changes is not discouraging; allowing for the provision of booster treatments as needed (see, for example, Marks et al., 1975), the therapeutic improvements are stable. The successful modification of the main obsessional problems often is followed by improvements in social and vocational adjustment. . . . In all the [clinical] series and controlled studies reported so far, some clear failures occurred—the failure rate ranges between 10% and 30%. The reasons for such failures are not known. (p. 148)

DEPRESSION

Depression is another clinical disorder for which promising cognitive–behavioral treatment techniques have been recently developed. For example, Beck's (1976) cognitive therapy, which I am including under the loosely defined rubric of behavior therapy, has yielded particularly encouraging results. Rush, Beck, Kovacs, and Hollon (1977) compared this approach to pharmacotherapy (imipramine) in the treatment of depressed patients who had been continually or intermittently depressed for about nine years, 75% of whom reported suicidal ideas. The majority had had previous psychotherapy with success, and 22% had been hospitalized on account of their depression. Treatment for both groups averaged eleven weeks.

Depression was substantially reduced by both treatments; however, cognitive therapy produced significantly greater improvement on self-ratings and clinical ratings of depression. Of the clients in the cognitive therapy condition, 79% underwent marked improvement or complete remission, as compared to 23% of the clients in the pharmacotherapy condition. These treatment differences were maintained at three- and six-month follow-ups. Aside from being more effective, cognitive therapy was associated with a significantly lower dropout rate over the course of the study. This is an important finding, since there is good evidence that clients who drop out of treatment are almost inevitably treatment failures. If statistical analysis of outcome results are based only on those clients who complete treatment, a biased picture may emerge.

In this study by Rush and others (1977), cognitive therapy was superior to pharmacotherapy, regardless of whether the dropouts were included in the analysis—an impressive finding. Consistent with these results, McLean and Hakstian (1979) found that a multifaceted therapy program, consisting of both behavioral and cognitive components, was more effective than drug (amitriptyline) therapy and short-term psychotherapy in the treatment of clinically depressed clients. Moreover, the combined cognitive–behavioral treatment resulted in significantly fewer dropouts from therapy.

These initial findings do not permit us to conclude definitively that cognitive–behavioral methods are superior to drug therapy, even when applied to the selected depressive patients in these two studies (e.g., Becker & Schuckit, 1978). Nonetheless, they strongly suggest the likely efficiency and efficacy of these methods.

SEXUAL DYSFUNCTION

Masters and Johnson's (1970, 1979) two-week rapid treatment program is the best-known example of short-term behavioral treatment of sexual dysfunction in heterosexual and homosexual men and women. The details of their approach need not be repeated here. Suffice it to state that successful results, comparable to those of Masters and Johnson, have been reported by other groups of investigators using these and other brief behavioral methods (see reviews by Franks & Wilson, 1977, 1978, 1979; Marks, 1978; Rachman & Wilson, 1980). In many cases of sexual dysfunction that are uncomplicated by interpersonal and communication problems, brief self-help behavioral programs, ranging from 6 to 15 sessions, with minimal therapist contact, have proved to be an efficient and cost-effective treatment strategy (e.g., Mathews, Bancroft, Whitehead, Hackmann, Julier, Bancroft, Gath, & Shaw, 1976; McMullen & Rosen, 1979; Zeiss, 1978). In less straightforward cases requiring intensive behavioral marital therapy and/or other cognitive–behavioral interventions as a prelude to, or in addition to, specific sex therapy, treatment may take anywhere from 20 to 50 sessions (e.g., Brady, 1976).

Kaplan (1979) recently argued for the existence of a distinctive class of sexual dysfunctions that she calls inhibited sexual desire (ISD). According to Kaplan, patients suffering from ISD "have deeper and more intense sexual anxieties, greater hostility towards their partners, and more tenacious defenses than those patients whose sexual dysfunctions are associated with erection and orgasm difficulties" (p. 55). In these cases, Kaplan asserts that brief behavioral methods are relatively ineffective, because they do not address the deeper, unconscious psychodynamic conflicts that characterize disorders of desire. She advocates a lengthier treatment approach that combines features of traditional, psychodynamic insight therapy and behavioral sex therapy methods. Whether or not this combined approach, which she terms psychosexual therapy, is more effective than behavior therapy alone remains an open, empirical question. In the meantime, the total absence of any compelling clinical or controlled-research evidence that psychodynamic methods have been effective in treating sexual dysfunction before the advent of behavioral sex therapy inspires little confidence in the alleged superiority of psychosexual therapy for sexual disorders, as does the lack of data showing that a combined psychodynamic and behavioral approach confers any advantage over behavior therapy itself in the treatment of nonsexual disorders (Rachman & Wilson, 1980).

ADDICTIVE DISORDERS

Brief behavioral treatment programs for alcoholism, obesity, and cigarette smoking are now commonplace (e.g., Miller, 1980). An instructive example of the treatment of this class of disorders is provided by Sobell and Sobell's (1978) therapeutic program for alcoholism. Seventy male, chronic alcoholics, who were inpatients at a state hospital, were assigned to four different treatment conditions: a controlled-drinking experimental group (CD-E), a controlled-drinking control group (CD-C), a nondrinking experimental group (ND-E), and a nondrinking control group (ND-C). The two control treatment groups received conventional hospital treatment for alcoholics, such as large therapy groups, Alcoholics Anonymous meetings, and chemotherapy. The experimental groups received 17 sessions of a multifaceted, individualized behavior therapy program in addition to the routine hospital program. Aside from the first 2 sessions, which lasted 3 hours, all sessions took 90 minutes.

An important feature of this study was that detailed, comprehensive follow-up evaluations were obtained at each six-month interval during the first two years and then again three years after the end of therapy. Estimates of daily alcohol consumption were gathered, with every attempt made to corroborate subjects' reports by securing reports from significant others in the subjects' environments who could best substantiate their reports. For purposes of evaluating the results, abstinent and controlled drinking days (days during which 6 ounces or less of 86-proof liquor or its equivalent in alcohol content were consumed) were summarized as "functioning well"; drinking days (days during which 10 or more ounces of 86-proof liquor or its equivalent in alcohol content were consumed) or days during which subjects were incarcerated were summarized as "not functioning well."

Both experimental groups were found to be significantly superior to their respective control groups in terms of number of days functioning well at about the six-month and one-year follow-up evaluations. At the two-year mark, the CD-E group was significantly different from the CD-C group. For the entire second year of follow-up, the CD-E subjects functioned well for an average of 89.61% of all days, as compared to a mean of 45.10% of all days for the CD-C subjects. The differences between the ND-E and ND-C subjects approached but did not reach significance at either the eighteen-month or two-year follow-ups. Over the entire second year of follow-up, ND-E subjects functioned well for a mean of 64.60% of all days, while ND-C subjects functioned well for a mean of 45.13% of all days. Differences between experimental and control group subjects were found not only for drinking behaviors but for other adjunctive measures of functioning as well. An evaluation of adjustment to interpersonal relationships and problem situations revealed the same pattern of results as for drinking. Subjects in the CD-E group were classified as significantly more improved than CD-C group members at each follow-up over the two-year period. Subjects in the ND-E group were rated as significantly more improved than ND-C subjects during the first year but not during the second year of follow-up.

Unlike the one- and two-year follow-ups, which were conducted by the original investigators, the three-year evaluation was an independently conducted, double-blind follow-up (Caddy, Addington, & Perkins, 1978). The results are strikingly consistent with those of the previous two years and are summarized by these researchers as follows:

> Comparison of the controlled drinking experimental group with its control group showed the significantly better functioning of subjects in the experimental condition on a number of drinking and other life functioning measures. Comparison of the non-drinking groups indicated only one possible difference on the drinking related measures involving a trend for subjects in the experimental condition to abstain more than those in the non-drinker control group. On other life functioning measures, however, subjects in the non-drinking experimental condition showed consistent improvement over their respective control subjects. Both of the controlled drinking groups reported more controlled drinking days than the non-drinking groups throughout the third year follow-up period. (p. 345)

The Sobells' (1978) study is not without its shortcomings (see Kazdin & Wilson, 1978b; Nathan & Briddell, 1977); however, the replicability of the treatment methods, the use of specific, multiple measures of outcome relating not only to direct alcohol consumption but also to non-drinking facets of the patients' lives, and the long-term follow-up with the extraordinary accomplishment of contact with over 90% of the original 70 patients are all exemplary features. Significant, too, is the fact that the regular and intensive follow-up assessments of the original investigators apparently served as a sort of maintenance strategy or continuing care service (Sobell & Sobell, 1978). No matter how effective any short-term treatment is in arresting addictive disorders, long-term durability of that treatment-produced success will depend on the development of effective maintenance strategies. Finally, the success of behavior therapy in this study is not unique. Azrin (1976) reported significant success in helping alcoholics achieve sobriety; his study used concentrated behavioral treatment, averaging 30 hours per patient, and a two-year follow-up.

THE BROAD APPLICABILITY OF BEHAVIOR THERAPY

These few examples must suffice in conveying a sense of the application and effects of behavior therapy to different clinical disorders. Considerations of space prevent me from citing numerous other illustrations of the application of behavioral methods to a wide range of diverse psychological, medical, and educational problems. (Details of this broad applicability of behavior therapy can be found in Brigham & Catania, 1979; Franks & Wilson, 1973, 1974, 1975, 1976, 1977, 1978, 1979; Kazdin & Wilson, 1978b; Rachman, 1977.) I do wish to emphasize, however, this point about the unusually broad applicability of behavior therapy to so many different problems and to reject what I hope is the now antiquated notion that behavior therapy is appropriate primarily for the treatment of monosymptomatic phobias and simple habits! Indeed, it can be argued convincingly that behavior therapy is far more broadly applicable to a wider range of clinical disorders than alternative forms of traditional psychotherapy—particularly the brief psychodynamic therapies, which, as other chapters in this volume show, are deemed appropriate only for a relatively small number of select patients.

Behavior therapy research is often faulted for what is said to be a disproportionate emphasis on the treatment of minor problems in the laboratory setting. Although this laboratory-based research is often faulted on highly debatable grounds (Borkovec & Rachman, 1979; Kazdin & Wilson, 1978b), it must be conceded that long-term investigations of complex clinical disorders have been far fewer than would be desirable. Agras and Berkowitz (1980) have summarized the current limitations of clinical research in behavior therapy as follows: "The difficulty is quite clear: the limitation of research to issues of generalization, maintenance, and the dissemination of results to the practicing clinician, as well as an examination of the effectiveness of therapeutic procedures in actual clinical practice." (p. 483).

These limitations notwithstanding, the few illustrations of the clinical evaluation of behavior therapy that I have presented above amply demonstrate that the approach goes well beyond the treatment of merely mild or minor problems in relatively well-adjusted individuals. In the terms of some critics of analogue research in behavior therapy, the examples I have discussed involve "real" people with "real" disorders treated by "real" therapists—that is, unless the entire exercise is viewed as "unreal."

TECHNICAL CHARACTERISTICS OF BEHAVIOR THERAPY AS SHORT-TERM TREATMENT

BRIEF VERSUS LONGER-TERM BEHAVIOR THERAPY

Not all behavior theapy, of course, is short-term treatment. Therapy lasting from 25 to 50 sessions is commonplace, and still longer treatment is not unusual. Therapy in excess of 100 sessions, however, is relatively rare. Although not necessarily representative of the clinical practice of behavior therapy elsewhere, an evaluation of the functioning of the Institute of Behavior Therapy in New York City over its first four years of operation (1971–1975) indicates that treatment takes an average of approximately 50 weekly, one-hour sessions (Fishman & Lubetkin, 1980). There are no established guidelines for deciding on the length of therapy in any a priori fashion. Many applied research programs are explicitly time limited. The basis for the particular number of treatment sessions in these research studies is not entirely clear. In some cases, as in the treatment of phobic and obsessive–compulsive disorders, enough evidence exists to allow reasonable projections of how many sessions are required to obtain treatment effects. In other instances, as in research on the treatment of obesity, however, nontherapeutic considerations of convenience and habit often dictate treatment length and format, as I indicate below.

The typical approach in clinical practice is to carry out a detailed behavioral assessment of the problem(s) and to embark upon an intervention as rapidly as possible. Assessment is an ongoing process, as the consequences of initial treatment interventions are evaluated against therapeutic goals. In principle, unless treatment is explicitly time limited from the start, the length of therapy and the scheduling of the treatment sessions are contingent upon the patient's progress (or lack thereof) toward treatment objectives that have been mutually negotiated between therapist and patient. (See Wilson & Evans, 1977, and Wilson & O'Leary, 1980, for a discussion of how treatment goals are chosen.)

In my own case, which I take to be fairly typical, my initial, working contract with the patient is to pursue a treatment plan for two to three months (approximately 8–12 sessions) and reevaluate progress at that point, assuming that the problem has not been solved. If we both agree that progress is being made, we continue. The relative absence of any discernible improvement is cause for reevaluating (a) whether I have conceptualized the problem accurately, (b) whether I am using the appropriate techniques or need to switch tactics, (c) whether there is some personal problem with me as the therapist rather than with the general approach, or (d) whether a referral to another therapist or another form of treatment might be called for.

In terminating a successful case, the behavior therapist usually avoids an abrupt end to treatment. A typical procedure, for example, is to lengthen gradually the time between successive therapy sessions, from weekly to fortnightly to monthly and so on. These concluding sessions which, progressively phase out the therapist's active involvement, may be shorter than earlier ones, with telephone contacts occasionally interspersed among them. This strategy derives from the need to facilitate the generalization and maintenance of therapeutic change, as discussed below.

A common occurrence in behavior therapy is for the patient to consult the therapist on periodic occasions in the months or even years following termination of treatment. For example, in the much discussed Sloane, Staples, Cristol, Yorkston, and Whipple (1975) comparative outcome study of the effects of short-term behavior therapy and psychoanalytically oriented psychotherapy, approximately half the patients in the behavior therapy treatment condition requested and received small amounts of additional therapy (an average of 10 sessions) during the year following the end of time-limited (an average of 13 sessions over a four-month interval) therapy. Usually, patients seek "follow-up" consultations to obtain guidance or clarification about coping with new, emerging difficulties they begin to encounter following the therapeutic changes they made during treatment. In short, people continue to grow and change following a course of successful therapy, short-term or otherwise, and occasionally need brief therapeutic assistance during the course of this continuing evolvement of lifestyle changes. In most instances, these subsequent contacts are not to be taken as signs of failure or even incomplete treatment; neither can they be rationalized in terms of the now discredited notion of "symptom substitution." In clinical practice, these sporadic, posttreatment contacts with the therapist are usually unscheduled and initiated by the patient. Behavior therapists often deliberately schedule posttreatment maintenance or booster sessions, however, as an integral part of the overall treatment program, as I elaborate below.

FACTORS AFFECTING DIFFICULTY AND LENGTH OF TREATMENT

What determines the difficulty of producing targeted therapeutic change and, by extension, usually dictates the length of treatment? No simple answer to this question can be given. What we can say with some confidence is that the descriptive nature of the target problem alone cannot serve as a basis for accurate prediction. Thus, as illustrated in the examples of brief behavior therapy in the beginning of this chapter, even complex agoraphobic disorders, chronic obsessive–compulsive conditions, and moderate to severe depressive reactions can be treated effectively and efficiently by short-term treatment. On the other hand, ostensibly uncomplicated problems may often appear intractable despite lengthy interventions. Why therapy is successful in some but not other instances is not always known. Yet, assuming reasonable technical competence and clinical skill on the part of the behavior therapist, some of the factors that influence treatment difficulty can be identified.

Foremost is the patient's motivation, his or her willingness to cooperate in what can be the arduous and challenging task of making significant changes in psychological functioning. Resistance to change or lack of motivation are frequent reasons for treatment failures in behavior therapy. Contrary to some proponents and opponents of behavior therapy alike, this approach does not reduce to an all-powerful system of unilateral control in which the "therapist" (?) can impose change on unsuspecting or unwilling "patients." The therapist's influence may be considerable, but it is far from total. (See Davison, 1973, and Wilson & Evans, 1977, for a fuller discussion of the ways in which the therapist may influence the client, how unilateral therapist control is limited, and why self-regulated change is preferable to external influence.) It is more realistic, not to mention more humble, to note that the therapist is more a consultant than a controller, skillfully directing consciously involved clients in active, self-regulated, problem-solving strategies.

Perhaps more than any other form of psychological treatment, behavior therapy involves asking a patient to *do* something—to practice relaxation training, self-monitor daily caloric intake, engage in assertive acts, confront anxiety-eliciting situations, refrain from carrying out compulsive rituals, and so on. The degree to which behavior therapists emphasize the importance of the client's activities and experience in the real world *between* therapy sessions (in other words, the degree to which they go beyond the more traditional method of focusing primarily, if not exclusively, on the client's functioning *during* treatment sessions) is one of the distinctive features of the behavioral approach. Behavior therapists have devoted less time to developing effective strategies for prompting adherence to these critical therapeutic instructions and homework assignments than to refining the formal treatment techniques themselves.

The patient's degree of social and family support is often a key factor in facilitating or hampering treatment success. To the extent that a spouse and/or other family members are contributing—directly or indirectly, deliberately or unwittingly—to the patient's problems, therapy must be addressed to changing these social support systems. This, then, raises the questions of the willingness or ability of the spouse or family to cooperate with the treatment plan.

Finally, while it is usually not the particular problem per se but the specific nature of the relevant maintaining variables that determines the ease of behavior change (Bandura, 1969), complex, multifaceted disorders almost invariably necessitate a broad-spectrum treatment approach—and this takes time. Consider, for example, Barlow, Reynolds, and Agras's (1973) unprecedented success in producing gender identity change in a young male transsexual using a multifaceted behavioral treatment approach over the course of more than a year's intensive therapy. It is difficult to see how so complex a disorder, requiring so many focal interventions, could have taken less time. Noteworthy, too, is Fishman and Lubetkin's (1980) report, based on their clinical practice, that their initial average of sessions per client increased from roughly 20 to 25 sessions to an average of 50 sessions as they increasingly were called upon to treat more complex cases.

THERAPY FORMAT

Behavior therapy has helped to demonstrate the feasibility and, in some instances, the necessity of expanding treatment services in ways that are more flexible and versatile than the traditional 50-minute hour with the expensively trained professional therapist. The application and evaluation of self-help manuals, involving minimal therapist contact and the use of "psychological assistants" (O'Leary & Wilson, 1975), including the patient's family member, psychiatric aides, peer group members, teachers, parents, and others, improves the cost effectiveness of treatment. Yet, much still remains to be done.

For the most part, behavior therapists have emulated the treatment format and scheduling of the more traditional psychotherapies in sticking to the standard 50- to 60-minute session on a weekly basis. I am unaware of any compelling theoretical or empirical rationale for this practice. More plausible but less defensible reasons for this conformity with past practice are the facts that it was, and still is, the "done thing", and that it cannot be beat in terms of convenience (the therapist's!) in making for a predictable and orderly week's work schedule. Put bluntly, we have been relatively unimaginative in creating treatment formats and schedules, although there is evidence that alternative arrangements might produce better results.

For example, the data show that in the treatment of phobic disorders, the technique of flooding becomes significantly more effective the longer the duration of the session. Stern and Marks (1973) found that two hours of continuous, *in vivo* exposure to the phobic situation produced greater change than four separate, half-hour sessions. Similarly, Rabavilas, Boulougouris, and Stefanis (1976) showed that in the treatment of obsessive-compulsive patients, 80 minutes of continuous, *in vivo* exposure was significantly superior to four separate, 20-minute sessions. The greater effectiveness of longer durations of exposure to feared situations is consistent with findings from the animal-conditioning laboratory and the predictions of two-factor learning theory, on which flooding was originally based (Levis & Hare, 1977; Wilson & Davison, 1971).

We do not know what the optimal parameters of *in vivo* exposure methods are, however, nor can we yet be sure of the theoretical mechanisms responsible for the success of these *in vivo* exposure techniques (Marks, 1978). What is known is that flooding, with its emphasis on exposure to high-intensity anxiety stimuli, may enhance rather than reduce phobic sensitivity under conditions in which patients do not receive exposure of sufficiently long duration (Stone & Borkovec, 1975). This disturbing possibility, allied to the difficulty of deciding what sufficient exposure is across different patients and problems (Gauthier & Marshall, 1977), suggests that a graduated form of *in vivo* exposure treatment, one that does not elicit such intense anxiety yet appears to be equally effective (e.g., participant modeling), may be the preferred method.

Are massed treatment sessions, namely, more frequently scheduled sessions, more effective than distributed or less frequently scheduled sessions? What advantage, if any, is there to Masters and Johnson's (1970) treatment format of daily treatment sessions over a brief, two-week period versus the same therapy conducted on an outpatient basis with weekly treatment sessions? The intensive, massed-treatment format of Masters and Johnson might be predicted to facilitate treatment outcome by minimizing distraction and competing activities that are more likely to complicate treatment spread out over a number of weeks or months; it might also ensure greater cooperation and adherence to therapeutic instructions, since the failure to engage in any particular homework assignment would be that much more salient and less easily explained away by appeals to "being too busy" or being preoccupied with other matters.

In discussing the advantages of intensive, brief treatment, Masters and Johnson have the following to say:

> When treatment crises occurred (and they occurred regularly), the clients were never more than 24 hours away from active professional support. Therapy crises can be turned into important teaching opportunities rather than thera-

peutic setbacks if faced in the relative immediacy of their onset. The two-week rapid-treatment format with daily therapy sessions conducted on a seven-day-a-week basis inevitably provides an opportunity to approach treatment crises in the relative immediacy of onset that a once- or twice-a-week therapy format cannot provide. Even if the crisis cannot be resolved satisfactorily, immediacy of therapeutic effort usually eases the severity of the trauma experienced by the distressed couple, and, of course, lessens the hazards to the therapeutic regime. In addition, the importance of continuing therapeutic reinforcement and modeling is maximized in a daily treatment format, drawing upon the underlying principles of social learning theory in a most efficient manner." (pp. 258-259)

The relative merits of alternative treatment schedules remain to be evaluated. In an initial study along the lines I am proposing here, Ersner-Hershfeld and Kopel (1979) compared "massed" versus "distributed" treatment sessions in the treatment of women with orgasmic dysfunction. Despite overall treatment success, they found no differential efficacy of the two formats. Comparing a schedule of 2 per week for five weeks with a schedule of weekly sessions, however, does not constitute an adequate test of massed versus distributed treatment.

Elsewhere (Wilson, 1980), I have criticized the typical treatment format in the behavioral treatment of obesity, where a schedule of fixed weekly sessions for a period of approximately 10 weeks has been virtually standard practice. This practice, however, seems arbitrary. In view of the refractory nature of a chronic disorder like obesity, a more plausible treatment format might require more frequent, intensive treatment sessions several times a week, at least at the start of therapy, followed by a different schedule of maintenance sessions to consolidate or continue weight loss. It is not without interest that Stuart (1967) used this more flexible scheduling of treatment sessions in his initial report of unprecedented success in the treatment of obese clients. While his principles and procedures have been widely adopted, his innovative treatment format has been overlooked. In sum, we have few, if any, clinical guidelines for deciding upon the duration or frequency (spacing) of treatment sessions. Of course, optimal combinations of these technical parameters of therapy will vary, depending upon the particular patient, problem, and treatment procedure(s).

INDIVIDUALIZATION OF TREATMENT AND THERAPEUTIC VERSATILITY

A distinguishing characteristic of behavior therapy is its emphasis on tailoring treatment strategies to the individual client. Behavior therapy is not a grab bag of techniques, although it has generated a great number of specific treatment techniques, but a problem-solving approach, in which the therapist draws upon a broad range of psychological principles and procedures. These principles and procedures are primarily derived from, or at least consistent with, the content and method of experimental–clinical psychology in general and social learning theory in particular (Agras, Kazdin, & Wilson, 1979). Different techniques and clinical strategies are required for different problems across diverse patient populations. This emphasis on specificity, versatility, and flexibility in clinical assessment and treatment is consistent with the all-important outcome question that therapists of all theoretical persuasions have to face, namely, *"what* treatment, by *whom,* is most effective for *this* individual with *that* specific problem and under *which* set of circumstances?" (Paul, 1967, p. 111). We should also add "on *what* measures" and "at *what* cost" to round off this appeal to specificity of therapy outcome evaluation (Kazdin & Wilson, 1978b; Rachman & Wilson, 1980).

Not only are some techniques and strategies more appropriate with some problems and patients than with others, but behavior therapy techniques are also differentially effective across different clinical disorders. For example, *in vivo* exposure methods that are performance based (e.g., participant modeling) have been shown to be more effective than methods that rely upon symbolic operations (e.g., imaginal systematic desensitization or flooding) in the treatment of phobic, obsessive–compulsive, and sexual disorders (e.g., Bandura, 1977a; Kazdin & Wilson, 1978b; Marks, 1978). As another example, covert sensitization has been demonstrated to be effective in the treatment of specific forms of sexual deviation, such as exhibitionism and transvestitism but has proven ineffective in the modification of addictive disorders, such as alcohol abuse and overeating.

There is no monolithic system of "behavior therapy" in the sense of a uniform technique that can be compared to another approach. Rather, there are several different techniques that collectively can be referred to as behavior therapy. Many behavior therapy techniques are based on different assumptions and therapeutic procedures. Of course, the same reasoning applies to the ill-defined global concept of "psychotherapy." This fact, among others, makes nonsense out of reviews of the comparative treatment literature, such as that of Luborsky, Singer, and Luborsky (1975), who attempted to justify their comparative evaluation of "behavior therapy" and "psychotherapy" by claiming that different behavioral treatment techniques do not differ from each other in terms of relative efficacy (see Rachman & Wilson, 1980).

DISTINGUISHING BETWEEN THE INITIAL TREATMENT-PRODUCED CHANGE
AND ITS SUBSEQUENT MAINTENANCE OVER TIME

Conceptually, most conventional outcome research has been influenced by the psychodynamic or quasi-disease model of psychological disturbances. In this model, clinical disorders are considered to be a function of intrapsychic conflicts. If internal conflicts are resolved through therapy, the person is said to be cured. A recurrence of the disorder is referred to as a relapse. Both cure and relapse are qualitative concepts that have tended to discourage the analysis of specific psychosocial variables that maintain treatment-produced improvement. Specifically, they tend to ignore or downgrade the influence of the social environment on the client's behavior following therapy.

From the perspective of behavior therapy, outcome evaluation must distinguish among the initiation of therapeutic change, its transfer to the natural environment, and its maintenance over time. It is important to distinguish among these different phases of treatment, since they appear to be governed by different variables and require different intervention strategies. Generalized behavior change, for example, should not be expected unless specific steps have been taken to produce generalization. Several strategies have been demonstrated to facilitate generalization of treatment-produced improvement (e.g., Bandura, Jeffery, & Gajdos, 1975; Stokes & Baer, 1977).

With respect to maintenance of therapeutic improvement, Kazdin and Wilson (1978b) have stated:

> A given treatment might produce highly significant improvement at posttreatment compared to appropriate comparative control groups, but show no superiority at a subsequent follow-up owing to the dissipation of the initial therapeutic effect over time. It would be premature to conclude that such a treatment method is ineffective; a more specific analysis may indicate that it is effective in inducing change, but fails to maintain change. It may be that by complementing the treatment method with strategies designed to facilitate maintenance of change, long-term improvement may be effected. Within this expanded framework it may be that a specific treatment technique and a specific maintenance method are both necessary although neither may be sufficient for durable therapeutic change. (p. 63)

Within a behavioral model, most abnormal behavior is seen as a function of antecedent and consequent environmental events and cognitive mediating processes that may vary in different situations, in different people, and often at different times in the same person. Behavior is neither a product of autonomous internal forces nor a simple function of external environmental contingencies. Psychological functioning involves a reciprocal interaction between a person's behavior and the environment: the person is both the agent and the object of environmental influence. In this analysis, maintenance will depend on a number of factors, including the problem being treated and the circumstances under which it occurs (Marlatt & Gordon, 1979; Wilson, 1979).

I have already noted that it is common practice for behavior therapists to provide booster or follow-up sessions for their clients at varying intervals following treatment termination. Some clinical disorders are characterized by higher rates of relapse than others, and in these cases, specific, long-term maintenance strategies are a necessary and integral part of the overall treatment approach. Addictive disorders, for example, and other psychological problems that resemble them highlight the need for effective maintenance strategies, if long-term success is to be achieved. Newly acquired self-control capacities, whether they involve eating less, quitting smoking, ceasing alcohol consumption, or desisting from compulsive gambling, have few, if any, immediately strong positive consequences, in contrast to the instant gratification afforded by eating and alcohol consumption. These newly acquired behaviors appear to be highly vulnerable to disruption, at least in their initial stages, a theoretical prediction that is amply borne out by the clinical evidence (e.g., Hunt, Barnett, & Branch, 1971). In most of these instances, short-term therapy may effect behavior change (e.g., abstinence in the alcoholic), but long-term sobriety will depend heavily on the degree to which adequate maintenance strategies are implemented to bolster self-regulatory skills.

The majority of clients who seek treatment for obesity, for example, cannot be helped to lose weight and keep it off on the basis of short-term therapy of any kind, behavior or otherwise, unless initial changes in eating and exercise patterns (producing weight loss, as a rule) are followed by a program of effective maintenance strategies (Stuart, 1979; Wilson, 1980). Emphasizing the importance of distinguishing between the initial treatment-produced change and its maintenance over time is the fact that posttreatment weight loss has usually been unrelated to weight loss at long-term follow-ups (e.g., Jeffery, Wing, & Stunkard, 1978). Detailed social learning analyses of "the relapse problem" in addictive and other clinical disorders have been presented by Marlatt and Gordon (1979), Stuart (1979), and Wilson (1979). Specific maintenance strategies have been developed that focus on the person's self-regulatory skills, cognitive coping competencies, and social support systems. Evaluation and refinement of these maintenance strategies is one of the major areas of research in behavior therapy today.

HOW EFFECTIVE IS BEHAVIOR THERAPY?

The examples of short-term behavior therapy that I have briefly described, many of them involving well-controlled treatment outcome research, provide some idea of the efficacy of behavior therapy with different clinical disorders, such as agoraphobia, sexual dysfunction, depression, and alcoholism. There is a steadily increasing body of evidence that bears on the efficacy of specific behavioral methods compared to appropriate control groups and on their comparative efficacy in relation to other forms of therapy. Even a cursory review of these data is beyond the scope of the present paper. In two recent books, Alan Kazdin, Jack Rachman, and I have analyzed in detail the evidence on the efficacy of behavior therapy (Kazdin & Wilson, 1978b; Rachman & Wilson, 1980). In short, there is persuasive evidence of the efficacy of some behavior therapy methods, when compared to the most stringent control groups, in the treatment of several clinical problems.

The comparative research data, however, reveal a paucity of studies that are sufficiently well controlled to allow unequivocal interpretations of the findings. Basic shortcomings in design and measurement are evident in the vast majority of studies. Many are completely uninterpretable and convey no useful information. Yet, it is apparent that despite the seriously flawed nature of these studies, conclusions are being drawn from this data base that may have a major impact on both future research and clinical practice. Thus, we are forced to take account of these fundamentally flawed studies, the findings of which Kazdin and I have summarized in the following four points:

1. Not a single comparison showed behavior therapy to be inferior to psychotherapy. On the contrary, many studies showed that behavior therapy was either marginally or significantly more effective than the alternative treatment.
2. No evidence of symptom substitution following behavior therapy was obtained, even in studies explicitly designed to uncover negative side effects. Typical of the findings in this respect is the comment by Sloane *et al.* (1975, p. 100) that not a single patient whose

original problems had substantially improved reported new symptoms cropping up. On the contrary, assessors had the informal impression that when a patient's primary symptoms improved, he often spontaneously reported improvement of other minor difficulties.

3. Behavior therapy is capable of producing broadly based treatment effects on specific target behaviors and related measures of general psychological functioning. A frequently voiced speculation is that behavior therapy might have greater effects on symptom-outcome measures than on more important or fundamental processes related to general adjustment. This suggestion reflects the traditional view that behavior therapy is best regarded as a limited and relatively superficial form of treatment that may be useful as an adjunct to conventional psychotherapy. The available data render this notion untenable.

4. Behavior therapy is far more applicable to the full range of psychological disorders than is traditional psychotherapy. Sloane *et al.* (1975), for example, concluded that "behavior therapy is clearly a *generally* [italics in original] useful treatment," and I have commented on the broad-ranging applicability of behavior therapy earlier in this paper.

EVALUATING THE OUTCOME OF SHORT-TERM THERAPY

Rather than belabor the manifold shortcomings of conventional comparative outcome research (see Kazdin & Wilson, 1978b; Rachman & Wilson, 1980), I wish to emphasize a few points about how behavior therapy, indeed any short-term therapy, should be evaluated if meaningful data are to result. First, we have to inquire about the specific effects of particular, carefully specified, replicable treatment techniques on operationally defined measures. There appears to be a general consensus on this point (e.g., Bergin & Lambert, 1978; Parloff, 1979), but actual research addressed to these issues has lagged behind. When all is said and done, more has been said than done! An obstacle to progress, in my opinion, has been the relative vagueness and absence of concrete alternatives with which many reviewers of psychotherapy outcome research have coupled their calls for action and the need for new directions in research.

MULTIPLE, PROBLEM-SPECIFIC RESEARCH STRATEGIES

One of the great contributions of behavior therapy has been the development of innovative research strategies for the study of treatment development and outcome. These methodological strategies range from single-case experimental designs to a variety of different group designs, including highly controlled, laboratory-based studies, more applied evaluations of complex treatment packages, and comparative outcome evaluations. As we will see, these different methodological strategies go well beyond conventional research methods and permit more refined empirical analyses of specific treatment questions. Nor are they confined to the evaluation of behavioral methods: they can be applied to all psychological treatment methods. Related to this expansion of research method are significant advances in the measurement of treatment outcome. The development of multiple subjective and objective measures of therapeutic outcome, which have been extensively assessed in terms of reliability, validity, and utility, has opened new frontiers of outcome research.

BROADENING THE CRITERIA FOR EVALUATING PSYCHOTHERAPY

Aside from the critically important issue of the efficacy of particular treatments using multiple subjective and objective measures to assess both treatment-specific effects and possible side effects (positive or negative), evaluation of treatment outcome must be broadened to include assessment of efficacy, various cost considerations, disseminability, and consumer satisfaction (Kazdin & Wilson, 1978a). If two contrasting treatments are equally effective, but one takes considerably less time than the other, the criterion of efficiency clearly dictates the preferred method. As I have made clear, I believe that behavior therapy has much to recommend it in this regard. Attempts to develop more efficient behavioral and nonbehavioral methods should be a priority for clinical researchers and funding agencies alike.

Aside from the amount of time required to administer treatment, efficiency can be measured by how treatment is administered. The examples of group treatment and the use of spouses or family members and nurse-therapists as part of the therapeutic program, as I have mentioned above, illustrate the rich potential of exploring these sources of "psychological assistants" to enhance efficiency.

In addition, the extent to which a technique can be widely disseminated is also a measure of efficiency. Thus, a technique that can be widely disseminated but is only moderately effective may have greater impact on client care than a technique that is more effective but less easily disseminated. Behavior therapy techniques have, as a whole, been carefully specified, easily replicable, and thus disseminable.

One of the most efficient means of disseminating treatment is through the use of self-help manuals. Glasgow and Rosen (1977) distinguished among self-administered programs, in which the written manual constitutes the sole basis for treatment; programs involving minimal contact, in which there is some contact with the therapist, such as phone calls or even periodic meetings; and therapist-administered programs, in which there is regular contact with the therapist, who guides the client in the use of the manual. Which of these different degrees of therapist involvement is appropriate for a particular client will depend on a number of factors, including the nature and severity of the problem and the type of self-help manual. There is, at present, no convincing evidence of the efficacy of totally self-administered programs or manuals, a disturbing finding in light of the fact that this is precisely the context in which most are likely to be used. Manuals with minimal contact, however, do have some empirical support and may offer the most prudent savings in professional time (e.g., Zeiss, 1978).

Several different costs are important in evaluating therapy techniques. One such cost, which is rarely discussed, is the amount of professional training required of the therapist. Traditionally, becoming a therapist, whether within psychiatry or psychology, entails lengthy and expensive training. Untrained or moderately trained individuals, however, frequently do just as well as professionals in effecting change in particular problems.

Consumer evaluation of therapy has also been conspicuously neglected in therapy outcome research. Different treatments for a given problem may not be equally acceptable to prospective clients. The acceptability of treatment is presumably influenced by the cost considerations mentioned above. Even effective treatments may not be acceptable to clients, however, if specific aspects of the procedures are objectionable.

It would seem premature to make definitive claims about the relative efficacy or utility of different treatments before a broad evaluation of therapy outcome has been made. Quite possibly, treatments will fare differently across diverse outcome criteria; thus, the superiority of one technique may be limited to a few criteria. The treatment of choice for a given patient may vary according to the outcome criterion best suited to the individual client's problem.

COMMONALITIES AND DIFFERENCES BETWEEN BEHAVIOR THERAPY AND NONBEHAVIORAL SHORT-TERM TREATMENTS

Most therapists, including behavior therapists, would agree that there are important therapeutic elements that are common to all forms of psychological treatment. It seems entirely reasonable to assume that these commonalities will be most pronounced among different short-term therapies with their inevitable time constraints. For example, Butcher and Koss (1978) stated that "regardless of therapeutic orientation, most brief therapists are directive in their approach to patients . . . in order to make more efficient use of time and keep the session content on track" (p. 748). Aside from directiveness of the therapist, other common characteristics of short-term therapies that Butcher and Koss list include the following:

- Goals are limited and are chosen, at least in part, by the patient.
- Therapy is focal in nature.
- Interviewing is "focused" with "present centeredness."
- The therapist is active and flexible in the use of diverse techniques.
- Assessment and intervention are prompt, with no lengthy psychometric evaluation.
- "Behavioral practice" is recommended.

At first blush, all these characteristics would seem to be emphasized in textbook descriptions of behavior therapy. Assuming that Butcher and Koss are accurate in their characterization of common ingredients among theoretically disparate short-term psychotherapies, the appearance of such powerful procedural similarities must lead one to ask whether or not behavior therapy is as distinctive an approach as it is usually depicted. What differences are there? How important are they? Do they provide a basis for the rational or empirically based selection of treatment methods for specific problems? While I concur with the view that there are significant process and procedural variables that are common to different treatment approaches, I believe that there are also fundamental differences, with major implications for clinical practice and treatment outcome. To illustrate the differences in approach that I am suggesting, following Butcher and Koss's synthesis, I wish to discuss briefly the nature of behavioral practice and the therapist's contributions to treatment.

BEHAVIORAL PRACTICE

I have always been struck by the following piece of "common-sensical" clinical wisdom concerning the desirability of what the author refers to as "extratherapeutic experiences," or what the contemporary behavior therapist would know as performance-based methods of psychological change:

> Like the adage nothing succeeds like success, there is no more powerful therapeutic factor than the performance of activities which were formerly neurotically impaired or inhibited. No insight, no emotional discharge, no recollection can be as reassuring as accomplishment in the actual life situation in which the individual failed. Thus the ego regains that confidence which is the fundamental condition, the prerequisite, of mental health. Every success encourages new trials and decreases inferiority feelings, resentments, and their sequelae—fear, guilt, and resulting inhibitions. Successful attempts at productive work, love, self-assertion, or competition will change the vicious circle to a benign one; as they are repeated, they become habitual and bring about a complete change in personality. . . . Fostering favorable experiences in the actual life situation at the right moment in the treatment tends to make for economical psychotherapy, bringing it to an earlier conclusion than otherwise. The therapist need not wait until the end of treatment but . . . should encourage (or even require the patient) to do those things which he had avoided in the past, to experiment in that activity in which he had failed before. (pp. 40–41)

You will recognize this advice as that of Franz Alexander (Alexander & French, 1946). From my perspective, the failure of psychodynamically oriented psychotherapists to act seriously on this admonition, to focus systematically on behaviorally based experiences in the patient's current natural environment (at least in addition to, if not instead of, the concern with the hypothesized reliving and modification of childhood emotional conflicts within the transference relationship), has been one of the major weaknesses of this approach. It may be that psychodynamic therapists, particularly those who practice short-term treatment, do, on occasion, recommend some form of extratherapeutic experience outside of the transference relationship, but I questions whether this feature of psychodynamic approaches can be likened seriously to the highly structured, explicitly scheduled, and systematically checked technique- and even problem-specific nature of *in vivo* homework assignments in behavioral assessment and therapy. Sloane *et al.* (1975), for example, showed that behavior therapists were significantly more directive than their psychoanalytically oriented counterparts, exercised more control over the content of the therapy sessions, and prescribed more courses of action.

Recently, Goldfried (1980), in the *American Psychologist,* attempted to illustrate basic commonalities among diverse therapeutic approaches by arguing that most, if not all, approaches advocate corrective or extratherapeutic experiences. Cited in support of this view are isolated statements by Freud (1924) himself, Fenichel (1941), and other psychoanalytic authorities about the desirability of having patients try new ways of behaving in the extratherapeutic environment. Gestalt therapy (Polster & Polster, 1973), encounter groups (Schutz, 1973), and other approaches are similarly said to include an emphasis on specific behavior change. Yet this sort of scholarly scanning of the vast literature on psychotherapy establishes only the most superficial commonality among diverse therapeutic approaches with respect to behavioral practice.

It is not just the structure and systematic nature of homework assignments in behavior therapy (e.g., daily self-monitoring records of operationally defined target thoughts, feelings, or behaviors that must be returned to the therapist by a certain date) that make it distinctive. The substantive nature of these assignments is also characteristically different. Consider, for example, the highly specific nature of behavioral assignments in sex therapy, such as sensate focus exercises, the "squeeze" or "stop–start" technique to eliminate premature ejaculation, masturbatory programs for primary orgasmic dysfunction, and so on. These procedures have revolutionized the treatment of sexual dysfunction and deviance. There had not been anything like this before Masters and Johnson (1970), building on the prior work of Wolpe and Lazarus (1966) and others, developed their methods. Nor had there been anything like the success that is now routinely recorded. This is the telling point. Other obvious examples could be culled from virtually any major neurotic disorder, but the point has been made.

Self-monitoring, a backbone of so much assessment and treatment in behavior therapy, is seen by Goldfried (1980) as one aspect of the purportedly common clinical strategy of providing the patient with *direct feedback.* But self-monitoring is surely not directly comparable to having the therapist reflect clients' thoughts back to them (in client-centered therapy) or having the clients receive feedback (in other humanistic–existential therapies, such as Gestalt therapy or encounter groups). Among other factors, look at the specific knowledge we now have about the particular parameters of self-monitoring. Research has shown that it matters a great deal precisely *what* people self-monitor (e.g., Green, 1978; Romancyzk, Tracey, Wilson, & Thorpe, 1973), *when* they self-monitor (e.g., Green, 1978), and *how* (e.g., Bandura & Simon, 1977). The conceptualizations that spurred this research, the methodology that facilitated it, and the clinical imperative of specifying antecedent and consequent variables that result in the significant use of self-monitoring in clinical practice are the dimensions that are important, and they serve to differentiate among competing therapeutic philosophies, despite what may appear to be surface similarities in approach.

One final point in this connection: Alexander (Alexander & French, 1946), in the essay to which I have already alluded, went on to declare:

> While it is important not to urge the patient prematurely, the therapist's fear that his patient will fail is usually stronger than it should be. The therapist must prepare the patient for failure, explaining that they are unavoidable and the most important thing for him is to be always ready to try new experiments. Moreover, failures can be turned to advantage when they are carefully analyzed and their cause thoroughly understood by the patient. (p. 41)

This is eminently sound advice and, at an abstract level, conceptually close to the formal cognitive–behavioral models of preventing relapse in substance abuse that Bandura (1977a), Marlatt and Gordon (1979), and Wilson (1979) have detailed. This general sense of the significance of coping with failure experiences, however, which I believe went largely ignored, is a far cry from the specific theoretical analyses of relapse and the particular maintenance strategies that have been devised to reduce the adverse impact of inevitable "slips" or failures in the treatment of addictive and other disorders (see Marlatt, 1978).

The specification of *what* actions the patient should engage in to cope with problems has been a strong suit of behavior therapy; however, we know less about *how* to ensure that patients comply with the therapist's prescriptions. The problems of overcoming patient resistance to change, which is part of the broader problem of facilitating adherence to the therapist's instructions, have, to date, received relatively little formal attention in the behavior therapy literature, although some initial formulations have been advanced (Davison, 1973; Lazarus & Fay, in press; Mahoney, 1974; Weiss, 1979; Wilson & Evans, 1977). This is one area in which behavior therapists would seem to be well advised to familiarize themselves with the eminently compatible, artful strategies of motivating patients to cooperate in therapy, strategies that are such prominent features of the problem-solving or systems theory approach to therapy (e.g., Haley, 1976; Sluzki, 1978).

Behavior therapists increasingly attend to the psychological significance of the performance of homework assignments for the patient. In contrast to earlier behavioristic approaches, with their reliance on automatic conditioning processes and the establishment of stimulus–response or response–reinforcement bonds or contingencies, the social learning approach emphasizes the importance of using behavioral procedures to alter cognitive mediating processes, which will then influence subsequent generalization and maintenance of behavioral change (Bandura, 1977b; Marlatt & Gordon, 1979; Rosenthal, in press; Wilson & O'Leary, 1980). In this formulation, the meaning patients attach to their behavioral successes or failures—that is, how they perceive, interpret, encode, and remember their experiences—is critically important. This is particularly evident in cognitive–behavioral approaches. In these treatments, the therapist is guided in the use of behavioral assignments by theoretical considerations of how behavioral performance affects specific attributional processes, by the patient's sense of personal efficacy, and by other cognitive processes (e.g., Bandura, 1977a; Beck, 1976).

THE THERAPEUTIC RELATIONSHIP

As Butcher and Koss (1978) observed, the therapeutic relationship is of seminal importance in all forms of short-term treatment. Behavior therapy is no exception, although this particular aspect is often ignored or downplayed in much of the behavioral literature. With a few particularly powerful techniques (e.g., participant modeling) and with straightforward, well-defined problems (e.g., simple phobias), the influence of the therapist relationship is usually less crucial. With more complex problems, however, particularly those in which interpersonal factors predominate and the patient may be resistant to change, the role of the therapeutic relationship becomes increasingly important. In this sense, the behavior therapist's personal contribution to treatment inevitably overlaps with that of therapists of alternative theoretical persuasions. Yet, the conceptualization of the therapeutic relationship and the way in which it is used to foster progress can be differentiated from most nonbehavioral approaches.

Discussed elsewhere are specific ways in which behavior therapy differs from other treatments in terms of the nature and use of therapeutic interpretations and the response to patient resistance to change (Goldfried & Davison, 1976; Weiss, 1979; Wilson & Evans, 1976, 1977). It is sufficient to note here that in adopting an active, directive, and selectively self-disclosing stance, as opposed to a more neutral and detached posture, the behavior therapist is a problem solver, a coping model who tries to instigate behavioral change in the patient's natural environment, and who serves as a source of social support and influence. In this process, the therapist's skill in overcoming resistance to change and prompting adherence to behavioral prescriptions can often decide the outcome of treatment. In contrast to classical psychodynamic views of the transference relationship, an emotion-laden interaction between the therapist and patient, in which critical unconscious, childhood conflicts are worked through, is not seen as a necessary or primary vehicle for therapeutic change, although the learning that may take place in interactions with the therapist is more important in some cases than in others.

Whereas procedural differences between behavior therapy and other forms of brief, directive psychotherapy, such as Haley's (1976) problem-solving therapy, are often blurred, the distinction between behavior therapy and brief psychodynamic therapy seems clear. If the actions of the therapists in Sloane *et al.*'s (1975) comparative outcome study of behavior therapy and brief, psychoanalytically oriented psychotherapy are at all representative of therapists in general—a reasonable assumption, I believe—then therapists from these two contrasting approaches not only talk differently about therapy but also do it differently. As Staples, Sloane, Whipple, Cristol, and Yorkston (1975) concluded on the basis of their study:

> Differences between behavior therapy and analytically-oriented psychotherapy . . . involved the basic patterns of interactions between patient and therapist and the type of relationship formed. Behavior therapy is not psychotherapy with special 'scientific techniques' superimposed on the traditional therapeutic paradigm; rather, the two appear to represent quite different syles of treatment although they share common elements. (p. 1521)

The behavior therapists were more directive, more open, more genuine, and more disclosing than their psychoanalytically oriented counterparts. Both sets of therapists used a similar number of interpretations during therapy, but the quality of these interpretations differed predictably, with the psychotherapists "focusing psychodynamically on feelings and the behavior therapists concentrating on behavior."

Whether or not behavior therapists, who differ from psychoanalytically oriented psychotherapists in "almost every obvious way imaginable," are, nonetheless, "fundamentally saying the same thing" and hence achieving comparable results, as Staples *et al.* (1975) suggest and Frank (1974) has long proposed, is the proper subject of well-controlled comparative outcome research that avoids the conceptual and methodological flaws that complicate the interpretation of the Sloane *et al.* (1975) study itself (see Kazdin & Wilson, 1978b). The available data, such as they are, indicate not only that behavior therapy and psychodynamic therapy differ procedurally, but also that they yield differential success across specific target problems (Rachman & Wilson, 1980).

SUMMARY

Behavior therapy is a flexible and versatile form of brief treatment, in which the therapist draws upon a range of different principles and procedures in tailoring treatment to each individual and his or her problem. Behavior therapy has broad applicability to diverse clinical, medical, and educational problems, and there is evidence indicating that specific methods are effective with particular problems. This success cannot be attributed to the adventitious role of "nonspecific factors" common to all forms of psychotherapy, as is popularly but erroneously thought.

By using self-help programs with minimal therapist contact and with nonprofessional, psychological assistants (such as family members), behavior therapy has expended the scope of treatment services, although still conforming, to a large extent, to the format of weekly, one-hour sessions. Alternative treatment formats and schedules might provide for more effective or efficient treatment.

A distinction is made between the initial therapeutic change and its maintenance over time in different situations. For some problems, such as addictive disorders, regardless of the initial efficacy of short-term treatment, durable success will depend largely upon appropriate maintenance strategies.

Behavior therapy has much in common with other forms of brief psychotherapy, but it is still a distinctive approach in terms of basic assumptions and specific treatment strategies.

REFERENCES

Agras, W. S., & Berkowitz, R. Clinical research in behavior therapy: Halfway there? *Behavior Therapy*, 1980, *11*, 472–487.

Agras, W. S., Kazdin, A. E., & Wilson, G. T. *Behavior therapy: Towards an applied clinical science.* San Francisco: Freeman, 1979.

Alexander, F., & French, T. M. *Psychoanalytic therapy: Principles and applications.* New York: Ronald Press, 1946.

Azrin, N. H. Improvements in the community-reinforcement approach to alcoholism. *Behaviour Research and Therapy,* 1976, *14,* 339–348.

Bandura, A. *Principles of behavior modification.* New York: Holt, 1969.

Bandura, A. Self-efficacy: Toward a unifying theory of behavioral change. *Psychological Review,* 1977, *84,* 191–215.(a)

Bandura, A. *Social learning theory.* Englewood Cliffs, N.J.: Prentice-Hall, 1977.(b)

Bandura, A., Jeffery, R. W., & Gajdos, E. Generalizing change through participant modeling with self-directed mastery. *Behaviour Research and Therapy,* 1975, *13,* 141–152.

Bandura, A., & Simon, K. M. The role of prosocial intentions in self-regulation of refractory behavior. *Cognitive Therapy and Research,* 1977, *1,* 177–193.

Barlow, D. H., Reynolds, E. J., & Agras, W. S. Gender identity change in a transsexual. *Archives of General Psychiatry,* 1973, *28,* 569–576.

Beck, A. T. *Cognitive therapy and the emotional disorders.* New York: International Universities Press, 1976.

Becker, J., & Schuckit, M. A. The comparative efficacy of cognitive therapy and pharmacotherapy in the treatment of depressions. *Cognitive Therapy and Research,* 1978, *2,* 193–198.

Bergin, A. E., & Lambert, M. J. The evaluation of therapeutic outcomes. In S. L. Garfield & A. E. Bergin (Eds.), *Handbook of psychotherapy and behavior change* (2nd ed.). New York: Wiley, 1978.

Borkovec, T., & Rachman, S. The utility of analogue research. *Behaviour Research and Therapy,* 1979, *17,* 253–262.

Brady, J. P. Behavior therapy and sex therapy. *American Journal of Psychiatry,* 1976, *33,* 896–899.

Brigham, T., & Catania, A. C. *Handbook of applied behavior research: Social and instructional processes.* New York: Wiley, 1979.

Butcher, J. N., & Koss, M. P. Research on brief and crisis-oriented psychotherapies. In S. L. Garfield & A. E. Bergin (Eds.), *Handbook of psychotherapy and behavior change* (2nd ed.). New York: Wiley, 1978.

Caddy, G. R., Addington, H. J., & Perkins, D. Individualized behavior therapy for alcoholics: A third year independent double-blind follow-up. *Behaviour Research and Therapy,* 1978, *16,* 345–362.

Davison, G. C. Counter-control in behavior modification. In L. A. Hamerlynck, L. C. Handy, & E. J. Mash (Eds.), *Behavior change: Methodology, concepts, practice.* Champaign, Ill.: Research Press, 1973.

Ersner-Hershfeld, R., & Kopel, S. Group treatment of preorgasmic women: Evaluation of partner involvement and spacing of sessions. *Journal of Consulting and Clinical Psychology,* 1979, *47,* 750–759.

Eysenck, H. E. *Behaviour therapy and the neuroses.* Oxford: Pergamon Press, 1960.

Fenichel, O. *Problems of psychoanalytic technique.* Albany, N.Y.: Psychoanalytic Quarterly, 1941.

Fishman, S., & Lubetkin, B. Personal communication, 1980.

Foreyt, J., & Rathjen, D. *Cognitive behavior therapy: Research and application.* New York: Plenum Press, 1978.

Frank, J. D. Therapeutic components of psychotherapy: A 25-year progress report of research. *Journal of Nervous and Mental Disease,* 1974, *159,* 325–342.

Franks, C. M., & Wilson, G. T. (Eds.). *Annual review of behavior therapy: Theory and practice* (Vol. I). New York: Brunner/Mazel, 1973.

Franks, C. M., & Wilson, G. T. (Eds.). *Annual review of behavior therapy: Theory and practice* (Vol. II). New York: Brunner/Mazel, 1974.

Franks, C. M., & Wilson, G. T. (Eds.). *Annual review of behavior therapy: Theory and practice* (Vol. III). New York: Brunner/Mazel, 1975.

Franks, C. M., & Wilson, G. T. (Eds.). *Annual review of behavior therapy: Theory and practice* (Vol. IV). New York: Brunner/Mazel, 1976.

Franks, C. M., & Wilson, G. T. (Eds.). *Annual review of behavior therapy: Theory and practice* (Vol. V). New York: Brunner/Mazel, 1977.

Franks, C. M., & Wilson, G. T. (Eds.). *Annual review of behavior therapy: Theory and practice* (Vol. VI). New York: Brunner/Mazel, 1978.

Franks, C. M., & Wilson, G. T. (Eds.). *Annual review of behavior therapy: Theory and practice* (Vol. VII). New York: Brunner/Mazel, 1979.

Freud, S. *Collected papers* (Vol. 2). London: Hogarth Press, 1924.

Gauthier, J., & Marshall, W. L. The determination of optimal exposure to phobic stimuli in flooding therapy. *Behaviour Research and Therapy*, 1977, *15*, 403–410.

Gelder, M. G., Bancroft, J. H. J., Gath, D., Johnston, D. W., Mathews, A. M., & Shaw, P. M. Specific and non-specific factors in behaviour therapy. *British Journal of Psychiatry*, 1973, *123*, 445–562.

Glasgow, R. E., & Rosen, G. M. Behavioral biblio-therapy: A review of self-help behavior therapy manuals. *Psychological Bulletin*, 1978, *85*, 1–24.

Goldfried, M. R. Toward the delineation of therapeutic change principles. *American Psychologist*, 1980, *35*, 991–999.

Goldfried, M. R., & Davison, G. C. *Clinical behavior therapy*. New York: Holt, Rinehart & Winston, 1976.

Green, L. Temporal and stimulus factors in self-monitoring by obese persons. *Behavior Therapy*, 1978, *9*, 328–341.

Haley, J. *Problem solving therapy*. San Francisco: Jossey-Bass, 1976.

Hand, I., Lamontagne, Y., & Marks, I. M. Group exposure (flooding) *in vivo* for agoraphobics. *British Journal of Psychiatry*, 1974, *126*, 588–602.

Hodgson, R., Rachman, S., & Marks, I. The treatment of chronic obsessive–compulsive neurosis: Follow-up and further findings. *Behaviour Research and Therapy*, 1972, *10*, 181–189.

Hunt, W. A., Barnett, L. W., & Branch, L. G. Relapse rates in addiction programs. *Journal of Clinical Psychology*, 1971, *27*, 455–456.

Jeffery, R. W., Wing, R. R., & Stunkard, A. J. Behavioral treatment of obesity: The state of the art. *Behavior Therapy*, 1978, *9*, 189–199.

Kaplan, H. *Disorders of sexual desire*. New York: Brunner/Mazel, 1979.

Kazdin, A. E., & Wilson, G. T. Criteria for evaluating psychotherapy. *Archives of General Psychiatry*, 1978, *35*, 407–418.(a)

Kazdin, A. E., & Wilson, G. T. *Evaluation of behavior therapy: Issues, evidence and research strategies*. Cambridge: Ballinger, 1978.(b)

Lazarus, A. A. *Behavior therapy and beyond*. New York: McGraw-Hill, 1971.

Lazarus, A. A. *Multimodal behavior therapy*. New York: Springer, 1976.

Lazarus, A. A., & Fay, A. *Resistance or rationalization? A cognitive behavioral perspective*. Unpublished manuscript, Rutgers University, 1980.

Levis, D. J., & Hare, N. A review of the theoretical rationale and empirical support for the extinction approach of implosive (flooding) therapy. In M. Hersen, R. M. Eisler, & P. M. Miller (Eds.), *Progress in behavior modification* (IV). New York: Academic Press, 1977.

Luborsky, L., Singer, B., & Luborsky, L. Comparative studies of psychotherapies: Is it true that "everyone has won and all must have prizes"? *Archives of General Psychiatry*, 1975, *32*, 995–1008.

Mahoney, M. J. *Cognition and behavior modification.* Cambridge: Ballinger, 1974.

Marks, I. Behavioral psychotherapy of adult neurosis. In S. L. Garfield & A. E. Bergin (Eds.), *Handbook of psychotherapy and behavior change* (2nd ed.). New York: Wiley, 1978.

Marks, I. M., Hallam, R. S., Connolly, J., & Philpott, R. *Nursing in behavioural therapy.* London: Royal College of Nursing, 1977.

Marks, I., Hodgson, R., & Rachman, S. Treatment of chronic obsessive–compulsive neurosis by *in vivo* exposure. *British Journal of Psychiatry,* 1975, *127,* 349–364.

Marlatt, G. A. Craving for alcohol, loss of control, and relapse: A cognitive–behavioral analysis. In P. E. Nathan, G. A. Marlatt, & T. Toberg (Eds.), *Alcoholism: New directions in behavioral research and treatment.* New York: Plenum, 1978.

Marlatt, G. A., & Gordon, J. R. Determinants of relapse: Implications for the maintenance of behavior change. In P. Davidson & S. Davidson (Eds.), *Behavioral medicine: Changing health lifestyles.* New York: Brunner/Mazel, 1979.

Masters, W., & Johnson, V. *Human sexual inadequacy.* Boston: Little, Brown, 1970.

Masters, W., & Johnson, V. *Homosexuality in perspective.* Boston: Little, Brown, 1979.

Mathews, A. M., Bancroft, J., Whitehead, A., Hackmann, A., Julier, D., Bancroft, J., Gath, D., & Shaw, P. The behavioural treatment of sexual inadequacy: A comparative study. *Behaviour Research and Therapy,* 1976, *14,* 427–436.

Mathews, A., Teasdale, J., Munby, M., Johnston, D., & Shaw, P. A home based treatment program for agoraphobia. *Behavior Therapy,* 1977, *8,* 915–924.

McLean, P. D., & Hakstian, A. R. Clinical depression: Comparative efficacy of outpatient treatments. *Journal of Consulting and Clinical Psychology,* 1979, *47,* 818–836.

McMullen, S., & Rosen, R. C. Self-administered masturbation training in treatment of primary orgasmic dysfunction. *Journal of Consulting and Clinical Psychology,* 1979, *47,* 912–918.

Meichenbaum, D., & Cameron, R. Cognitive behavior modification: Current issues. In G. T. Wilson & C. M. Franks (Eds.), *Handbook of behavior therapy.* New York: Guilford Press, in press.

Miller, W. R. (Ed.). *The addictive behaviors: Treatment of alcoholism, drug abuse, smoking and obesity.* New York: Pergamon Press, 1980.

Nathan, P. E., & Briddell, D. W. Behavioral assessment and treatment of alcoholism. In B. Kissin & H. Begleiter (Eds.), *The biology of alcoholism* (Vol. 5). New York: Plenum Press, 1977.

O'Leary, K. D., & Wilson, G. T. *Behavior therapy: Application and outcome.* Englewood Cliffs, N.J.: Prentice-Hall, 1975.

Parloff, M. B. Can psychotherapy research guide the policymaker? A little knowledge may be a dangerous thing. *American Psychologist,* 1979, *34,* 296–306.

Paul, G. L. Outcome research in psychotherapy. *Journal of Consulting Psychology,* 1967, *31,* 109–118.

Polster, E., & Polster, M. *Gestalt therapy integrated.* New York: Brunner/Mazel, 1973.

Rabavilas, A. D., Boulougouris, J. C., & Stefanis, C. Duration of flooding session in the treatment of obsessive–compulsive patients. *Behaviour Research and Therapy,* 1976, *14,* 349–355.

Rachman, S. (Ed.). *Contributions to medical psychology* (Vol. I). Oxford: Pergamon Press, 1977.

Rachman, S., & Hodgson, R. *Obsessions and compulsions.* Englewood Cliffs, N.J.: Prentice-Hall, 1980.

Rachman, S., & Wilson, G. T. *The effects of psychological therapy.* Oxford: Pergamon Press, 1980.

Romancyzk, R. G., Tracey, D. A., Wilson, G. T., & Thorpe, G. L. Behavioral techniques in the treatment of obesity: A comparative analysis. *Behaviour Research and Therapy*, 1973, *11*, 629–640.

Rosenthal, T. L. On the significance of differences between social learning theory and cognitive–behavioral conceptions: Type I and type II errors. In G. T. Wilson & C. M. Franks (Eds.), *Handbook of behavior therapy*. New York: Guilford Press, in press.

Rush, A. J., Beck, A. T., Kovacs, M., & Hollon, S. Comparative efficacy of cognitive therapy and pharmacotherapy in the treatment of depressed out-patients. *Cognitive Therapy and Research*, 1977, *1*, 17–37.

Schutz, W. C. Encounter. In R. Corsini (Ed.), *Current psychotherapies*. Ithaca, Ill.: Peacock, 1973.

Skinner, B. F. *Science and human behavior*. New York: Macmillan, 1953.

Sloane, R. B., Staples, F. R., Cristol, A. H., Yorkston, N. J., & Whipple, K. *Psychotherapy versus behavior therapy*. Cambridge: Harvard University Press, 1975.

Sluzki, C. Marital therapy from a systems theory perspective. In T. Paolino & B. McCrady (Eds.), *Marriage and marital therapy from three perspectives*. New York: Brunner/Mazel, 1978.

Sobell, M. B., & Sobell, L. C. *Behavioral treatment of alcohol problems*. New York: Plenum Press, 1978.

Staples, F. R., Sloane, R. B., Whipple, K., Cristol, A. H., & Yorkston, N. Differences between behavior therapists and psychotherapists. *Archives of General Psychiatry*, 1975, *32*, 1517–1522.

Stern, R., & Marks, I. Brief and prolonged flooding. *Archives of General Psychiatry*, 1973, *28*, 270–276.

Stokes, T. F., & Baer, D. M. An implicit technology of generalization. *Journal of Applied Behavior Analysis*, 1977, *10*, 349–368.

Stone, M., & Borkovec, T. D. The paradoxical effects of brief CS exposure in analogue phobic subjects. *Behaviour Research and Therapy*, 1975, *13*, 51–54.

Stuart, R. B. Behavioral control of overeating. *Behaviour Research and Therapy*, 1967, *5*, 357–365.

Stuart, R. B. Weight loss and beyond: Are they taking it off and keeping it off? In P. Davidson & S. Davidson (Eds.), *Behavioral medicine: Changing health lifestyles*. New York: Brunner/Mazel, 1979.

Weiss, R. Resistance in behavioral marriage therapy. *American Journal of Family Therapy*, 1979, *3*, 3–6.

Wilson, G. T. On the much discussed nature of the term "behavior therapy." *Behavior Therapy*, 1978, *9*, 89–98.

Wilson, G. T. Cognitive factors in life-style changes: A social learning perspective. In P. Davidson & S. Davidson (Eds.), *Behavioral medicine: Changing health lifestyles*. New York: Brunner/Mazel, 1979.

Wilson, G. T. Behavior therapy and the treatment of obesity. In W. R. Miller (Ed.), *The addictive behaviors: Treatment of alcoholism, drug abuse, smoking and obesity*. New York: Pergamon Press, 1980.

Wilson, G. T., & Davison, G. C. Processes of fear reduction in systematic desensitization: Animal studies. *Psychological Bulletin*, 1971, *76*, 1–14.

Wilson, G. T., & Evans, I. M. Adult behavior therapy and the therapist–client relationship. In C. M. Franks & G. T. Wilson (Eds.), *Annual review of behavior therapy: Theory and practice* (Vol. IV). New York: Brunner/Mazel, 1976.

Wilson, G. T., & Evans, I. M. The therapist–client relationship in behavior therapy. In A. S.

Gurman & A. M. Razin (Eds.), *The therapist's contribution to effective psychotherapy: An empirical approach.* New York: Pergamon Press, 1977.

Wilson, G. T., & O'Leary, K. D. *Principles of behavior therapy.* Englewood Cliffs, N.J.: Prentice-Hall, 1980.

Wolpe, J. *Psychotherapy by reciprocal inhibition.* Stanford: Stanford University Press, 1958.

Wolpe, J., & Lazarus, A. A. *Behavior therapy techniques.* New York: Pergamon Press, 1966.

Zeiss, R. A. Self-directed treatment for premature ejaculation. *Journal of Consulting and Clinical Psychology,* 1978, *46,* 1234–1241.

CHAPTER 7
FOCUSED SINGLE-SESSION THERAPY: INITIAL DEVELOPMENT AND EVALUATION

Bernard L. Bloom

Focused single-session therapy examines the concept of planned short-term therapy by deliberately creating and evaluating the limiting case—an encounter designed to provide a significant therapeutic impact in a single interview. Because its theoretical base is psychodynamic in character, some of my colleagues have suggested that I call it focused analytic single-session therapy. I have resisted that suggestion, in part because the resulting acronym would seem shamelessly contrived. Before describing my initial experiences with this form of psychotherapy, it will be useful to put this effort into its ideological and conceptual context and then to review the existing single-session therapy literature.

Until quite recently, the conventional American wisdom put the prevalence of psychological disorder at about one case in ten; that is, in any given year, about 20 million people in the United States could be identified as having some form of significant psychopathology. Recent studies (Regier, Goldberg, & Taube, 1978) have furnished us a bitter harvest. These studies have indicated that that figure is a substantial underestimate, and that in spite of our efforts during the past generation, 15% rather than 10% is a more accurate indication of the prevalence of emotional disorders in our country.

Needless to say, were these 30 million people to descend on the mental health service delivery system, we would witness a catastrophic traffic jam, just as would happen if our 200 million-plus Americans heeded the admonition to have an annual physical examination. But for those of us who still find validity and inspiration in the original hopes of the com-

BERNARD L. BLOOM. Department of Psychology, University of Colorado at Boulder, Boulder, Colorado.

munity mental health movement, the task of providing significant therapeutic help for all people, who seek it constitutes a challenge of the first
magnitude. That challenge is even more compelling when we realize that
any service delivery strategy must leave enough mental health resources
available to ensure that they will be able to work toward the more long-
term goal of successful primary prevention.

Clearly, in the public sector at least, planned short-term therapy must
be the treatment of choice. Treatment would then be feasible for larger
numbers of clients. Waiting lists—a source of chronic tension for staff,
clients, and the public—could be eliminated. Moreover, for many clients,
whether because of economic or sociocultural considerations, planned
short-term therapy is the only real alternative to no treatment at all.

While advocacy for planned short-term treatment flies in the face of a
deeply ingrained mental health professional value system, it is remarkably
syntonic with the results of evaluation studies. These studies are easy to
summarize. Of the dozen published investigations I have found comparing the effectiveness of planned, short-term outpatient therapy or hospitalization with open-ended, long-term therapy or hospitalization, where
there has been random assignment of patients to short-term and long-term
conditions, the short-term outcome has been equal or superior to long-
term care and treatment in every case (Bloom, 1980). I have yet to find a
single persuasive exception to this conclusion.

Aside from the issue of relative cost and effectiveness, planned short-
term therapy coincides with the most common anticipations of therapy
clients and with the facts of therapeutic life. When representative samples
of therapy applicants are surveyed before the inauguration of therapy,
they typically indicate that they would expect evidence of significant improvement within five sessions and virtual recovery from their presenting
complaints within ten (Coleman, 1962; Garfield, 1978; Garfield & Wolpin, 1963).

Finally, those studies that survey typical patterns of psychotherapeutic care have consistently revealed that median length of therapy nation-
wide is five to six interviews (Lorion, 1974). Hoffman and Remmel (1975),
noting that most treatment is short-term, have concluded that "long-term
psychotherapy is indicated . . . only if the client both wants and needs it.
Experience shows that the overwhelming majority of the clients do not
want it" (p. 267). The therapy evaluation literature I have reviewed indicates, in addition, that the overwhelming majority of clients do not need
it.

In the process of examining the planned short-term therapy literature, I found my attention drawn to occasional references to the incidence or effects of a single therapeutic interview. Most of the references are in parenthetical phrases, and I hope the following review will help give that literature greater salience. The remainder of the first half of this paper presents a review of that literature on single therapeutic interviews.

THE FREQUENCY OF SINGLE-SESSION EPISODES OF CARE

Occasional reports have appeared in the literature during the past 30 years that provide information as to the frequency with which clients in mental health and family casework agencies have one-session episodes of care. Professional attitudes toward these single contact episodes can be quickly discerned when it is noted that such clients are virtually always referred to as "dropouts."

One prevalent finding is that such episodes are unusually common in lower social classes. Lazare, Cohen, Jacobson, Williams, Mignone, and Zisook (1972), summarizing the research of the prior 15 years concerned with outpatient treatment among persons in the lower socioeconomic class, noted that these studies report dropout rates of over 50% after the first interview (see also Fiester & Rudestam, 1975). These authors (Lazare et al., 1972) believed that "patients seemed to want the therapists to give practical advice, medications, and warmth—expectations that clearly differed from those of the therapists" (p. 882). We will meet this assertion of therapist–client mismatch again.

Social workers, particularly those identified with family service agencies, have long been interested in the "short-contact case"(Frings, 1951). Such cases have been defined as those having a maximum of one planned intake appointment but including all telephone calls and letters. In 1948, the Family Service Association of America conducted, in 64 cooperating agencies, a one-month survey of cases that had been closed after having had one in-person interview (see Shyne, 1957). Such cases constituted about one-third of all cases in any given time period. Kogan (1957a, 1957b, 1957c), in an effort to learn more about short-term cases in a family agency, examined the records of all new clients in the Division of Family Services of the New York Community Service Society for one month in late 1953. During that month, 250 new cases had a first in-person interview. Of these 250 cases, 141 (56%) were closed after one interview.

More recent surveys in community mental health centers have reported similar findings. Ewalt (1973) reported that half the client families at the Framingham (Massachusetts) Youth Guidance Center ceased clinic contacts before treatment could be begun. Spoerl (1975) reported that in 1972, 39% of the 6780 clients seen at his clinic (a clinic that functions as part of a private, prepaid, nonprofit health maintenance organization) were seen only once, even though these clients had full financial coverage for the first ten visits. Reed, Myers, and Scheidemandel (1972) indicated that in 1969, 27% of the Kaiser Foundation Health Plan of Southern California clients ($n = 1892$) were seen for only one visit; in 1970, 39% of the clients of the Detroit Community Health Association Program for federal employees were seen only once. More recently, Sue, Allen, and Conaway (1978) reported that during a three-year period, 30% of the Anglo-Americans, 42% of Chicanos, and 55% of native Americans were seen only once in 17 community mental health facilities in the Seattle area.

Bloom (1975) described a number of characteristics of the mental health service delivery system in Pueblo, Colorado, for a two-year period during 1969–1971. Length of episodes of care (i.e., time between admission and discharge) were calculated for the 1572 first admission outpatients and for the 280 outpatients with prior histories of psychiatric care. Of the first admissions, 505 (32%) had episode lengths of one week or less, as did 55 (20%) of the repeat admissions. Virtually all these one-week episodes in outpatient settings involved cases where clients were seen only once. About 30% of these outpatients were seen in the private sector. The proportion of clients seen only once was not significantly different when public and private sector clients were contrasted.

Fiester and Rudestam (1975) reported that in their studies conducted in three urban community mental health centers, "between 37% and 45% of eligible adult outpatients 'drop out' after the first or second session" (p. 528). Similar figures are reported by Hoffman and Remmel (1975). Littlepage, Kosloski, Schnelle, McNees, and Gendrich (1976) studied a sample of 349 patients—all the outpatients who terminated from a community health center during 1974. Of this group, 75 (21%) had had only one contact with the center prior to termination. Of a total of 735 clients seen at the Benjamin Rush Center in Los Angeles (an early-access brief treatment facility) during an 18-month period, Jacobson, Wilner, Morley, Schneider, Strickler, and Sommer (1965) reported that 192 (26%) were seen only once.

Single-session episodes of care seem slightly less common in university mental health facilities, although there appear to be few published reports of treatment duration. Sarvis, Dewees, and Johnson (1959) described a form of time-limited psychotherapy employed at a university student health facility. Of the more than 800 clients who were seen during 1955 and had not returned to the clinic as of 1957, 10% were seen only once. The authors pointed out that patients seen for brief therapy were not "rejects." They indicated that "the length of a given therapeutic transaction was considered to be either optimal or useful at the time for the patient" (p. 285). Speers (1962) undertook brief psychotherapy with 68 college students in his capacity as a part-time psychiatric consultant to a neighboring women's college during the academic year 1958–1959. Of these women, 18 (26%) were seen only once.

Conservative general figures that seem appropriate on the basis of these reports are as follows: in family agencies, 30–35% of clients are seen only once; in community mental health centers, 25–30% of clients are seen only once; in university-based mental health programs, perhaps 15% of clients are seen only once.

EARLY TERMINATION AND CLIENT SATISFACTION

There is no question but that mental health professionals tend to view early and unilateral termination by clients as a sign of therapeutic failure and client dissatisfaction. Thus, it may be reassuring to know that empirical studies of client satisfaction and length of treatment (with particular reference to single-session therapy), consistently fail to support this view.

Of Kogan's (1957a) 141 one-interview cases, 42 (30%) were considered to be unplanned closings, by virtue of the fact that the client failed to keep subsequent, agreed-upon appointments. Kogan was able to interview, either in person or by telephone, 80% of these 141 cases between three months and one year after the case was closed; he had similar success in contacting cases with planned and unplanned closings. In addition, therapist evaluations prepared at the time of case closings were analyzed. Kogan's results are illuminating. In the majority of cases, therapists attributed unplanned closings to client resistance or lack of interest. Follow-up interviews with these single-session clients revealed that reality-based factors preventing continuance and improvements in the problem situations may have accounted for a substantial proportion of these unplanned closings.

About two-thirds of all clients felt they had been helped. There was no difference in this proportion when clients with planned closing were compared to clients with unplanned closings. In contrast, therapists considered that clients were, in general, helped, but that those with planned closings were helped significantly more than those with unplanned closings. Therapists consistently underestimated the help which clients with unplanned closings judged they had received, and they consistently overestimated how helpful they had been to clients with planned closings.

Silverman and Beech (1979) successfully contacted by telephone 47 people out of a pool of 184 clients of a community mental health center who, in the past year, had been seen only once, and who were neither terminated nor referred elsewhere; that is, these clients had terminated their contact with the mental health center unilaterally. An effort was made to reach all the 184 clients, but many had disconnected telephones or had given wrong numbers, had moved, or could not be reached despite repeated efforts. Of the 47 persons who were reached, 70% expressed satisfaction with the services they had received, 79% reported that the problems which had brought them to the mental health center were solved (although in only half the cases did the ex-clients attribute those solutions to the center), and the majority indicated their expectations had been met. Thus, in the words of the authors, "the notion that dropouts represent failure by the client or the intervention system is clearly untenable" (p. 241).

Littlepage *et al.* (1976) assessed client satisfaction by contacting 130 former clients out of the 349 who had terminated during 1974. These clients had had from 1 to 24 contacts with the community mental health center where they had been enrolled. General level of satisfaction was high and was unrelated to the number of treatment contacts. Clients whose treatment terminated after only limited center contact evaluated their experiences just as highly as clients who had had extended contact with the center. Clients who dropped out of therapy did not evaluate their experiences differently than clients who attended their final scheduled therapy session. These authors concluded that their findings "are not consistent with the implicit assumption that persons with limited contacts terminate therapy because of dissatisfaction with the services," and that one should not "automatically assume that early client terminations reflect treatment failures" (p. 167).

In a more complex investigation, Fiester and Rudestam (1975) studied two different public-sector mental health programs and contrasted clients who unilaterally terminated after the first or second session with clients who remained for three or more sessions, regardless of final disposition.

Demographic information (e.g., age, sex, education, socioeconomic status, and history of prior psychiatric care) and an array of pretherapy expectations and posttherapy reactions were collected prior to and following the first session. In addition, some demographic and professional background information was collected from all therapists. Results of their analyses were not the same in the two settings, a finding attributed by the authors to differences in therapist characteristics.

In the facility where the therapeutic staff was older, more experienced, upper class, and psychodynamically oriented, the clients who dropped out early and unilaterally tended more often to be lower class people, who felt they had been attentive to the therapist, whom they found to be helpful and serious, but who found themselves angry during the interview without being able to talk about it. In this setting, clients who terminated early tended to be dissatisfied with the services they had received.

By way of contrast, in the other setting, where the staff was younger, less experienced, less doctrinaire, and of lower social class, very few clients who terminated early were dissatisfied. Rather, most reported benefiting from their brief therapy. Clients described themselves as serious, in need of answers to questions, and desirous of an opportunity to express their emotions and resolve their problems. Furthermore, they tended to see the therapist as providing just what they needed. In this setting, early termination was not usually equated with failure. Dropout rate was unusually high, however, in the case of seriously disturbed patients assigned to lower status therapists (students, paraprofessionals, and mental health technicians).

The authors suggested that higher dropout rates among lower class patients may take place primarily in settings where strict psychodynamic therapy is the treatment of choice; that is, that differential dropout rate is more closely related to therapist characteristics than to client characteristics. In the nondoctrinaire setting, "quite possibly, dropping out represents a problem primarily from the (rejected) therapist's perspective. This perspective is probably a corollary of clinical lore that asserts a direct relationship between length of treatment and patient improvement" (Fiester & Rudestam, 1975, p. 534).

THE EFFECTIVENESS OF A SINGLE THERAPEUTIC SESSION

If the reader is alert for assertions as to the effectiveness of single-session therapy, they can be found, often in the form of a side comment or parenthetical phrase. Here are some examples:

There is a tendency to overlook the fact that a *single interview* can have beneficial therapeutic consequences. . . . Even when further interviews are available, they may not be needed or wanted. (Barten, 1971, p. 17)

Even patients who have only one visit are under certain circumstances considered treated. Therapeutic intent is present from the start in a conscious and
systematic way, with no formal separation of treatment and diagnosis, and
each hour is considered as if it may be the last treatment opportunity. (Jacobson *et al.*, 1965, p. 1179)

So whether the therapy will be short or long really depends in the ultimate
analysis on the ego's integrative capacity, not what kind of symptoms or syn-
dromes the patient has. I have seen ulcer patients who reacted after ten interviews. One case which I saw, in one interview reacted beautifully. (Alexander,
1965, pp. 102–103)

Human warmth and feelings, experienced by a patient in one session with an
empathetic therapist, may achieve more profound alterations than years with
a probing, detached therapist intent on wearing out resistance. (Wolberg,
1965, p. 138)

Clearly, psychiatrists who undertake consultations should not automatically
assign patients to long-term psychotherapy or even to brief psychotherapy,
but should be aware of the possibility that a single dynamic interview may be
all that is needed. (Malan, Heath, Bacal, & Balfour, 1975, p. 126)

A full 80 percent of Crisis Psychotherapy clients return for additional interviews. And even among the 20 percent who do not return, there is reason to
believe that they have already been helped by a single session of Crisis Psychotherapy. (Ewing, 1978, p. 48)

If a patient is seen, even for a single interview, it should be a therapeutic experience. Sometimes it is not enough to offer the patient a mirror in which to see
himself; often he must be encouraged to open his eyes and be shown where to
look. . . . Psychiatrists are accustomed to a passive therapy lasting many
months, perhaps several years. But "brief psychotherapy" is brief only to the
psychiatrist. Except for those sophisticated in the ways of psychoanalysis,
most people have never had even a single personal, intensive, interrelated interview with a doctor . . . the interview becomes an awakening, an intense
stimulation of mind and spirit, and hopefully a corrective emotional experience. (Lewin, 1970, pp. 49, 69)

There can be little doubt that this rather large one-interview segment of the
population of many psychiatric clinics contains a sizeable percentage of dropouts from therapy, patients who did not make contact, who felt poorly understood by their therapists, mismatched, or put another way, people who in
some sense felt that they had not gotten what they had come for. But there are
also many patients in the one-visit category who, to a varying degree, did have
a meaningful and therapeutic experience and who did not return simply because they did not feel the need for further help. (Spoerl, 1975, p. 283)

At times, however, the therapeutic impact of the evaluation or of the first interview is such that there is no need for further psychotherapy, because in reality the patient's problem is actually being solved. (Sifneos, 1979, p. 70)

Actually, an incisive intervention in a single interview can contain more psychoanalytic orientation than a protracted series of sessions that merely imitates the external trappings of psychoanalysis but contains little of its essence. (Gillman, 1965, p. 601)

Treatment begins in the first interview, and the majority of work, in fact, may often be accomplished at that time. There are occasions when the client feels better after one session, and if this happens, the therapist need not feel like a failure for not involving him in continued treatment. (Hoffman & Remmel, 1975, p. 262)

From one contact, a client may get some feeling of release from the pressure of a problem which has never been fully articulated but has been merely mulled over with frantic reiteration in his own mind. . . . There may be a sense of sharing a problem. . . . Some placement of the problem may result so that the client sees what really is the disturbing element . . . some value might also come through the idea . . . that there is actually something he can do about it, should he ever want to. (McCord, 1931, pp. 191–192)

Duration . . . is de facto not the crucial variable. This has been well documented by the contributions of the "Chicago School of Psychoanalysis" . . . where a number of patients showed noticeable and lasting "improvement" after a single or a few treatment sessions. (McGuire, 1968, p. 218)

In addition to these assertions, a small number of successful single-session therapy case histories (sometimes including verbatim transcripts of portions of the interview) have appeared in the literature. The earliest one I have found was published over 80 years ago. In chronological order, these case histories include Freud in the 1890s (Breuer & Freud, 1957, pp. 125–134), Tannenbaum (1919), Groddeck in 1927 (Groddeck, 1951, pp. 90–95), Reider (1955, pp. 116–118), Kaffman (1963, pp. 223–225), Rosenbaum (1964, p. 511), Gillman (1965, pp. 603–604), Lewin (1970, pp. 88–93), and Sifneos (1979, pp. 70–73). These case histories are invariably presented as a way of illustrating how patients occasionally make significant changes in their own lives as a consequence of a single therapeutic intervention.

Such assertions and case histories do not, of course, substitute for more objectively conducted empirical research studies. A small number of such studies have been reported, however, and they uniformly support the conclusion that a single interview can have a significant therapeutic impact.

Getz, Fujita, and Allen (1975) sought evaluations of a single interview with a paraprofessional during a period of crisis. Their sample consisted of 104 patients who had made one-time use of a night crisis intervention service connected with a community hospital emergency room. The patients were contacted 6 to 12 months after their interview at the crisis program. (Interestingly, this sample comprised only 39% of persons who were eligible to be included in the study; the remaining 61% could not be located.) The patients generally felt that the crisis intervention service had been very helpful, exceeded in helpfulness only by the support provided by significant others in their lives. Degree of helpfulness was clearly related to the presenting problem, with patients whose complaint was depression or anxiety attributing twice as much helpfulness to crisis counselors as patients whose problems involved drug abuse or psychosis. The authors concluded that "timely intervention in crisis situations may have long-lasting effects on particular kinds of problems" (p. 143).

Malan *et al.* (1975) conducted two- through eight-year follow-up studies of 45 adult neurotic patients, who were seen for a one-interview consultation but, according to the authors, had never had psychotherapy. Prior to the follow-up interviews, no patients in this sample had been interviewed by a psychiatrist more than twice in their entire lives. These authors found that one-quarter of the patients had improved symptomatically, and another quarter had also improved dynamically, a type of improvement the authors call "genuine." On the basis of their careful clinical assessments, the authors concluded that "these single diagnostic interviews had some powerful therapeutic effects" (p. 122). Three of these patients had, in fact, written to their interviewing psychiatrist, saying that they felt better as a consequence of the acquisition of insight into their difficulties. These findings forced the authors to the realization that they "had not been studying spontaneous remission at all, but one-session psychotherapy" (p. 122).

Edwards, Orford, Egert, Guthrie, Hawker, Hensman, Mitcheson, Oppenheimer, and Taylor (1977) randomly assigned 100 male, married alcoholics to two treatment groups in London following an initial, three-hour physical, psychological, psychiatric, and social work assessment of the couple. Males were between 25 and 60 years of age and free of severe physical disease, psychosis, or gross brain damage. In the treatment group, both husband and wife were offered an initial counseling session followed by medical, psychiatric, and social work services; in addition, the husband was introduced to Alcoholics Anonymous, and inpatient services were made available as needed. The treatment period lasted one year. In the advice group, by way of contrast, couples were seen in one counseling session.

Assessments of progress were made at monthly intervals throughout the one-year period by means of brief interviews which social workers conducted with the wives. All the patients were seen by a psychiatrist at the one-year anniversary of the intake assessment.

As might be expected, there were dramatic differences in the amount of help obtained from all sources, both within and outside the project. Edwards et al. (1977) wrote that "although some advice-group patients sought help from other sources, and some treatment-group patients engaged in only a rather minimal degree of contact with the Clinic, the over-all between-group differences remained at a level which can leave no doubt that two very different types of therapeutic engagements are being compared" (p. 1012).

The findings can be briefly summarized. The authors could find no substantial differences between the two groups at the time of the one-year follow-up in terms of amount of alcohol intake, subjective ratings of the drinking problem, social adjustment, or other difficulties. Significant improvement was shown by 39% of the advice group as against 26% of the treatment group.

Perhaps most interesting were the patients' views on what was most helpful to them during the preceding year. In both groups, the three factors most commonly judged responsible for their improvement were unrelated to the treatment program: first, changes in external reality (e.g., work conditions, work settings, or housing); second, the single-session intake interview; and third, changes in self-appraisal or mood. With regard to the latter intrapsychic changes, the authors indicated there was no persuasive evidence that they were related to the therapeutic program.

Perhaps the most provocative findings reported in the literature are those linking a single therapeutic interview with dramatic subsequent reductions in the use of medical care. There is already a substantial body of literature showing that brief psychotherapy can have this effect (e.g., Goldberg, Krantz, & Locke, 1970; Jameson, Shuman, & Young, 1978; Rosen & Wiens, 1979) but to demonstrate it following a single interview is startling indeed.

Cummings and Follette (Cummings, 1977a, 1977b; Cummings & Follette, 1968, 1976; Follette & Cummings, 1967) undertook a series of studies in order to investigate the role of psychotherapy in reducing medical care utilization in a prepaid health plan setting. In such settings, they found that patients could easily somatize emotional problems and thus overutilize medical facilities. They estimated that "60% or more of the physician visits are made by patients who demonstrate an emotional, rather than an organic, etiology for their physical symptoms" (Cummings, 1977a, p. 711).

Among the groups they studied was a sample of 80 emotionally distressed patients, who were assigned to receive a single psychotherapeutic interview. They found, totally unexpectedly, that one therapeutic interview, with no repeat psychological visits, reduced medical utilization by 60% over the following five years, and that that reduction was the consequence of resolving the emotional distress that was being reflected in physical symptoms.

The results of two other studies provide additional, equally startling findings. Goldberg *et al.* (1970) studied the effect of short-term outpatient therapy on utilization of medical services. Their sample consisted of 256 people who were enrolled in the Group Health Association prepaid medical program in Washington, D. C., and who had been referred for and found eligible and in need of outpatient psychiatric care. In the year following referral for psychiatric care, this group showed an average reduction of 31% in physician visits and 30% in laboratory and X-ray visits compared to the previous year. But this reduction was independent of whether those referred for care actually received it. In fact, while the reduction in physician visits was 23% among those who had had ten or more sessions of psychotherapy, and 30% among those who had had between one and nine sessions, it was 39% among those who had had no psychotherapy at all.

In another study, Rosen and Wiens (1979) examined the same issue at the University of Oregon Health Sciences Center. Comparisons were made between four groups of patients: (1) those who received medical services but were not referred for psychological services, (2) those who were referred for services in the Medical Psychology Outpatient Clinic but never kept their scheduled appointments, (3) those who were referred for psychological services but received only an evaluation, and (4) those who were referred and who received both an evaluation and subsequent brief psychotherapy. Groups 1 and 2 (that is, those who were either not referred or who were referred but did not keep their appointments) showed no subsequent reduction in the utilization of medical care, including number of outpatient visits, emergency room visits, days of hospitalization, diagnostic procedures, and pharmaceutical prescriptions. Groups 3 and 4, those receiving only an evaluation or an evaluation and brief psychotherapy (averaging seven interviews), showed significant subsequent reduction in the utilization of medical care, but the group receiving only the evaluation demonstrated the most consistent reduction in, among other things, medical outpatient visits, pharmaceutical prescriptions, emergency room visits, and diagnostic services.

The one fact that links the findings of all these studies is that a single contact, virtually regardless of the nature of that contact, appears to have salutary consequences. That is, it appears to make no demonstrable difference whether the contact is designed to serve a primarily evaluative function, or whether its purpose is primarily therapeutic in intent. Under these circumstances, it would be very helpful to know exactly what went on during these contacts. In the case of the Rosen and Wiens (1979) study, that evaluation was quite extensive. The clients "experienced a comprehensive social, personality, and intellectual evaluation that ordinarily takes 3–5 hours" (p. 427). Furthermore, the evaluation often involved family members and other individuals associated with the client and often included detailed feedback to the client. In the case of the British study of alcoholics conducted by Edwards and his colleagues (1977), the counseling session included considerable advice and admonition: "the advice-group couples were told that responsibility for attainment of the stated goals lay in their own hands rather than it being anything which could be taken over by others, and this message was given in sympathetic and constructive terms" (p. 1006). In the case of the Goldberg, Krantz, and Locke (1970) study, no information was provided regarding the psychiatric screening procedure that resulted in the referral being made for outpatient psychiatric therapy. Notes prepared by the screening psychiatrists were not part of the client's medical record and were not made available to the authors. Similarly, little information has been provided in the other studies as to the nature of the consultation, crisis intervention, or single-session psychotherapy.

An alternative explanation of these findings is that they are flawed, either in terms of experimental design or in the failure to examine alternative explanations. It should not be surprising that startling results, such as these, would receive the most careful scrutiny. Olbrisch (1977) examined the critiques that have been advanced regarding these types of studies and indicated that one rival hypothesis, that of statistical regression, has yet to be ruled out. With particular reference to the Cummings and Follette studies, Olbrisch noted that "only a small percentage of high utilizers of medical care remain high utilizers over an extended period of time . . . and the group of high utilizers comes from the average utilization population and returns to it after about 5 years" (p. 767). That is, it is quite likely that these high utilizers would have become average utilizers of medical services as a function of the normal reduction in utilization of medical care that takes place without any special intervention, simply as a function of time. In spite of this hypothesis, however, Olbrisch concluded that "research with inappropriately high utilizers of medical services is quite promising, and further evidence, perhaps even generated on the basis of true experiments, will be helpful in making the case for its effectiveness" (p. 774).

In summary, single-session encounters between mental health professionals and their clients are remarkably common. Not only is their frequency underestimated, but more importantly, their therapeutic impact appears to be underestimated as well. Such encounters appear to have positive consequences, whether their primary objective is therapy or evaluation, and as Rubin and Mitchell (1976) recently reported, interviews whose primary purpose is research may have profound clinical impact on subjects as well. To the extent that the deliberate use of single therapeutic interviews can be appropriately implemented, we may be able to increase our abilities to be of assistance to an entire community of clients without requiring a parallel increase in personnel or funds.

FOCUSED SINGLE-SESSION THERAPY:
A PRELIMINARY REPORT

Most of my limited experience in focused single-session therapy has taken place in our local community mental health center where, for a couple of months at a time, I spend one-half day per week seeing clients who are referred to me. There have been two series of such clients: the first consisted of 13 cases seen about three years ago, the second of 10 cases seen during the fall and winter of 1979. The most important difference between the two series was the length of the appointments. In the first series, the appointments were one hour long; in the second series, they were two hours long. This change was inaugurated because I was often unable to limit the intervention to one session in the first series. In fact, on the average, I saw each client in the first series for two separate interviews. In the second series, all cases were satisfactorily concluded in a single, two-hour interview.

After introducing myself, getting the client's permission to tape-record the interview, and explaining my volunteer status at the mental health center, the contractual agreement I made with each client was that I was assuming that a single appointment will be sufficient. If, at the conclusion of the interview, we both felt that another appointment was necessary, we would schedule it for the following week. If not, I would give the client my card and invite him or her to call me if there was a need to get in touch with me for any reason—with a problem or a progress report, for example. Finally, I said that if the client did not contact me in a couple of months, I would call to see how he or she was getting along. I have called every one of the clients I saw, in this very primitive type of evaluation, and have heard the following report: nearly all are doing well; nearly all found the intervention helpful; and with one exception, they have not sought additional help.

I want to assure you that I do not believe I have any remarkable therapeutic skills other than those that may be associated with age and experience. I believe any reasonably skilled therapist would get the same results. I also believe, however, that we all sell or give our time, our most precious resource, far too easily, and that we can all accomplish far more in brief therapy than we realize, if we are deliberate and plan well.

I asked the staff in the adult outpatient unit of the mental health center to send me the widest possible variety of clients. What has happened, in fact, is that the clients I do see vary in the intensity and severity of their problems as a function of how busy the professional staff are. If the staff have some vacant hours, I get the least disturbed cases or none at all; if they are swamped, I get more difficult cases. Most of the time, with the exception of the obligatory paperwork that the clients complete with the assistance of the clerical staff immediately prior to their appointments with me, I am the only person they see at the mental health center. Appointments are made by the appointment secretary over the phone, usually at the time the client first calls the center, and all clients are told that it is a single appointment: "Dr. Bloom will have a couple of hours to spend with you next Friday morning at 8:15." I complete a short note and the necessary forms on each client before leaving the center and arrive back in my university office ready to listen to the tapes and to try to figure out what went well, what went badly, and what I have learned.

Now, let me outline a dozen different technical principles of focused single-session therapy that seem valid to me as of today. All of them are presented very tentatively. Most apply to long-term therapy as well as to single-session therapy. They are all subject to revision, and I am sure that many will be extensively modified as I gain additional experience. I hope, of course, that others might undertake to treat a series of clients in this way, because I am sure that our collective experiences will function synergistically.

IDENTIFY A FOCAL PROBLEM

It is my hope in every focused single-session therapy to listen hard enough and explore skillfully enough to be able to identify a piece of psychological reality that is pertinent to the client's presenting problem, below the client's initial level of usable awareness, and yet acceptable to the client in the form of an interpretation or observation. In doing so, I am careful not to focus too early or foreclose too quickly. The success of the session seems to depend, in part, on my ability to identify and focus on one salient and relevant issue. I find myself feeling good about interviews when they are over if I can summarize that issue to myself in a very few words, for example, "I think you are going to have to forgive your father"; "you won't be able to decide what to do about your marriage until you figure out why you think you are such a terrible person"; "you are going to have to learn to communicate with your wife with words instead of with actions"; "you seem to be willing to let fate determine what happens to you in life."

Identifying a salient issue is facilitated when the therapist has a workable theory of personality and psychopathology that can serve as a template for the interview. The concept of a salient issue is similar to French's notion of a focal conflict (see Balint, Ornstein, & Balint, 1973, pp. 10–11). French distinguished between what he termed a "nuclear" conflict, that is, a dormant and repressed conflict originating during crucial developmental periods in early life, and a "focal" conflict, by which he meant a preconscious derivative of these deeper and earlier nuclear conflicts, which is able to explain much of the clinical material in a therapeutic interview.

DO NOT UNDERESTIMATE CLIENTS' STRENGTHS

I think of the therapy session as having the potential for breaking through an impasse in the client's psychological life, so that the client can resume the normal process of growth and development. I count on clients' abilities to work on an identified issue on their own, particularly if I can be helpful in identifying what that issue might be. I count on clients' ego strengths and their abilities to mobilize their strengths. Trying to identify *the* impasse in a client's life or, more realistically, *an* impasse in the client's life is an intellectually and technically challenging task and is what makes focused single-session therapy so exciting for me. It is as if I am trying to answer the question, "What have these clients failed to understand about their lives that could make a difference in how they are conducting themselves now and how they might manage their lives in the future?"

Without adequate ego strengths on the part of the client, focused single-session therapy will have only limited effectiveness. Thus, severely depressed clients or clients whose thought processes are significantly disordered will probably gain little from this therapy. But I should add two comments. First, these are the very same clients who present serious problems for the long-term therapist; that is, these limitations are not unique to focused single-session therapy. Second, to say that our therapy will have limited effectiveness with severely disturbed clients is not to say that it will have no effectiveness. The clinical literature is replete with examples of remarkably effective short-term therapy with psychotic or near-psychotic clients. I do not believe we have begun to tap the ways in which psychotherapy can be of significant help to such clients, but I do know that a great deal of short-term therapy is provided to very disturbed clients, often in the public sector, and often with excellent results. I suspect we can underestimate the abilities of our clients to change, just as much as we can underestimate the power of psychotherapy to effect such changes and to effect them promptly.

BE PRUDENTLY ACTIVE

I have found it useful to be more active than I have been accustomed, but active in specific ways. I ask questions rather than make statements. I try not to make speeches or lecture. I do virtually no self-disclosure. I avoid asking questions that have yes-or-no answers. When necessary, I give information, but in the context of the client's presenting problem, and I keep it simple. I use the client's language, but making sure first that I understand what is meant by the key words and phrases he or she uses.

Most people who write about planned short-term therapy seem to agree that it requires a higher level of activity on the part of the therapist than is typically reported in long-term therapy. I have listened to some early single-session therapy tapes of mine, however, in which I was entirely too active, particularly by sharing my own experiences and opinions.

While these interviews were reasonably helpful, in some of them the client learned as much about me as I learned about the client. I know that self-disclosure is one of the principal ways in which day-to-day encounters between good friends turn out to be therapeutic, and that self-disclosure should not be dismissed out of hand as not being a legitimate and important short-term strategy. But I find myself reacting negatively to my own interviews in which I talk a great deal in the process of giving advice, support, information, and ideas or engage in excessive self-disclosure at the apparent cost of reducing the opportunities clients might have to learn more about themselves.

Helping clients understand themselves requires that we learn about them and, in particular, that we learn their language, that is, how they use words. Michael Balint (Balint *et al.,* 1973) once described being supervised by Max Eitington and remembered Eitington saying to him, "Every new patient must be treated as if he had come directly from Mars; and as no one has met a Martian, everything about each patient must be considered as utterly unknown" (p. 126).

Thus, while I am somewhat more active in single-session therapy than I would be in long-term therapy, I now tend to be quite parsimonious and disciplined. My interactions are, more often than not, designed to help me learn about clients and to help clients learn something about themselves, rather than to simply be supportive; furthermore, I want clients to learn more about their own personal psychodynamic predicaments rather than about the general human existential predicament.

EXPLORE, THEN PRESENT INTERPRETATIONS TENTATIVELY

In my interpretations, I try to do all the necessary exploration first and then tentatively present an idea in such a way that it is persuasive yet may be disagreed with without jeopardizing my potential effectiveness: "Do you think it is possible that . . ."; "I wonder if . . ."; "I'm beginning to think that . . ."; "Have you ever wondered why . . ."; and so on. While it is possible to provide a genuinely therapeutic experience in a single interview, I would urge that the therapist not move too quickly. It is, in fact, because having seen how easy it is to work too fast, I now schedule two-hour rather than one-hour appointments. I have become very conscious of the steps I must take to get from an idea in my head, however valid, to that same idea, in useful form, in the client's head. Like a good computer programer, I now automatically subdivide those ideas into their elemental component points and then very deliberately try to gain credibility for those components, one at a time and in proper sequence, in order to build toward the acceptance of the more complex concept.

Thus, for example, before dealing with *why* an obviously depressed client may be depressed, it is necessary to establish that the client is aware of *being* depressed. In turn, that may mean helping the client discover that he or she is sad, blue, down in the dumps, or whatever label the person is willing to tolerate—all of which add up to the somewhat more complex concept of "depressed." And sometimes, before clients can consider the possibility that they feel sad, they have to come to accept the more elementary possibility that they have feelings of any kind.

Knowing when and how to label or confront or interpret is, in part, a matter of experience and, in part, a matter of style. Reading the literature on planned short-term therapy provides a startling range of therapeutic styles, and there are enough good verbatim or near-verbatim illustrations in that literature to provide sound examples of a number of very different strategies. Therapists vary in their willingness to take risks, in the rapidity of their pace, and in their incisiveness, as examining that literature will dramatically attest.

ENCOURAGE THE EXPRESSION OF AFFECT

I encourage and explicitly recognize the expression of affect and use its expression as a way of pointing to important life events or figures. "It's okay to cry." "That really upsets you, doesn't it?" Similarly when it seems timely, I point out incongruities in affect: "You're laughing, but there doesn't seem to be anything to laugh about." In my limited experience with focused single-session therapy, I have not found any more effective technique than the explicit and accurate recognition of the feelings that the client is carrying around. Those feeling states, whether of sadness or anger or frustration or disappointment or loneliness or desperation, are usually easy to recognize and label, and in my experience, identifying them often has very salutary consequences. In these instances, the ability to be empathic has an enormous payoff. One of the things I have learned by listening to the tapes of my own interviews and those of colleagues and students I supervise is to expect the appearance of new and important material immediately after an accurate, sincere, and timely empathic statement on the part of the therapist.

These three characterizations of empathic remarks—accuracy, sincerity, and timeliness—are not to be taken lightly, however. A client may laugh but laugh bitterly. It is the bitterness rather than the amusement that must be labeled. Many of you have heard the therapist with the reflexive, nonspecific, generic empathic grunt or short phrase. It does not take clients very long to sense that that therapist does not really understand them and, in fact, may not even be listening to them. Sometimes, clients will react to that lack of sincerity without being able to point to what exactly they are reacting to. Such clients are often vaguely dissatisfied with their experiences in therapy without knowing why. Proper timing is the final characteristic of an effective empathic remark, given that it is accurate and sincerely felt. While it is not a fatal error to return to a client's earlier display of affect, to recognize it when it happens seems far more effective.

USE THE INTERVIEW TO START A PROBLEM-SOLVING PROCESS

I try to identify important life figures in relation to unresolved issues and start or encourage a process of getting some of that unfinished business taken care of. "Have you ever told your mother that when you were a little girl you used to be so frightened of her?" "Have you ever talked with your sister about that?" "Do you think your father could shed some light on why you used to do that?" "Does your mother know how upset you are about her divorce?" In a way, this effort gives the single session some increased longevity by attempting to internalize a process that can continue for a period of time.

It is important to identify the types of unfinished business that can be finished. Two judgments have to be made: first, what myths or false beliefs do clients carry around regarding themselves and important figures in their lives, and second, can additional experiences with these important figures convert those myths or beliefs into a less distorted appreciation of reality? In a way, this strategy is a kind of behavior modification. The repertoire—talking, sharing, questioning—exists; it need only be employed with appropriate targets.

The development of a plan for problem solving in this manner ties in with the follow-up procedure I have developed. If the client does not call me following the single-session therapy interview, I call the client. The plans we made or talked about for dealing with unfinished business can then be one of the matters discussed in the brief follow-up conversation. The conversation is not a request for a recital of accomplishments, nor does it attempt to instill a sense of obligation in undertaking a process that the client may not be ready for. But it can be couched in terms of, "Did it make sense to you to try to do what we talked about?" If the client indicates that it did, we can talk about how it went and what the client learned. If not, the client can be reminded that finishing that unfinished business can be something the client can keep in mind for the future, whenever the time seems right.

KEEP TRACK OF TIME

I keep track of time. There is a tempo, a pacing, to a two-hour interview. It is enough time so I do not feel rushed, yet I have to keep aware of the passing time and keep planning how to use it. Sometimes I make a few notes to myself, jotting down topics I want to make sure to talk about. More often, I do not need to keep notes, but either way, it is important to estimate how much time will be needed to discuss a particular topic and to make sure that there is a reasonably good match between the needed and the available time.

In addition to the question of making sure of the availability of time, there is also the issue of the phases through which the interview passes. I have begun to think about the introductory material, the middle identification and development of important themes, the planning period (if that is appropriate), and the gradual closing of the interview. It is something of an exaggeration, to be sure, but in a way, I think of minutes the way I used to think about hours.

Similarly, I tend to judge how heavy or light the interview is, and how much or little anxiety clients brought with them to the interview versus how much seems to be generated by the interview. I act accordingly, now exploring in a way I know will raise anxiety, now modulating the anxiety, now introducing humor, now being very serious—all this in an effort to keep the interaction at its optimal level—enough anxiety to assure progress but not so much as to be disabling.

DO NOT BE OVERAMBITIOUS

I try not to do too much. If I can find just one issue, just one idea, just a teaspoonful, that is useful to the client, the intervention can be a successful one. My experience, from listening to both my own interviews and those of others, is that it is very hard for clients to make real use of more than two or three ideas in a single interview. As a consequence, the choice of which ideas to elaborate on when exploring an issue is very important. But in addition, it is important to keep the ideas simple. My personal rule of thumb is that if I cannot express a fundamental issue of concern to the client in ten words—ten *short* words—or less, I do not understand the issue.

I find it very easy to demonstrate to students whose therapy I supervise (nearly always be listening to tape recordings or watching video recordings) that the effectiveness of an interview is negatively correlated with the number of different issues raised during the interview; that is, more issues make for less effectiveness.

What seems absolutely counterproductive in focused single-session therapy is to leave the client reeling from fifteen different interpretations, however accurate the interpretations might be. On the other hand, to leave the client stunned with the power and salience of a single observation is quite a different matter. A client can chew on that observation for weeks and continue to make use of it long after the interview is over. But the more interpretations one offers, the more the likelihood that the client will have no alternative other than to dismiss the entire interview as useless, even though the client may have a nagging feeling that there might have been something to those interpretations, if he or she only remembered and understood them.

KEEP FACTUAL QUESTIONS TO A MINIMUM

I avoid collecting demographic information or doing a traditional mental status examination. It is my experience that the answers will nearly always be forthcoming without my having to ask. I rarely ask age or number of siblings or information about parents or children. Asking such questions can be intrusive, and the most important information will emerge in the normal course of the interview. In arriving at this simple principle, I have had to overcome a very powerful need for orientation. Part of that came from my training; part is characterological. But I am getting better at waiting for demographic information to appear on its own. On the other hand, it is folly to be unaware of what you do not know, and absent or delayed information can help identify salient issues.

Sometimes it is useful to ask for identifying information as a way of reducing a momentarily excessive level of anxiety, but except for this occasion, the quest for demographic information about the client and significant people in the client's life seems a poor use of time. I am virtually always sorry when I go on a quest for such information, since it seems to produce so little therapeutically useful data.

DO NOT BE OVERLY CONCERNED ABOUT THE PRECIPITATING EVENT

Focused single-session therapy is not crisis intervention, so I feel no necessity to identify a crisis or event that precipitated a client's coming to the mental health center. In many cases, clients seem not to know exactly why they came in. So I simply begin an interview by asking, "What can I do to be helpful?" There was a time when I felt that asking clients about precipitating events would provide very important information, particularly for those people interested in the development of preventive intervention programs. I am still curious about those precipitating events, and sometimes it is clear what those events are. But more often, clients have only the vaguest idea about why they came looking for help now rather than a month earlier or a month later.

In undertaking focused single-session therapy, one can never overestimate the therapeutic leverage in the setting. The question, "What can I do to be helpful?" says it all. The client has come in because something is wrong for which help is needed, not because he or she has a regular appointment at that time every week. Since the client has inaugurated the therapeutic encounter, the therapist has every right to expect the client to get to work, to describe the problem, and to begin moving toward its solution. No interview has more leverage in this regard than the first interview, and that leverage is further enhanced by the fact that both client and therapist know that it is likely to be the only interview.

AVOID DETOURS

I have had to learn to avoid attractive detours and to remain single-minded about what I am trying to accomplish. There are numerous occasions in every intervention when I find myself wishing I could explore some little phrase for just a few minutes, but such diversions have nearly always turned out to be technical errors. Initially, of course, I have no idea where I am heading, so I keep all my options open. I try to narrow the domain of inquiry in proportion to what I am learning about the client, and I do not single out a particular issue or conflict to concentrate on until I have every reason to believe that it is an appropriate target for investigation and clarification. All this means that not only is there no time to explore side issues, but that such exploration detracts from the potential effectiveness of the therapy.

DO NOT OVERESTIMATE A CLIENT'S SELF-AWARENESS

Finally, I am continuing to learn not to overestimate how much clients know about themselves. Clients may be totally oblivious of something about themselves that seems perfectly obvious to me and would, I believe, be perfectly obvious to everyone who knows them. I have had clients scream at me that they are not angry and tearfully tell me they are not sad. I have had to learn that a PhD in chemistry does not guarantee any wisdom in psychology, and, in fact, that a person with a PhD in psychology can be very unaware of his or her own psychology. Thus, very often, when I find myself saying, for example, "This client *must* know that his actions are driving his wife and children away from him," I am wrong. While it is obvious to me and undoubtedly to the client's wife and children, the client, whatever his IQ, has to discover it. In fact, I have found, more often than not, that in Boulder's heady environment, a graduate education can be a hazard to psychotherapy. All too often, such clients use their well-developed vocabularies defensively and offensively.

While clients, in one sense, are expert on what is going on inside them, they are very often unable to label, acknowledge, or use that knowledge effectively. Increasing a client's useful self-awareness, even in only one critical area, can have an important impact on the adequacy of his or her functioning. In working toward that objective, an accurate appraisal of what clients do or do not know about themselves is critically important.

FOCUSED SINGLE-SESSION THERAPY: A CASE EXAMPLE

The best way of illustrating these tentative principles is to see them in the context of a focused single-session therapy interview. What follows is a verbatim transcript of one such interview, along with some comments that try to capture what was going on in my thinking as the interview took place. This interview lasted just under one hour (the client came in during her lunch hour), and the transcript begins from the time the tape recorder was activated. Before that time, I explained to the client my interest in trying to be helpful in a single session, and I obtained her permission to make a tape recording of the interview.

I think this interview had the potential for being a useful one. But there was a lot of material to keep track of, and I made a number of errors, particularly in the last few minutes of the interview, as I was trying to finish on time. If we had had two hours available, we could have gone into one or two areas that we were unable to in the one hour, and I could have concluded the interview in a more unhurried fashion.

THERAPIST (*activating the telephone-answering machine*): Okay, we shouldn't be disturbed by the telephone with that machine turned on. Tell me what I can do to be helpful.

CLIENT: Well, initially I called you because a friend of mine had come to see you, I guess when the Separation and Divorce program was still . . . you were still interviewing people or something. And, she wasn't married but she said she had come to talk with you and that she had found it helpful. So, I was recently discussing with her the situation that I was in, and I had been to see a lawyer to get a divorce and the lawyer found that I was kind of like hemming and hawing whether I wanted really wanted to do it or not and thought it would be better if I saw a psychiatrist or someone before I spent a lot of time and money on him, and then not going through with it, or something like that. So he recommended a couple of psychiatrists in town and then I found out they cost $75 an hour and . . . the thing I found out then was that insurance pays for it, but I'm losing my job and I didn't want to depend on my husband's insurance to pay for something that I needed for myself since I wanted to divorce myself from him, you know. So, I thought there's gotta be something else I can do, that I don't have to be dependent on him for that. She had suggested I call you, that's why I came. I found myself in a situation recently that . . . it shouldn't have surprised me, actually, but I just allowed myself to realize that my husband was an alcoholic. And, I've only been married four months, and I just, I started going to this Al-Anon group and my husband has joined AA since we started having a whole lot of problems. But . . . it didn't . . . we separated before we came to this conclusion that we ought to be doing something more positive, you know, than separating. But we were apart for about a week, and then it was a big crisis and I started going to Al-Anon and he started going to AA and we talked about it and decided we'd come back together and everything and we came back together, and then, I was trying to learn about what he was gonna be going through and problems because he did quit drinking and then we started having severe problems again, and we split up again (*Laughs nervously.*), and he was gone for a week, and it was just pretty much of a disaster and he was telling me, ya know, I'm not gonna go to a lawyer, if you wanna go to a lawyer you go, and then I finally decided to go to a lawyer and get some information, and when I was there I found out that my husband had a lawyer. *(Laughs.)* And I just went through, I don't know, just a big emotional crisis in the past month about this, and then . . . my husband and I've talked a lot since and he has decided that he figured once he gave up drinking that all his problems would go away and that's why he wasn't able to deal with anything because he didn't even know why they were still there. So, you know, we seem to be able to communicate better now, but I've just, I have . . . I just, I have a lot of fears in the relationship wondering whether I'm doing the right thing, you know, all the time whether. . . . Well, Al-Anon tells you not to feel that you're going to cause him drinking because he doesn't, you're not the cause, but you know, I'm so used to living with him and feeling . . . we were living together before we got married . . . living together and feeling that if I say the wrong thing it's gonna bring on a drunk, because I've been in that mold, thinking that for some time. If I, now knowing that he doesn't drink, I still feel I'm gonna bring on this violent anger that it kept coming on before and I don't know how to relax myself and feel that I can be comfortable in a relationship because I do want it, you know, not . . . not want it just to have a relationship but I do feel that we can communicate, that we can find new ways but I don't, I don't know, I don't even know where that feeling comes from. *(Laughs.)* You know, I don't know why I can feel positive about it if it hasn't been positive. We don't have anything real positive in the recent months to base being able to be positive now. Maybe in our early months of our relationship we can think back on that and hope we can get back there or something or not get back there but have something better again. I don't know. But being part of this group, this Al-Anon group and everything, helps to talk, helps to go, because everyone else talks about the resentments they have, and the anger they feel, and the difficulties they have. But I don't find that I am adjusting very well to the group, being in there, and I thought that the lawyer's suggestion that I seek someone out to talk to on an individual basis would probably be most helpful to me, since I have been involved in that group for a couple of months and I don't feel that I am facing the things that I am supposed to be or something.

THERAPIST: I am not sure what you are trying to decide.

[This seems like the best thing to say in response to the client's long speech that lasted more than six minutes. I have no way of knowing with suffi-

cient certainty what I should pick up on in the client's soliloquy, and at the same time I want the client to know that her speech is unclear enough to leave me unsure how to proceed. There are a number of comments I could have picked up on—her reluctance to pay for the time of a mental health professional (with the implication of an initial negative transference toward the helping process—I came recommended to her, but I don't charge a fee. How good can I or a single interview be?); her dependency—independency conflict with her husband; her marriage to a person she failed to recognize as an alcoholic; the basis for her thinking that she had a role in her husband's drinking; her obvious anxiety; or why she did not make full use of the Al-Anon group. Each of these topical candidates has something to recommend it, but in the end, it seems better to file them away for later use and, at this beginning stage in the interview, avoid premature closure on a topic.]

CLIENT: Well, a month ago I was trying to decide whether I could make it on my own or not, because we were definitely hitting rock bottom in our relationship, and *(Laughs.)* when I talked to my lawyer, he told me that I was having a hard time deciding between whether I wanted to separate myself from him totally or whether I really wanted the relationship. *[A very perceptive lawyer.]* And whenever he does something that, you know, leave the house and not come back for a week or talk to me like I am dirt, I feel like I definitely don't want the relationship, or whenever he is kind and loving and giving I definitely want it, so I am still, I am wondering how to deal with the situations that he is going through that makes him put these things on me, that make me feel like I am not a good person, without feeling that I don't want the relationship because those things happened. *[Her husband calls her dirt, and at some level she thinks he is right. But why?]* That's what I am feeling that I need to do, because I . . . in this group that I am in they tell me now that I am supposed to just take it easy and not get myself all concerned with the fact that he is having these bad times and that he wants to put the blame on me for what he is going through, and he wants to take out his violence on me and he wants to do all these things. I shouldn't take this personally, you know, but I do. I don't know how to sit there and go, "Okay, fine, yeah, okay, fine."

THERAPIST: So what he thinks about you is really . . . really very important?

CLIENT: Yeah, it is. *(Sighs.)* It is but I don't know if that is a bad thing or not. I don't know if I am supposed to feel like it doesn't matter what he thinks. That doesn't make sense to me. It makes sense that I am supposed to think well enough of myself to be able to, you know, stick this relationship out if I really want it, or walk out of it if I really don't want it. But, I don't think I know. I don't think that I think that well of myself to be able to sit there and take it and stay there even though that's what I want. And maybe I don't think well enough of myself to be able to walk out if that's what I want. I just don't know.

[Nearly nine minutes have elapsed since the interview began. It already seems clear that this client thinks badly of herself and that her dependence on her husband and her inability to decide whether to leave him or not is, in part, a consequence of her low self-esteem. It will be useful to learn more about that low self-esteem and to try to discover how much of it relates to her current situation and how much is associated with earlier times in her life. At the same time, it will be important to find out more about the nature of her dependency on her husband. Yet, it is early in the interview, and some of these ideas may need to be discarded as new material emerges. But, for the moment, I will concentrate on the two interrelated issues of low self-esteem and dependency.]

THERAPIST: For how long have you not thought very well of yourself?

CLIENT: Oh, probably 27 years; that's how old I am. *(Laughs.) [The client tells me how old she is without my having to ask.]* I don't know. I just . . . I can't exactly say how long I have not . . . I go through phases of thinking, "I'm okay, I'm fine, I'm just as good as anybody else. I can do, I am strong, I can do everything that I am supposed to do to make my life the way it is supposed to be." And then I go through phases of having to lean on somebody really bad. I don't know when I turn it on and when I turn it off. I don't know.

THERAPIST: What's that mean, to lean on somebody?

CLIENT: I think I find myself getting really afraid of making decisions about certain things and then when I find myself in that situation, I find somebody who will make it so I don't have to. Leaning on somebody like that.

THERAPIST: You mean to be dependent on them?

CLIENT: Yeah.

THERAPIST: So you're really dependent on your husband?

CLIENT: At times.

THERAPIST: In ways you're not sure are wise?

[This comment represents a calculated risk, in the sense that I may be mov-

ing too quickly. It is one thing for the client to acknowledge her dependency on her husband and another to admit that she is too dependent on him. So I try to make the comment tentatively.]

CLIENT: Right . . . I mean, that is what confuses me. I don't think that it is a bad thing to be dependent on him but I think that it is a fault in my character in the ways sometimes that I am dependent on him. I think that all ties in together in why I don't know whether I am supposed to be walking out at certain times or not, or whether I am supposed to be just standing there and taking it.

THERAPIST: And that is connected up with feeling so badly about yourself as a person that you half-jokingly say has been true of you all your life. *[I want the client to know that I take seriously the long-standing nature of her problem.]*

CLIENT: One time I can remember my husband was putting me down, saying . . . when he was drinking he did it a lot. I don't know if he knew, he knows that much about me that he knew that would get me, you know, if that was why he doing it, not that he would do it intently to hurt me. But when people are drinking they do things that they don't intend to do. But, you know, he would call me dirt *[There is that word* dirt *again. My earlier speculation that she agrees with her husband's accusation must be correct.]* and he would tell me that he hated me, that I was no good anyway or something like that. And instead of standing there going, "He's wrong," I would stand there and go, "I know *(Laughs.),* I know I am no good." But then I would feel so much more like I had to live up to so much more because he would tell me that I was no good.

THERAPIST: Are you thinking about a particular time, when you are describing this conversation with your husband? *[The client is being very general about her problems. This question encourages her to be more specific.]*

CLIENT: Yeah, different evenings that he was on a drunk.

THERAPIST: So this is not a conversation you have had only once? You have had this a number of times?

CLIENT: Oh yeah. One that I can remember talking about.

THERAPIST: Tell me about it.

CLIENT: I was telling him that when he says certain things it makes me feel certain things. I wish that I didn't feel those things because I don't know how to deal with those things that I feel. I was just going through this big thing with him and he ends up getting really upset and I remember telling him about times when I was a kid that my parents would come down on me for doing certain things and how I ended up making lists of ways in which I was no good, that I had to correct all these faults in my life. I don't know at what point I gave it up, trying to correct all these things that they said were no good about me. I feel like I still live with them even though if I don't know what they are. *(Starts crying softly.)*

[The client now begins to describe the childhood origins of her low self-esteem, and as she does, the first overt signs of emotionality are seen. I want to make sure that the client knows that I am aware of her crying and that it is appropriate for her to do so. It looks like the message to get across to her is that the reason she cannot decide whether to stay with her husband or not is because that decision is entangled with feelings of low self-esteem that long predate her marriage.]

THERAPIST: It sounds like you haven't ever given them up.

CLIENT: It doesn't make sense though that I feel strong enough to walk out and do whatever I want sometimes and then other times I can't do anything.

THERAPIST: Do you think you are dirt? *(Long pause—client's crying increases.)* It's okay to cry.

CLIENT: It's not okay to cry. I can't talk when I am crying. *(Pause.)* I don't see any reason that I should be, but I don't just always find the confidence to convince myself that I shouldn't take the things that I take sometimes so personally and that I just don't find that I am not. . . . *(Pause.)* When this started happening, it was like I got really frightened because I understand that some of the hardest things that people deal with in life is changing jobs, changing relationships, changing location, and that kind of stuff, but when this started happening I thought, "I am getting laid off from my job at the end of this month—well fine—and I don't know where I am going to have money coming in"—so that frightened me. The prospect of looking for a job frightened me because I didn't think that with the self-image that I had built up with this relationship that I could take someone telling me, "No, you can't have a job here," so I thought how am I ever going to look for a job now. So it started to really frighten me. And then I thought, "I can't even handle my relationship. I am going to lose my husband because we can't communicate. I am going to lose my job and have to find a new one, and I don't know how I am going to do that. I am going to lose my house because I can't afford it. I'm so scared." All these things came down on me and I thought, "Okay, fine, I have to be able to find a job.'' And that's when it hit me—that staying in my relationship the way it was, and accepting the put-downs that I was accepting because I thought those were true, that I couldn't have a good self-image to find another job. I couldn't have it, and so I started to think that I have to do something for myself, I have to get out of this. Okay? But, since we separated and started to try to get back together I find that as much as he has put on me, you know, I have put on him—blame on him for the way I feel, because I don't want to feel what I feel, I don't want to feel low, so I blame him all the time, you know? And I feel that getting out of the relationship is not the answer to my feeling better about myself, I mean, just as much as drinking for him—not drinking doesn't cure all his problems. Getting rid of him doesn't cure all mine either. He doesn't put me down any more. He stopped drinking, you know, and that's stopped and I'm still with him, and I don't feel like I need to get rid of the relationship. But I feel like during the relationship, when there was drinking involved in it, maybe I kept it going—his drinking—because it gave me an excuse to think of why I was so low. I don't know, I just don't know. So that's why I feel like going to this group, this Al-Anon group, makes me be able to deal with my husband's irritability, my husband's change in lifestyle as far as not drinking. But they're not able to tell me why I feel so badly about myself. I don't know either. *(Crying continues but has diminished.)*

THERAPIST: But you think it long predates your relationship with your husband—thinking so badly about yourself?

CLIENT: Yeah, I do.

THERAPIST: Tell me something about you and your parents.

[I think the client recognizes her low self-esteem and her excessive dependency on her husband and, at the same time, her possible role in her marital difficulties. It seems timely now to learn more about the client's current and past relationships with her family. At this point, the interview has been going on for 19 minutes.]

CLIENT: *(Pause.)* Um, I don't know what to tell you. I am more confused about my relationship with my parents now since either I have been going through this crisis with my husband, because I have come a lot closer to them than I have felt for a really long time. But . . . I don't know what to say about my parents. The thing that sticks out in my mind that happened most recently, as far as the decision I made regarding my parents, is when I moved from their house because I felt like I was depending too much on them and I was getting too old to depend on them, so I left, and I didn't feel when I made the decision to leave their house that I could leave their house and live around the corner. They live back in _____. I just told them I had to—I was going to move out—I had lived in Colorado before, for part of my schooling, and so I told them I was going to be moving and that I was moving back here and I felt I had to—that's really strange to me, but I felt I had to live this far away to not depend on them. I had to find a way to make myself feel good about myself. *(Starts crying again.)*

THERAPIST: And you couldn't feel good about yourself around them? *(Pause.)* Why not?

CLIENT: I don't know. I don't know. I felt really good around them when they came to visit me, when we got married—we got married here you know, and so I was accommodating them and they were in my home, I felt real good. But I don't know why I couldn't feel good around them, when I was in their home. I don't know.

THERAPIST: But you really cry a lot about that. *[This is an explicit recognition of the pain associated with the client's relationship with her parents.]*

CLIENT: *(Pause.)* Before I moved out here—this was two years ago—I felt like I was going through a big crisis, you know. I had to decide whether I was going to continue living in _____. I had to decide whether I was going to leave my parents. I had to decide so many things you know, and all the petty things were even important you know, and I can remember going to—I belonged to the _____ Community Health Plan they had in _____, and they had a mental health center in there and I remember going in there and thinking, "Well, I'll just go in here 'cause I belong to this anyway so now I'll find somebody to talk to." And like I started talking to the person there, this woman—I only went one time—I started crying about the exact same things and I didn't know why then and I don't know now. *[So this is not her first single session, and in some ways, it is a repetition of the earlier therapy experience.]* All I know is when I walked out of there, I thought, "Well, I will just have to decide what to do and that's it." I couldn't figure anything out. I can remember starting to talk about my dad and talking about dependency to her and talking about my dad and I started crying and I thought, "I better get out." It was shortly after that that I moved out and I guess I thought, "Well, if I move away and I create my own environment where I am comfortable in and I'm . . . successful, so to speak, at being able to work things out someplace else, then everything will be okay." You know? *(Crying diminished.)*

[The move to Colorado represents a breaking away from her father. I now want to get to the low self-esteem issue and think the way to do it would be to pick up on the word dirt *that the client had used in describing her husband's description of her. But I do not know how successful I will be in getting the client to talk about her low self-esteem—that may be more than one should expect in this kind of interview.]*

THERAPIST: Yeah. What does your husband mean when he says you're dirt? That's quite a powerful accusation.

CLIENT: I don't know, I don't know what he's meant when he said that. It's hard to understand, because all the things that I have to base those things that he said on is when he was drinking, you know, and I don't know, I can't ask him why he said things because at the time when he was drinking, if I said, "Why do you say those things," he'd say, "Because I meant them." You know, he was very angry.

THERAPIST: What do you think he meant, though, when he said that he thought you were dirt?

CLIENT: I don't know.

THERAPIST: What does a person mean when he calls somebody else dirt? *[I persist.]*

CLIENT: I don't know. It made me feel very low, I don't know. Other than that he made me feel that I don't, I don't live up to expectations or something, or I don't . . . I guess more or less something like that, that I just don't live up to his expectations, you know, that I'm below him, you know, below his expectations. I don't know. It's the only thing I could think of.

THERAPIST: Do you think your parents thought you were dirt?

CLIENT: No, not really, I don't know where I got the feeling, I don't know where I got it, you know? I mean I know they love me very much, they never . . . they never did anything intentionally cruel or anything like that, I don't know where I got it. *[All these "I don't know" protestations by the client make it obvious that I am pushing too hard.]*

THERAPIST: Yet when you think about your father, it's hard to keep from crying. *(Pause.)* *[I give up, at least for the moment.]* Do you have brothers or sisters? Tell me about them. *[I do not know very much about her father, who is clearly a central figure in her dilemma. I probably would have done better to ask about her father.]*

CLIENT: I have an older sister, and a younger brother, and my younger brother, he went in the service when he got out of high school and he's, then he moved back to, to . . . _____ for a while, and then he went to school in _____ and now he just got a job in _____ and he works down there. And he's buying a home and he lives by himself and he's anxious to get married but he hasn't found the right person, and that's the kind of situation he's in. And my sister, she's older than I am, she was married for three years, she got married right after she got out of college, and she got divorced three years later, and she kept her home and lived there for about another couple years, and had a serious relationship with one person, and then had . . . broke off from that with a lot of regrets, and she recently got married and moved to _____. She's living up there, and that just happened a couple months ago, and she is up there now. That's pretty much what they've been . . .

THERAPIST: What do your folks think of your brother and sister? Do you have any idea?

CLIENT: Um *(Pause.)*, they worry a lot about my brother because he, they feel like he makes decisions that aren't, that aren't all that wise. He makes investments that they would never make. He takes risks that they would never do, and things like that. They worry about him for those reasons, but he seems to come through everything OK. Um, he doesn't, he's not at all dependent on them. *[The client describes her brother as very different from the way she is on the dependency dimension. But I may not be able to do much with that.]* If he's got something wrong, they might find out about it six months later, after he's settled it all, you know, or something. Or he might talk about it, but he doesn't talk about it in a way that he needs help, um, and my sister, um, I guess they're worried about her now just because she's never lived that far away from home, and she's 30 years old but they're still worried about it because she's always . . . my sister . . . it's funny to think about it . . . my sister doesn't think that much of herself either. *[The client discovers an important similarity with her sister.]* It just occurred to me because I just got a letter from my sister telling me that she just got married, she's been married a couple of months. A month after she was married she got pregnant, and she, she's happy and she thinks everything's going great, and all her new husband's relatives really like her, but she doesn't think she deserves it. *(Laughs.)* That's what she wrote and told me. And I thought, "How strange," and I thought, "She shouldn't feel like that," and then I thought, "I never thought about myself when I read it."

THERAPIST: So there's something surprisingly similar between the two of you. *[I pick up on the similarity with her sister, and I am thinking that it would be useful to have these sisters talk with each other about when they were children.] (Pause.)* Are your folks the kind of people who make it hard for you to feel good about yourself? There are folks like that, who seem to be awfully tough on their kids.

CLIENT: I never noticed it, I don't know what action they would have taken that would have, you know, that I could see as making things difficult for me. You know I always felt during the time that I was growing up that they did things to . . . to make me a stronger person, to make me take care of things myself so that I wouldn't be dependent on them. I always felt they did things like that.

THERAPIST: Yet you said you could make a whole long list of things that you needed to do to make yourself, in a way, more acceptable to your folks. *[I disagree with the client, but gently.]*

CLIENT: Yeah, that's when I was really little, I can remember that, I remember having lists in my top drawer that I'd look at when my mom made me cry, I'd think, "That's why, because I don't do this right, and that's why, because I don't do that right." But . . .

THERAPIST: Is that how she made you cry . . . by criticizing you?

CLIENT: I don't know, I don't remember things she used to say. All's I remember is having those lists, and I don't even remember what was on them anymore.

THERAPIST: Do you remember crying?

CLIENT: I remember that I would never let her see me cry because I didn't want her to think that she got me, you know, that she got the best of me. I used to want to go in my room and I'd hide. And then I'd come out and be strong and be really cool. *(Crying again.)*

THERAPIST: But that's not what was really going on? *[I label what she is saying, that is, that she hid her true feelings from her mother.]*

CLIENT: No, whatever it was that happened really hurt, and I'd go and hide it, and I don't know what it was, I can't remember what the things, that made me go do that, I don't know what they were. *(Pause.)* I'd go hide it all the time.

THERAPIST: Do you think moving to Colorado was hiding?

CLIENT: I don't know. I don't feel bad about having moved here, I feel like I've grown a lot since I've been here, you know, I mean it might be hiding something, I don't know.

THERAPIST: From them?

CLIENT: I don't know, I really don't . . . I don't feel . . . I don't really feel when I moved that I was running away. I felt that I was trying to do something for myself, I really felt that. I felt that I needed, you know, I needed to do something for myself, and that was the same kind of feeling I had when I needed to do something for myself then as when I thought that I needed to leave my husband.

THERAPIST: Do you still make lists? *[This question is an effort to lighten things up a little but, at the same time, to underline the continuity of the past with the present, in keeping with the client's similar linking of her past and present behavior.]*

CLIENT: *(Laughs.)* No . . . no.

THERAPIST: Now tell me, tell me how it happened you got married. I take it it didn't come to you as a surprise that your husband drank too much . . . you called him an alcoholic. You must have known that before you got married.

[The interview is now 35 minutes old, and we have to talk more about the immediate past and the current problem. I hope to get into the present by finding out about her husband's alcoholism and the circumstances of their marriage.]

CLIENT: No, I didn't know he was an alcoholic but I knew that he drank too much. You know, it's like the reason that I never really thought that it was serious was I was going through this thing where I felt like everything that happened was the reason that he was drinking. It wasn't an ongoing thing. It wasn't something he had done forever in the past or something he would do forever in the future. Like, his dad passed away last summer, and he drank a whole lot then, and I thought, "Well, when this goes, you know, when he . . ." I don't know what it's like to lose someone really close. I never lost anybody in my family so . . . I didn't know if that was what that was causing him to drink or not, you know. I know that's not a good excuse for drinking but, I figured maybe it was the only thing he could think of doing.

THERAPIST: How about before that? Why was he drinking?

CLIENT: Before that, I never thought he drank all that much. You know, see . . . I'd seen him drink a lot on occasion, but I never saw it on a continuous basis, you know. I mean he may have drank . . he may have drank when we went out, you know, but I never saw him in person in between to know he drank all the time in between that we weren't seeing each other, and it was around this time a year ago that his dad died that we started living together. And that's when I started to drink . . . *[I toyed with the idea of picking up this slip of speech, and then abandoned the idea.]* seeing him drinking all the time, and then after that, I don't know. He was married before, and he had one crisis after another with his . . . he's got kids, you know, and something would happen and I'd think, "Well, this upsets him, that upsets him," and I always . . . it just . . . *[New information here, but I did not see any feasible way of making use of it in the context of the interview.]*

THERAPIST: So you made excuses for him.

[This is a good illustration of the problem of theme selection in focused single-session therapy. It is already clear that there is much that can be learned regarding the relationship of the client and her father, but that there is not enough time. Now we learn that the client's husband had a prior marriage and has children from that marriage—again an issue that there is not enough time to discuss. I have to be very careful to stick with the developing plan for the interview, doing a more careful analysis of fewer themes rather than going off in all directions, however appropriate that might be for therapy that would be of far longer duration.]

CLIENT: Yeah, just all throughout that whole time I just thought, "Well, that's why he is drinking, that's why he is drinking."

THERAPIST: How long did you live together before you got married?

CLIENT: *(Pause.)* About nine months.

THERAPIST: And then how did you decide to get married? How did that come about?

CLIENT: Um . . . I don't know . . . it was before we started living together that he asked me to marry him. We had gone back to _____ and had met my folks and we had talked about it and everything, and came back and started planning it and um . . . I don't know. That's just more or less how we started doing it. I would just . . . *[It seems to me that the client does not present any clear rationale for her marriage.]*

THERAPIST: And is his drinking worse now than it was before you got married, or is it just . . .

CLIENT: Well, he doesn't drink at all now.

THERAPIST: But at the time that you said he was an alcoholic, which was, I take it . . .

CLIENT: It was a lot worse.

THERAPIST: His drinking got worse after you got married?

CLIENT: Yeah, and I made excuses for that, too, for a while, thinking, "Well, this is another adjustment, this is a new lifestyle."

THERAPIST: You mean your being married, you used married as a . . .

CLIENT: Yeah, and then I thought, "If I am going to use marriage for an excuse, that means that I have to stay in this and be in this excuse forever," and then I thought, "We got to do something about this," and that's when we had the first crisis, you know, as far as my saying, "I can't be in it, you know, I can't continue with it anymore." It's something that I learned about in the group I am in, and it's a merry-go-round that you get on, you know, with an alcoholic and, you know, it's up to you when you decide to get off, or if you want to stay with it or not, and I just decided to get off, you know. But it's . . . the drinking part I mean, I understand that he's going to have dry drunks, and that he is going to have problems adjusting to it, um . . . for the rest of his life or at least the next couple of years having a hard time. I didn't know how long he had been drinking, and I know now.

THERAPIST: And he's quit, at least . . . and for how long has it been since he's had a drink, how long has it been?

CLIENT: About a month . . . something like that.

THERAPIST: And the problems didn't disappear? The problems haven't disappeared . . . between the two of you.

CLIENT: No, not really. He started seeing a psychiatrist out at work, where he works, and he started going to an encounter group, and . . . it seems like he starts doing things after I say I am going to do them. If I say I am going to see someone, I am going to go to Al-Anon, he'll go to AA. If I say I am going to see a psychiatrist, he'll go. He finds the strength to go. So I say to myself, "Well, I'm not that weak a person." *[The client comes back to the self-esteem issue but now presents herself as far stronger than was the case earlier in the interview, as if she is working out this problem in the course of the interview.]* I must be pretty strong, because I am able to initiate all these things and do these things and, you know, plug on and do this, and now I find myself feeling like I can't really do them, you know? And, the ideas are there, creativity is in my mind to be able to live a better life but I don't feel like I carry on through with the right frame of mind. I feel like I am not going to make it all the time.

THERAPIST: Sure, sure . . . are you guys back together again now?

CLIENT: Yeah. We have been together for about a week now.

THERAPIST: Well, what do you want to do about that merry-go-round? *[Again, I deliberately use her picturesque word.]*

CLIENT: Well, something, you know, that I have realized since he's stopped drinking and I have been going to this group is the fact that . . . you know . . . the better a person you make yourself, the better you can make your relationship, you know, and everything, and I have always known that before. It's just that I never thought anything was really wrong with me, you know, that wasn't wrong with anybody else, you know. But I just think that I have to find a way to either find out why I go through such terrible lows, or before . . . before I start anything, you know, I mean, I guess before I could really start this marriage I had to put myself really low like I couldn't make it, you know, or something. Before I ever started anything in my life I went through crises of never thinking I could do it, and then I do it. But I always had to think that I could never make it, you know, and I don't know why I have to go through that. I want to find out why.

THERAPIST: That's like the way you define the word *dirt* . . . somebody who is really low.

CLIENT: *(Pause.)* I want to find out why I don't have a very good opinion of myself because I . . .

THERAPIST: Do you have a pretty good relationship with your parents now, would you say?

CLIENT: Yeah, I think it's pretty good. You know, I had a lot of long conversations with them about what I was going through in the past month and . . .

THERAPIST: Do you talk to each other on the phone?

CLIENT: Yeah, you know, it seems like . . . well . . . insecurity and independence and all those things seem to be a big things to me, and when, in the past, the first time I lived in Colorado, I can remember talking to my parents on the phone and saying, "I don't know if I will find a job or not," and my dad saying to me, "I think you ought to come home," and immediately I was home the next time, the first day I could get out, you know, I thought, "Well, he thinks I ought to come home, and I came home," *[I cannot do much with it, but we now have a clue as to her conflict with her father—he does not have much confidence in her.]* and in this crisis, living here and stuff, I mean it was really good because I felt like, I have established myself here, and everything, that when I talk to him about the crisis I was going through, instead of either one of them saying anything to me about "Why don't you forget everything out there and why don't you just come home," like they would have in the past, my mom said to me, "You've got a house out there, you've got commitments. You made a commitment to this relationship. Either you've got to work out what you want from it first, you have to figure out whether you want to keep the house, you got responsibilities, you figure them all out," and then she says, "If then you want to come home for a while, you tell us," but she said, "I don't think you ought to come home right now."

THERAPIST: That's a change in her behavior compared to when you were younger and your father's, too. *[That is a guess; there is no evidence for a change in her father's attitude. My guess is that the parents tend to speak with one voice on this issue.] (Pause.)* Well, it sounds like they want you to separate yourself from them. I guess separate yourself from them in the way a child would be connected to the parents . . . to be an adult with your parents. It sounds like they want the same thing you want, which is for you to be somewhat more independent. It sounds like you're not . . . you haven't quite done that. You still are tied to them, like you were when you were younger . . . their opinion . . . still can make you cry. *[This is a big speech, but I think it is not complicated and that the work of the previous 40 minutes makes this observation acceptable.]*

CLIENT: But I don't understand why, if I want independence from them, I am still seeking dependence on them. Why if I want that, why I don't give it up, you know, the dependence. And it's the same thing with my husband, you know, I want to be independent of him but I want to have a good relationship with him. I want to be independent of him but I still depend on him every way I can and I don't . . .

THERAPIST: So there's not that big a difference between the struggle you are having with your parents and the struggle you are having with your husband?

CLIENT: I don't think so, I think it's, you know, I think it's a lot the same. I have the same *(Pause.)* fears of being independent of him as I had of being independent of my parents. Not that I don't think I can make it on my own, but I don't want to let go either . . . you know. And I don't understand why I feel like that because I . . . *(Sighs.)*

THERAPIST: Well, I think it's frightening to be on your own . . . it would be frightening. It's scary.

CLIENT: But why should I let it affect me like this for the rest of my life, you know?

THERAPIST: Well, I guess I don't think that it will affect you the rest of your life. But I think you haven't separated yourself properly from your folks. That doesn't mean to be absolutely independent. I think children are always dependent on their parents, even when the children are 50 and the parents are 80. They are still dependent on their parents, in some ways. I guess you haven't figured out that balance yet of right ways to be dependent and the right ways to be independent. *[I am somewhat hortatory here —perhaps too much so.]*

CLIENT: How do you figure that out though? If I never figured that out with my parents, how am I going to figure it out with my husband?

THERAPIST: Well, I wish you would try to learn more about how it was with you and your parents when you were younger. I think maybe, it would be helpful. Have you ever told your mother that you went into the bedroom and cried? And that you made lists?

CLIENT: Oh, no. *(Laughs.)* No, I told my husband that just because I was trying to figure out what was going on.

THERAPIST: And that there were times that she made you feel very bad about yourself? *(Pause.)* Well, you might want to tell your mother and ask her to help you understand that. I guess I think you may have to make peace with your parents before you can be wise about what to do about your husband.

[This is the most overt instance of my effort at facilitating useful insight. And, at the same time, I am beginning to suggest a modest but constructive course of action that might make it possible for this client to disentangle the past from the present. I am clearly more active and directive now, trying to put into acceptable language what I think I have learned about this client.]

CLIENT: I wonder if it has anything to do with, you know, I feel that they made me feel bad so I depend on them to make me feel good again.

THERAPIST: That's like with your husband. You depend on him to make you feel good . . . what do you think?

CLIENT: I don't know. Maybe I should go to more Al-Anon groups so I can learn to feel better about myself by myself . . . not depend on somebody else to make me feel good.

THERAPIST: What does Al-Anon say about that merry-go-round, they say you have to decide.

CLIENT: Well, they don't tell you that you ought to split up or they don't tell you any of that stuff. They just tell you that . . . this is when I really start thinking about it. They tell you you have to be good to yourself, and so often in this relationship, in the past year, you know, if my husband really made me feel bad, that I wasn't a good partner, that I wasn't a good wife, in the few months that we have been married, instead of going out and saying, "I am going to make myself feel good because there is no reason I should feel like this," I would sit home and cry, you know, that I am not good, you know, and so since I have been in the Al-Anon thing, I feel like, "Okay, fine." There have been times that he has made me feel really rotten since we have started doing this, but, just because he's got these anxieties and he puts the blame on me for things, and so in those times, there was one time this weekend, I just, I was sitting home and I was feeling really bad, because he was saying, "I want to do this, no I don't want to do this, no, I don't want you to come with me," you know, and just making me feel really bad, and he left the house, and then I thought, "I feel really bad," and I sat there and I couldn't do anything, and then I thought, "I have to go out, I got to go do something and see that some . . . that I can have, you know, more positive rapport with something, because I can't feel like this because it's not . . . I'm not going to feel any better when he comes back," and so, you know, I went out and found a friend of mine who was broke down in a car and they found me . . . I was in the shopping center, and they asked me to help, and I helped them, and I thought, "Jeez, you can't be such all that bad a person, you know, you are helping somebody, what's wrong with you for thinking that," you know. And then I went back home and I felt better about myself, but I was still scared that I wouldn't be able to stand there and feel good, you know. And it's just that they teach you that in the group, you know, that you've got to think about what to do for yourself. Because, you can't help them, which is what you want to do in a situation like that, if you are not feeling good about yourself. You can't do anything positive for yourself if you are not feeling good about yourself, so . . .

THERAPIST: Are you surprised that you don't even really know why you got married?

CLIENT: Am I really surprised that I don't know why I got married? I don't feel like I don't know why I got married, I feel that I love my husband and he was someone that I thought that I could live my whole life with because we had a lot of good things going between us. And, I thought that we had a lot of the same goals and a lot of the same ambitions and a lot of . . . *[I have obviously made an error here. My assertion that she did not know why she got married is imprecise, if not completely wrong.]*

THERAPIST: I'm sorry, I asked you before why did you happen to get married and I thought you said you really didn't know, but now you are making a good list of reasons why people get married.

CLIENT: I thought the question you asked me before was why I got married when I knew my husband was an alcoholic or something like that. Why I would get married to an alcoholic . . . I don't know that except it might have something to do with the fact that I don't feel good about myself, you know, or I didn't, *[She is trying to put her low self-esteem into the past and remove it from the present.]* and alcoholics have a way of perpetuating that.

THERAPIST: Well, look, it sounds like your work with Al-Anon is paying off, slowly, but paying off. And if you can continue that, I think that is a really good idea. I think the lessons they are trying to teach I would applaud them . . . I think they are important lessons. I think it's hard to be really good to another person unless you feel pretty good about yourself. I agree with that. What do you think your husband's chances are of stopping drinking or cutting down . . . getting rid of that alcoholism?

CLIENT: I think his chances are good. I think it's as hard for him as it is for any other alcoholic because he is so much into his old friends who are all . . . who I think are all alcoholics.

THERAPIST: Does he think of himself as an alcoholic?

CLIENT: He's beginning to see himself as an alcoholic.

THERAPIST: Now I hear what you are saying as meaning that you certainly don't think today you want a divorce. *[There are only a few minutes left to bring the interview to a close.]*

CLIENT: No, I don't think today that I want a divorce.

THERAPIST: You may think that way a month from now. *[That is not a helpful remark, even if it might turn out to be correct.]*

CLIENT: Yeah, if I don't think good about myself, then I will think that I shouldn't be there.

THERAPIST: You certainly don't think that way now. So you think you would like to stay on the merry-go-round a while longer and see how it goes.

CLIENT: Well, the merry-go-round is involved with the drinking. I don't feel like I am on a merry-go-round right now. *[I used the phrase one time too often. Again, I am not sufficiently precise.]* I think that we're on the road to being able to communicate better together but, you know, he said to me, he's been wanting to get more involved with things together with me that bring us more able to communicate together, and one of the things was this retreat that he had heard about that he thought would be good if we went to, but he had prefaced it by telling me he had heard that it is something we ought to really think about before we do because we have to be totally honest with each other. And I thought, "Well, that's fine, I am totally honest with you, it's fine." Then I started getting scared thinking, "Well, am I? I mean, do I know all that much about myself that I am?"

THERAPIST: Do you think it is realistic to try to raise some of the issues that we talked about with your mother, with your parents? Is that a possibility? *[It is entirely possible that what I am suggesting this client do is beyond her capacities at the present time.]*

CLIENT: I think it's a possibility. I don't know if at this distance we'd be able to get that much accomplished.

THERAPIST: You know, sometimes you can do some nice things with letters.

CLIENT: That's true.

THERAPIST: Sometimes, maybe a letter is better than even with a phone call . . . that you have been thinking about some things that were true of you when you were a child, and you feel like you would like to share some of them with your mother, in particular, maybe even with both of your parents. And that you wonder what light they can shed. Maybe they might be able to tell you things that might give you a better understanding of those days.

CLIENT: The only person who used to make me feel like I wasn't crazy for feeling like this was my sister, because we used to communicate about the feelings that we had that were similar.

THERAPIST: It sounds like your sister is prepared to get into a nice correspondence with you, too. It sounds like she's telling you quite openly some things about herself that are personal and that you notice are similar to you. I guess, if I could make a suggestion, one of them obviously is to continue the Al-Anon and see how that goes. The other is to see if there is any way in the world that you can enter into a kind of dialogue with your folks and with your sister, too, about earlier days, and I . . . if you are able to do that and you learn some things about yourself, I'd appreciate it if you would give me a call and we could chat over the phone or you might want to come in again. I'd like to hear more about what you are learning about yourself. I think it is clear to you, you are carrying with you a big load of issues that you haven't resolved yet with your folks, and that's what you are crying about. And it's hard to deal in the here and now when you still have that load you are bearing. It sounds like whatever you could do to lighten that load would really pay off. *(Pause.)* You know how to get hold of me, so I really wish you might, if you think it is something you could manage skillfully, see if you could get into closer touch with your folks and with your sister . . . by letter is fine. Sometimes it works very well by letter. See if you can get a better perspective on why you felt so badly about yourself and maybe why your sister felt so badly about herself when you were younger. See if you can get that into the past instead of keeping it in the present. Then I wish you would call me and let me know how you are doing. *[I deliberately give her an assignment and a chance to tell me how the task went.]*

CLIENT: I would like to reach some peace of mind about this.

THERAPIST: I'd like to try to help and also learn a little bit about that process you'd be going through.

CLIENT: It is important now that I do it because my husband is going through something trying to, you know, straighten himself out, and if we are going to stay together in any way at all, I better straighten myself out, too, and I don't know. Maybe it would be a good idea to try to communicate with my folks and see what their response is. As to doing that, I don't know what it will be. I think my sister is more willing to do it because she is wanting to find out why, too. *[She sounds very tentative about engaging her parents in a discussion of her childhood.]*

THERAPIST: Well, look, why don't you think about that? I don't want you to do anything unless you think about it and it seems like a good idea, and please let me know how that process goes. I would like to have a chance to learn more about it from you. Is this something you think you might be able to do?

CLIENT: Well, I would like to at least be able to get to the point where I can discuss problems with people without crying.

THERAPIST: Good . . . good . . . good. Okay, well, please keep in touch; let me know how it goes. I appreciate your coming in and I hope you found it useful.

CLIENT: Oh yeah. *(Pause.)* Do you work here throughout the year?

THERAPIST: Yeah, I am in the department almost all the time. You can always get ahold of me, and when I'm not here, my machine will answer.

CLIENT: Yeah, I talked to that once.

THERAPIST: You can leave your name, phone number, and of course, I will call you back. All right?

CLIENT: I will write down our appointment time if we need one and I won't end up having to call . . . *[This is a reference to the fact that the client had to call me prior to this interview because she had forgotten what day the interview appointment was scheduled.]*

THERAPIST: It's a deal. No problem at all.

CLIENT: Thanks a lot.

THERAPIST: You're really welcome.

CLIENT: Do you know the time?

THERAPIST: Yes, it's just about one o'clock.

CLIENT: Okay, thanks a lot.

THERAPIST: Bye-bye.

INTERVIEW FOLLOW-UP

I have had three brief telephone conversations with the client since this interview—one month, two months, and nearly five months after the interview took place. She is still working on keeping her marriage together and has begun what she reports as very helpful conversations with her sister and her parents.

One month after the focused single-session therapy interview, I called her and found that she had begun to discuss her childhood recollections with her sister and parents. Her sister was not able to be very helpful, because she was in the midst of her own marital difficulties and had gone home to her parents for a visit. Conversations with her parents had just begun. The client mentioned that she is recognizing more and more that her problems with her husband come out of her own past and, in particular, arise because she does not feel good about herself. Her husband has stopped drinking but is going through periods when he is pessimistic about the marriage and when he withdraws and won't talk with her. I suggested that she could call me in a month or so to let me know how she is getting along, if she cared to do so.

One month later, the client called me. She was very discouraged. Her husband had started drinking again and was talking about wanting a divorce, saying that things would never work out. The client indicated that she did not know if she wanted to stay in the marriage—it seemed to be destroying her. Her husband was still calling her "dirt," but she was saying to herself that those things were not true. She was trying to persuade her husband to enter an alcoholism recovery program, and she had spoken with a priest about her difficulties, a conversation she found helpful. The client has continued the dialogues with her sister and her parents. Her sister is back with her husband and appears happier. The client envies her and has recalled that same feeling of envy toward her sister when she was younger. Conversation with her parents had resulted in her realization that, as a child, she felt that her father did not love her as much as he loved her sister. As a consequence, she now believes, she looked for a husband who could love her unconditionally. The fact that he does not is leaving her feeling demolished.

Nearly three months after this conversation, I called her again and found that she was considerably happier. Her husband had completed a one-month alcoholism recovery program, and as part of the program, the client met with other spouses of alcoholics in a one-week retreat. There she learned that she held a lot of resentments and that it was difficult for her to forgive her husband. She came away feeling better about herself and more hopeful. The client and her husband visited her parents, and she spent a good deal of time with her parents talking about the origins of her envy of her sister. The client still feels uncertain about her marriage and is, along with her husband, somewhat optimistically living one day at a time.

CONCLUDING REMARKS

Many mental health practitioners seem to subscribe to two beliefs that are virtually unknown in the rest of the healing arts: first, in order to get better, it will take a long time; and second, once you are better, you probably will never need to come back. Most human service providers hold an alternative point of view, one that seems more persuasive in the context of short-term therapy: first, let us try to help you as quickly as possible; and second, something might very well go wrong in the future, in which case come back and we will try to help you once again.

With the latter orientation, commitment to the client can be seen from a very different point of view than that typically considered by the mental health professions. Rabkin (1977) described the short-term therapy orientation to that commitment very well when he wrote:

> Under the best of conditions, relationships with professionals other than psychotherapists are not regarded as terminating at all. They are seen as intermit-

tent. For example, the accountant, lawyer, family doctor, or barber may have permanent relationships with clients and perhaps their families, although the actual face-to-face contacts occur only for specific tasks or problems. Particularly in relationships of confidence, as in the case of the accountant and the physician, the tie may last a lifetime. (p. 211)

I believe that focused single-session therapy can be an effective and responsible form of psychotherapy if we remember that the relationship between client and therapist and between client and agency can be lifelong but intermittent.

REFERENCES

Alexander, F. Psychoanalytic contributions to short-term psychotherapy. In L. R. Wolberg (Ed.), *Short-term psychotherapy.* New York: Grune & Stratton, 1965.

Balint, M., Ornstein, P. H., & Balint, E. *Focal psychotherapy: An example of applied psychoanalysis.* London: Tavistock Publications, 1973.

Barten, H. H. The expanding spectrum of the brief therapies. In H. H. Barten (Ed.), *Brief therapies.* New York: Behavioral Publications, 1971.

Bloom, B. L. *Changing patterns on psychiatric care.* New York: Human Sciences Press, 1975.

Bloom, B. L. Social and community interventions. *Annual Review of Psychology,* 1980, *31,* 111–142.

Breuer, J., & Freud, S. *Studies on hysteria.* New York: Basic Books, 1957.

Coleman, J. V. Banter as psychotherapeutic intervention. *American Journal of Psychoanalysis,* 1962, *22,* 69–74.

Cummings, N. A. The anatomy of psychotherapy under national health insurance. *American Psychologist,* 1977, *32,* 711–718. (a)

Cummings, N. A. Prolonged (ideal) versus short-term (realistic) psychotherapy. *Professional Psychology,* 1977, *8,* 491–501. (b)

Cummings, N. A., & Follette, W. T. Psychiatric services and medical utilization in a prepaid health plan setting: Part II. *Medical Care,* 1968, *6,* 31–41.

Cummings, N. A., & Follette, W. T. Brief psychotherapy and medical utilization. In H. Dorken & Associates (Eds.), *The professional psychologist today: New developments in law, health insurance and health practice.* San Francisco: Jossey-Bass, 1976.

Edwards, G., Orford, J., Egert, S., Guthrie, S., Hawker, A., Hensman, C., Mitcheson, M., Oppenheimer, E., & Taylor, C. Alcoholism: A controlled trial of "treatment" and "advice." *Journal of Studies on Alcohol,* 1977, *38,* 1004–1031.

Ewalt, P. L. The crisis-treatment approach in a child guidance clinic. *Social Casework,* 1973, *54,* 406–411.

Ewing, C. P. *Crisis intervention as psychotherapy.* New York: Oxford University Press, 1978.

Fiester, A. R., & Rudestam, K. E. A multivariate analysis of the early dropout process. *Journal of Consulting and Clinical Psychology,* 1975, *43,* 528–535.

Follette, W. T., & Cummings, N. A. Psychiatric services and medical utilization in a prepaid health plan setting. *Medical Care,* 1967, *5,* 25–35.

Frings, J. What about brief services? A report of a study of short-term cases. *Social Casework,* 1951, *32,* 236–241.

Garfield, S. L. Research on client variables in psychotherapy. In S. L. Garfield & A. E. Bergin (Eds.), *Handbook of psychotherapy and behavior change: An empirical analysis* (2nd ed.). New York: Wiley, 1978.

Garfield, S. L., & Wolpin, M. Expectations regarding psychotherapy. *Journal of Nervous and Mental Disease*, 1963, *137*, 353–362.

Getz, W. L., Fujita, B. N., & Allen, D. The use of paraprofessionals in crisis intervention: Evaluation of an innovative program. *American Journal of Community Psychology*, 1975, *3*, 135–144.

Gillman, R. D. Brief psychotherapy: A psychoanalytic view. *American Journal of Psychiatry*, 1965, *122*, 601–611.

Goldberg, I. D., Krantz, G., & Locke, B. Z. Effect of a short-term outpatient psychiatric therapy benefit on the utilization of medical services in a prepaid group practice medical program. *Medical Care*, 1970, *8*, 419–428.

Groddeck, G. *The unknown self.* New York: Funk & Wagnalls, 1951.

Hoffman, D. L., & Remmel, M. L. Uncovering the precipitant in crisis intervention. *Social Casework*, 1975, *56*, 259–267.

Jacobson, G. F., Wilner, D. M., Morley, W. E., Schneider, S., Strickler, M., & Sommer, G. J. The scope and practice of an early-access brief treatment psychiatric center. *American Journal of Psychiatry*, 1965, *121*, 1176–1182.

Jameson, J., Shuman, L. J., & Young, W. W. The effects of outpatient psychiatric utilization on the costs of providing third-party coverage. *Medical Care*, 1978, *16*, 383–399.

Kaffman, M. Short term family therapy. *Family Process*, 1963, *2*, 216–234.

Kogan, L. S. The short-term case in a family agency: Part I. The study plan. *Social Casework*, 1957, *38*, 231–238. (a)

Kogan, L. S. The short-term case in a family agency: Part II. Results of study. *Social Casework*, 1957, *38*, 296–302. (b)

Kogan, L. S. The short-term case in a family agency: Part III. Further results and conclusion. *Social Casework*, 1957, *38*, 366–374. (c)

Lazare, A., Cohen, F., Jacobson, A. M., Williams, M. W., Mignone, R. J., & Zisook, S. The walk-in patient as a "customer": A key dimension in evaluation and treatment. *American Journal of Orthopsychiatry*, 1972, *42*, 872–883.

Lewin, K. K. *Brief encounters: Brief psychotherapy.* St. Louis: Warren H. Green, 1970.

Littlepage, G. E., Kosloski, K. D., Schnelle, J. F., McNees, M. P., & Gendrich, J. C. The problem of early outpatient terminations from community mental health centers: A problem for whom? *Journal of Community Psychology*, 1976, *4*, 164–167.

Lorion, R. P. Patient and therapist variables in the treatment of low-income patients. *Psychological Bulletin*, 1974, *81*, 344–354.

Malan, D. H., Heath, E. S., Bacal, H. A., & Balfour, F. H. G. Psychodynamic changes in untreated neurotic patients: II. Apparently genuine improvements. *Archives of General Psychiatry*, 1975, *32*, 110–126.

McCord, E. Treatment in short time contacts. *Family*, 1931, *12*, 191–193.

McGuire, M. T. The instruction nature of short-term insight psychotherapy. *American Journal of Psychotherapy*, 1968, *22*, 218–232.

Olbrisch, M. E. Psychotherapeutic interventions in physical health: Effectiveness and economic efficiency. *American Psychologist*, 1977, *32*, 761–777.

Rabkin, R. *Strategic psychotherapy: Brief and symptomatic treatment.* New York: Basic Books, 1977.

Reed, L. S., Myers, E. S., & Scheidemandel, P. L. *Health insurance and psychiatric care: Utilization and cost.* Washington, D.C.: American Psychiatric Association, 1972.

Regier, D. A., Goldberg, I. D., & Taube, C. A. The de facto U.S. mental health services system. *Archives of General Psychiatry*, 1978, *35*, 685–693.

Reider, N. A type of psychotherapy based on psychoanalytic principles. *Bulletin of the Menninger Clinic,* 1955, *19,* 111–128.

Rosen, J. C., & Wiens, A. N. Changes in medical problems and use of medical services following psychological intervention. *American Psychologist,* 1979, *34,* 420–431.

Rosenbaum, C. P. Events of early therapy and brief therapy. *Archives of General Psychiatry,* 1964, *10,* 506–512.

Rubin, Z., & Mitchell, C. Couples research as couples counseling. *American Psychologist,* 1976, *36,* 17–25.

Sarvis, M. A., Dewees, S., & Johnson, R. F. A concept of ego-oriented psychotherapy. *Psychiatry,* 1959, *22,* 277–287.

Shyne, A. W. What research tells us about short-term cases in family agencies. *Social Casework,* 1957, *38,* 223–231.

Sifneos, P. E. *Short-term dynamic psychotherapy: Evaluation and technique.* New York: Plenum Press, 1979.

Silverman, W. H., & Beech, R. P. Are dropouts, dropouts? *Journal of Community Psychology,* 1979, *7,* 236–242.

Speers, R. W. Brief psychotherapy with college women: Technique and criteria for selection. *American Journal of Orthopsychiatry,* 1962, *32,* 434–444.

Spoerl, O. H. Single session-psychotherapy. *Diseases of the Nervous System,* 1975, *36,* 283–285. (Abstract)

Sue, S., Allen, D. B., & Conaway, L. The responsiveness and equality of mental health care to Chicanos and Native Americans. *American Journal of Community Psychology,* 1978, *6,* 137–146.

Tannenbaum, S. A. Three brief psychoanalyses. *American Journal of Urology and Sexology,* 1919, *15,* 145–151.

Wolberg, L. R. The technic of short-term therapy. In L. R. Wolberg (Ed.), *Short-term psychotherapy.* New York: Grune & Stratton, 1965.

SECTION III
THEORETICAL ISSUES IN FORMS
OF BRIEF THERAPY

CHAPTER 8
TOWARD THE REFINEMENT
OF TIME-LIMITED DYNAMIC
PSYCHOTHERAPY

Hans H. Strupp

Short-term psychotherapy—and the subform, time-limited dynamic psychotherapy, which will be the primary focus of this chapter—is a product of our time, and the developments that will occur in this area in the foreseeable future are a reflection of society's current concerns: to evolve forms of treatment for specific disorders that are efficient, cost effective, and applicable to the largest possible number of patients. In other words, the developments that are being sought are technological; they are not principally aimed at the advancement of knowledge, such as the etiology of neurotic disorders, the basic ingredients of psychotherapy, and so on. Increments in scientific knowledge may, of course, occur as a result of improvements in technology, but they are clearly seen as secondary. Instead, the emphasis is pragmatic: "does it work?" not "why does it work?"

The distinction impresses me as important, because the contemporary thrust appears to be based on the assumption that available knowledge is sufficient to support technological developments. In my view, serious questions must be entertained whether this is, in fact, the case. It can be argued, of course, that the two positions are not mutually exclusive, and the history of science is replete with instances where attempted solutions to practical problems have given rise to significant advances in scientific knowledge. My concern is with the inordinate emphasis on technology, the furor with which "horse races" between seemingly divergent forms of psychotherapy are currently being implemented, and the relatively scant attention accorded the necessarily slow and painstaking efforts aimed at achieving a better understanding of the dynamic forces con-

HANS H. STRUPP. Department of Psychology, Vanderbilt University, Nashville, Tennessee.

fronting the psychotherapist. Modern psychotherapy, in general, has become or is threatening to become a field "in a hurry." It remains to be seen whether a more orderly, scientific development can be short-circuited or bypassed. My comments suggest that I have doubts on that score. The danger lies in the preoccupation with gimmicks rather than technologies that are based on solid knowledge and understanding.

In this chapter, I discuss a number of basic issues confronting psychotherapy. Whether or not they are explicitly recognized in technological developments, they are, nonetheless, real, and they will eventually have to be faced. In my view, it is unlikely that we shall achieve victories on the frontiers of technology without addressing ourselves to these core problems, which will remain with us. Nonetheless, time-limited dynamic psychotherapy may provide us with golden opportunities to examine in greater detail and depth why, in a given case, we succeed or fail and to open the doors to a better scientific understanding of the process of psychotherapy in general.

Let us start with the following questions: How can therapeutic outcomes be improved in the shortest possible time? There are several possible options:

1. We can select patients whose presenting difficulties and personality makeup is such that relatively minor interventions will guarantee good therapeutic results.
2. We can scale down the therapeutic goals we wish to achieve and declare that we shall be satisfied with relatively circumscribed improvements.
3. We can seek to improve the therapeutic technology, such that therapeutic change occurs more rapidly. A distinction must be made here between rapid improvement and lasting improvement. Furthermore, questions must be entertained as to whether a particular approach is humane, is in keeping with the patient's best interest (however this may be defined), is consonant with reasonable demands on the therapist (time, effort, commitment, etc.), and addresses other *practical considerations.*

If we examine the state of the art in time-limited dynamic psychotherapy (notably the work of Alexander & French, 1946; Davanloo, 1978; Malan, 1976a, 1979; Mann, 1973; and Sifneos, 1972, 1979), we find that major efforts in this area have been directed at the foregoing issues, and that solutions have been sought through a better alignment between patient selection, goals, and appropriate technology. In this chapter, I attempt to illuminate these issues in somewhat greater detail, particularly with reference to tasks to be accomplished in the future. Such an exploration may prove useful in highlighting the potentialities as well as the limits of time-limited dynamic psychotherapy and may help sharpen the thinking of the clinician and the researcher. It may lead to the implementation of much-needed empirical research, which may tell us more about who can help whom and how. Finally, it may enable us to provide legislators, policymakers, and the public at large with better and more precise information on what may be expected from psychotherapy under particular conditions. As we all know, the challenge is great.

PATIENT SELECTION

One of the notable ways in which modern proponents of time-limited dynamic psychotherapy have sought to improve therapeutic outcomes has been to select patients who are most likely to benefit from what the therapist has to offer. This approach follows the classical psychoanalytic tradition of a method in search of patients. Not surprisingly, the selection criteria formulated by contemporary workers in the time-limited area show a remarkable resemblance to those invoked by classical analysts (Bachrach & Leaff, 1978; Freud, 1905/1953, 1913/1958). It is well to remember here that Freud, in his earlier writings, viewed psychoanalysis as a last resort (1905/1953), and although his practice did not seem fully in keeping with his pronouncements on this subject, he defined the radius of psychoanalysis in rather narrow terms (the so-called transference neuroses) (1917/1958). Butcher and Koss (1978), in their admirable review of the literature, considered the following "types of patients" optimally suited for time-limited psychotherapy:

1. those in whom the behavioral problem is of acute onset
2. those whose previous adjustment has been good
3. those with a good ability to relate
4. those with high initial motivation

The foregoing variables are, of course, complex and far from independent. If one attempted to bring them under a common denominator, "strong ego resources" might be the most suitable term. This would include a relatively high level of emotional maturity, responsibility, autonomy, success in mastering and adapting to life's challenges (including stability in interpersonal relations), and ability and commitment to work collaboratively with a therapist, whose major tool is the facilitation of understanding and insight into intrapsychic conflicts. Conversely, patients who are unsuitable for time-limited dynamic psychotherapy can be characterized as showing profound dependency, persistent acting out (impulse disorders), self-centeredness, masochism, and self-destructiveness (Butcher & Koss, 1978, p. 739). In the Vanderbilt Project (Strupp & Hadley, 1979; Gomes-Schwartz, 1978), we identified additional contraindications: pervasive characterological disturbances, profound negativism, and rigidity. Our findings also lend weight to the overriding importance of motivation as a key variable (Keithly, Samples, & Strupp, 1980).

These criteria are obviously in need of further refinement, but our research provided strong evidence that the patient's suitability can be determined fairly readily in the first three interviews—and often in the course of a single assessment interview. If these results can be replicated, we might soon have a rather powerful tool for identifying those persons who are well suited for time-limited dynamic psychotherapy. Malan's (1976a) concept of a "focal conflict," which allows the formulation of a "dynamic focus" in therapy, appears to be another important criterion for patient selection.

We have, as yet, little evidence on the degree of departure from these criteria that can be tolerated before time-limited dynamic psychotherapy is definitely contraindicated, and it is clear that few patients are ideally suited on all counts. We must also be prepared to adduce further evidence to answer the criticism that (a) time-limited dynamic psychotherapy, as currently practiced, is appropriate only for a very small percentage of the total patient population, (b) the patients selected by these criteria might be the ones who improve "spontaneously" without therapeutic help, and (c) such patients may improve with almost any kind of therapeutic help (i.e., there is noting unique about time-limited dynamic psychotherapy that conduces to the improvement of such patients). In this connection, the finding from the Vanderbilt Project that the most suitable patients showed the greatest improvement when treated by a highly experienced professional therapist may suggest that optimal matching between patient and therapeutic method results in the greatest payoff. Conversely, neither experienced therapists nor untrained college professors were impressively successful with patients who fell short of the major selection criteria.

Among the key prognosticators for short-term therapy, acute onset appears to be the most controversial and perhaps the least important. It is reminiscent of a maladaptive stress response in a previously well functioning personality. It is quite plausible that such patients may be unsuitable on other grounds. Malan (1976b) provided evidence that acute onset is not necessarily a good prognostic sign. He also showed that persons with relatively severe character pathology may profit from time-limited psychotherapy, thus refuting the widely held misconception that time-limited psychotherapy is most helpful to those who may need it the least.

At the same time, one of the best established findings, corroborated in a number of the better studies, points to severity of the disturbance as one of the key variables for predicting success in almost any kind of psychotherapy, both time-limited and long-term. This result constitutes powerful evidence against the traditional claim of psychoanalysis that long-term, intensive psychotherapy can be instrumental in producing a radical reorganization of the personality. I know of no hard evidence that such reorganization occurs with a high degree of frequency. Obviously, this is not to say that it never occurs. The selection criteria traditionally invoked by psychoanalysts, however, probably contain a highly valid core. That core again points to the presence of a constellation of strong ego resources, which despite the presence of significant psychopathology, allow the patient to become engaged in a meaningful and productive relationship with a therapist, which, in turn, leads to significant amelioration.

One might say that good prognosis depends markedly on the extent to which a patient's difficulties are intrapsychic as opposed to "behavioral." That is, the best candidates for psychotherapy of all kinds are those individuals who suffer more or less silently while at the same time being able to discharge their day-to-day adult responsibilities. An unfortunate corollary of this hypothesis is that, by superficial standards, these patients also *appear* least disturbed. Conversely, those persons whose disturbance is of the impulse-dominated, acting-out variety are far more difficult to help via psychotherapy. Thus, we may have come full circle: psychotherapy is, indeed, what it originally was intended to be, namely, a treatment for basically intrapsychic disturbances. These disturbances obviously have their manifestations in the patient's intimate relationships with significant others, but they are not typically the kind of disorders of which society, rather than the patient, complains (e.g., antisocial behavior, drug addiction, delinquency, and the like).

Another critical implication of the selection criteria for time-limited psychotherapy is their striking lack of congruence with the diagnostic categories set forth in such systems as DSM-III. I believe it is highly significant that the clinical experience of time-limited dynamic psychotherapists points to the importance of "person" variables rather than "pathology" variables. Previous adjustment, ability to relate, and motivation are variables that point to particular personality organizations rather than to discrete symptoms or "disorders." By the same token, it is probably no accident that practitioners of time-limited psychotherapy have not focused on the development of specific treatments for depression, phobias, and the like. Instead, time-limited therapists seem to say that they can help individuals with particular kinds of personality structures, and that those with other kinds of personality organizations are more or less unsuitable.

To be sure, we need to explore much further what is meant by "more or less," but the thrust of the evidence throughout psychotherapy research strongly supports this viewpoint. Correspondingly, the beacon for future research points toward the identification of people with particular personality organizations rather than the treatment of specific disorders. This suggests that greater effort should be invested in studying which people rather than which disorders can be treated. To be sure, there tend to be certain correlations between the two; however, the direction of investigative work will be quite different, depending on which viewpoint one adopts. The findings of time-limited psychotherapy may prove a most important guide. As we shall see, there are also important implications for technique development in terms of the extent to which it is realistic and fruitful to devise specific techniques for specific disorders.

This point impresses me as so critical that I would like to highlight it from another perspective. What contemporary time-limited psychotherapists have done is to attempt an articulation between a particular form of diagnostic assessment and therapeutic operations; that is, they have begun to make clinical determinations that have a more or less direct bearing on what needs to be done in psychotherapy. Conversely, assessments of the degree, extent, and severity of a symptom (e.g., depression, anxiety, etc.) are static; they may serve to pigeonhole a patient for "statistical" purposes, an activity that may help insurance companies in determining a patient's eligibility for benefits, but they do not point to ways in which a therapist can help a patient via psychotherapy. We may need both static and dynamic assessments, perhaps to assess the locus and function of the patient's disturbance in his current adaptation; but from the standpoint of technique development in psychotherapy, dynamic assessments will be infinitely more useful. So far, we have made only modest strides in that direction, and much greater refinement of selection criteria, as well as studies to determine precisely where the dividing lines between suitability and unsuitability lie, are needed. There is no doubt in my mind, however, that this is the road we need to travel if psychotherapy is to become a more refined art and science.

THERAPEUTIC GOALS

Closely related to problems of patient selection is the stipulation of therapeutic goals. Again, this is an area in which clinical thinking and research are in need of much closer scrutiny by means of systematic research. In terms of selecting patients with impressive ego resources, it might be argued that the latter produce synergistic effects in the hands of a skillful therapist. In other words, the striving toward health in those patients who are judged as most suitable is so strong that impressive therapeutic results may be achieved with relatively little effort and in relatively short periods of time. Conversely, where a patient is markedly deficient in this area, either we will have to settle for much more modest achievements or the therapeutic effort will have to be intensified. With respect to the latter set of circumstances, this inevitably means longer periods of time.

The Vanderbilt Project again provides leads. We found that in the case of patients who were markedly hostile, negativistic, rigid, and resistant, none of the therapists—neither highly experienced professionals nor untrained college professors—was able to achieve impressive therapeutic results in 25 hours or less. To me, this signifies that, on the whole, therapeutic progress is severely circumscribed by the difficulties and obstacles posed by the patient's personality organization at the time of entering therapy. In much of the therapy literature, insufficient attention has been paid to the precise nature of the improvements achieved (or achievable) in a given unit of time. For example, if we are satisfied with a diminution of a patient's current depressive episode (measured by a drop in the MMPI D scale or similar measures), we have posited a very different goal than if we demand that sufficient reorganization of the personality should have occurred to lessen the likelihood of recurrences of depressive episodes. In short, symptom relief is a very different order of improvement than more pervasive personality reorganization.

The trouble is that we do not know exactly what the latter is. It could be asserted, perhaps with considerable validity, that symptom improvement almost always carries with it some degree of cognitive reorganization, and that improvements of all kinds must be reflected in some form of behavioral change. Stated otherwise, it is unlikely that improvement can be diagnosed in the absence of symptomatic and behavioral change. The distinction between "symptomatic improvement" and "character change" posited by classical psychoanalysis may be artificial. Again, we are faced with the extraordinary difficulties in measuring structural (intrapsychic) change in the absence of subjective and behavioral change. The former is always an inference from the latter, and apart from projective techniques which, at present, enjoy a low degree of popularity and credibility, I know of no highly satisfactory techniques which would allow us to reliably assess changes in personality organization.

We must also disabuse ourselves and our consumers of the notion that psychotherapy achieves cures "once and for all." All practicing clinicians have the experience of dealing with patients who, following a formal course of therapy, return at subsequent times in their lives to deal with difficulties that crop up as a result of new stresses. There are, in all of us, vulnerabilities and loci minoris resistentiae that may lead to the recrudescence of neurotic disturbances; in other words, a predisposition to neurotic disturbances may forever remain. This idea has already been enunciated by Freud (1937/1964) in "Analysis Terminable and Interminable," but I believe it has not been taken sufficiently seriously. I would strongly resist the allegation that patients of this kind are "failures."

We have not yet succeeded, however, in developing good indices that would allow us to assess that significant progress has been made, even though the patient may return at a later point for further therapeutic help. Somehow, we must develop better measures of adaptive functioning, which is not synonymous with the total absence of symptoms and invariably must differ from individual to individual. Nonetheless, I believe that the task is not insuperable. There are some reasonable practical indicators that might be adapted for this purpose. At the same time, I believe that we should not rest content with some minor improvements in functioning, The point is how to make these differentiations. When is an improvement a "real" improvement, and when is it an insignificant or transient change? These are real and important issues for time-limited psychotherapy as well as for any other form. To reiterate, our thinking on this point has been far from clear, with the result that outcome statistics may convey a misleading picture.

THERAPEUTIC TECHNOLOGY

The major objective of time-limited dynamic psychotherapists has been to adapt the therapeutic technology to the achievement of appropriate objectives. This has meant refining and sharpening the technology, a goal which, of course, also has broad implications for psychotherapy in general. It may be said that time-limited psychotherapy provides a unique proving ground for testing the efficacy and utility of techniques, something that is difficult to accomplish in open-ended approaches. Thus, it is no accident that innovations and experimentation with techniques have occurred chiefly in time-limited approaches. The research potential of time-limited psychotherapy, in this regard, is a fairly recent realization, and contemporary research on therapeutic techniques has found time-limited approaches particularly congenial and germane to systematic testing. To carry out the necessary tasks, close attention must be paid to the therapeutic process and the variables affecting it. As elsewhere in psychotherapy research, progress has been severely hampered by the crudeness of available tools to assess pertinent process variables. Nonetheless, advances have occurred, and we may look forward with considerable confidence to future developments.

In this connection, it is important to note that process research must be linked to outcome and cannot meaningfully be conducted in the absence of suitable outcome measures. To this end, we must, as a minimum, have complete process records as well as outcome measures. The latter provide important anchors for exploring whether particular process variables are meaningfully related to outcome. This strategy has been followed in several recent outcome studies, including the Temple study (Sloane, Staples, Cristol, Yorkston, & Whipple, 1975) and the Vanderbilt Psychotherapy Project (Strupp & Hadley, 1979).

As we have seen, even without tampering with the therapeutic technology, it is possible to improve therapy outcomes by selecting appropriate patients and delimiting therapeutic goals. In some sense, these stipulations may be seen as artificial, because, in themselves, they do not address the question of whether refinements in therapeutic technique produce better results. On the other hand, they can be viewed as genuine advances, because they are realistic attempts to determine the potentialities and limits of psychotherapy. In this respect, they are no different from exploring systematically under what conditions a particular drug or a surgical procedure is appropriate and effective. On the whole, such developments have been too slow in coming in psychotherapy, although they are precisely the direction in which the field must move.

Another logical move for improving therapeutic outcomes is to examine the technology itself for the purpose of achieving possible refinements. Major areas of possible technological advances seem to fall under the following rubrics, all of which are, of course, closely related to the therapist's attitude, stance, and activity: (1) management of the patient–therapist relationship, which subsumes issues of transference and countertransference, and (2) technical interventions, which include primarily interpretive activities (addressed often to a "dynamic focus"). I shall omit from consideration the setting of time limits, a maneuver which, in a number of studies, has been shown to accelerate therapeutic progress in itself.

MANAGEMENT OF THE PATIENT–THERAPIST RELATIONSHIP

The importance of focusing on the therapeutic relationship has been stressed since Freud's (1911–1915/1958) writings on technique. Indeed, Freud (1917/1958) stated forcefully that therapeutic progress occurs solely and uniquely through the patient's relationship to the therapist. Nonetheless, the bulk of the literature has been concerned with the technical management of the transference, that is, the patient's relationship to the therapist, rather than the interactional system. The fact that countertransference has been recognized as a weighty problem since 1910 does not mitigate this fact.

Only in relatively recent years has there been a resurgence of interest in the "therapeutic alliance" or "working alliance," particularly in the writings of Greenson (1967), who set the stage for the newer emphasis on what might be called a systems approach. Thus, it is characteristic of the literature on time-limited dynamic psychotherapy that major emphasis has been accorded the technical management of the transference and the nature of the therapist's interpretive activity. This emphasis on technical management is also manifest in the behaviorally oriented literature (e.g., Beck's, 1976, cognitive therapy). By its very nature, it tends to deemphasize the therapist's attitudes and stance at the expense of technical considerations.

In the following discussion, I propose to follow an approach that stresses the interactive aspects of the patient–therapist relationship. Within that context, particularly the quality of the relationship, technical features may exert a facilitative, perhaps even a synergistic, effect. As I have maintained for a number of years, however, technique, in and of itself, remains inert. I base my adoption of this position on accumulating research evidence—for example, the Temple Study (Sloane *et al.,* 1975), the Menninger Project (Kernberg, Burstein, Coyne, Appelbaum, Horwitz, & Voth, 1972), the Tavistock Studies (Malan, 1976a, 1976b), and the Vanderbilt Psychotherapy Project (Strupp & Hadley, 1979)—which has shown that the quality of patient–therapist interaction represents the fulcrum upon which therapeutic progress turns. The second source of evidence derives from the finding that, with very few exceptions, no specific techniques have been shown to be singularly effective (Bergin & Lambert, 1978; Frank, 1979).

The quality of the therapeutic relationship, as we were able to show, depends heavily on *(a)* the patient's character makeup, motivation, and readiness to enter and participate in a therapeutic relationship of a particular type (i.e., the kind offered by a particular therapist), and *(b)* the therapist's ability to capitalize on the patient's qualities just enumerated. In practice, the latter means a certain flexibility of approach, empathy, and skill in contributing to the formation of a productive therapeutic alliance; most importantly, it means the therapist's ability to control and effectively channel his or her countertransference reactions. In addition to this ability to neutralize the patient's negative transference (hostility, negativism, resistance, and other obstacles which are part and parcel of the patient's problems), the therapist must also be able to resist his or her own ambition, which may be manifested by a furor sanandi, a tendency to mount frontal attacks on the patient's defenses, and impatience with what the therapist may experience as slow progress.

THE ROLE OF INTERPRETATION

Interpretive activity has been one of the major emphases of time-limited dynamic therapists. Sifneos (1972) stressed interpretations of Oedipal conflicts; Malan (1976a, 1976b) gave great weight to interpretations linking the conflicts which come alive in the patient–therapist relationship to the patient's parent figures; Mann (1973) placed interpretations dealing with separation in the forefront of his scheme; and Davanloo (1978) advocated frontal attacks on obsessional defenses. To a greater or lesser extent, all these activities presuppose the identification of a "dynamic focus" or a "core conflictual theme" (Luborsky, 1977). In other words, it seems clear that any interpretive activity can become effective only to the extent that a conflict becomes "alive" in the transference, that is, sufficient affect has been mobilized, and the patient is actively struggling with a painful conflict in the here and now.

This requirement cannot be overemphasized, because it relates crucially to what every therapist knows—the *timing* of an interpretation. Unless the timing is right, interpretations have no more effect upon producing a dynamic reorganization of a cognitive–affective structure than reading a menu satisfies a starved person. I place so much emphasis on these facts because they appear to have weighty implications for what might be done to accelerate progress in time-limited therapy (or any other form) and the obstacles impeding progress. I perceive the following issues:

Context versus Content

Although the proponents of different approaches to time-limited dynamic psychotherapy have made claims for the unique effectiveness of particular kinds of interpretations, there is, as yet, no convincing evidence that such specific classes of interpretations (or, for that matter, any other technical maneuver) produce *unique* therapeutic results. These findings might be coupled with a previously cited result from the Vanderbilt Project, that professional therapists appeared to be particularly effective (more effective than untrained counselors) with patients possessing the highest levels of ego resources, including motivation. On the other hand, none of the therapists (either experienced professionals or lay counselors) was notably effective with patients showing marked resistance, negativism, rigidity, and hostility. This suggests that the effectiveness of dynamically oriented time-limited psychotherapy does not depend upon particular *kinds* of interpretations offered by the therapist, but rather upon the *quality* of the therapeutic relationship existing between the two participants.

The latter is a reasonably well documented finding also obtained by other investigators. It may be possible, however, to specify its significance more sharply: Interpretive activity of a particular kind may be notably effective, provided there exists a good therapeutic alliance, which, in turn, is determined by particular qualities preexisting in the patient and coming to fruition in the therapeutic process. Stated somewhat differently, interpretations of a particular kind may be highly effective, provided they happen to be the kind of interventions that appeal and make sense to the patient and to which he or she can positively resonate.

In this connection, it is important to mention that in the Vanderbilt

Project, therapists tended to be relatively invariant in their use of techniques (Strupp, 1980). Again, this means that if the patient was able to "use" the therapist's particular interpretive approach, therapeutic movement occurred. If, on the other hand, the therapist's approach remained alien to the patient, if resistances and other impediments in his psychological makeup prevented him from taking advantage of what the therapist had to offer, the effect of interpretations or similar activities was essentially nil.

To reiterate, I continue to be skeptical that particular kinds of interpretations per se exert a mutative effect; instead, they are effective if, like a piece in a jigsaw puzzle, they happen to constitute an important missing piece. This is not to say that one interpretation is as good as another (e.g., whether it deals with current interpersonal relationships or a classic childhood conflict), but it does say that, first and foremost, it must be personally meaningful to the patient in the context of the cognitive and affective constellation of the particular moment in therapy.

Technical Flexibility

Proponents of time-limited psychotherapy have traditionally stressed the need for flexibility on the therapist's part. In the Vanderbilt Project, we found little evidence that such flexibility existed in our therapists; on the contrary, their approach tended to be rather rigid. We can only speculate whether therapists in general possess the kind of "flexibility" apparently demanded by short-term approaches. It is more likely that some degree of flexibility exists in most therapists, but it may not be nearly as great as one might like to believe. The term "flexibility," of course, is in need of better definition.

One of the questions raised is the extent to which individual therapists can adopt a "special" therapeutic stance (even if it were clearly indicated on technical grounds) without sacrificing their authenticity, ceasing to be spontaneous, and becoming "gimmicky," none of which may remain hidden from sensitive patients. I believe that there is a distinct affinity between therapist and technique, and it is no accident that particular therapeutic approaches are uniquely congenial to particular therapists. If this is so, one might ask if it is possible for a therapist, who, for example, has gravitated toward a therapeutic model in which the gradual emergence of latent themes is stressed, to comfortably adopt the role of, say, a "relentless therapist" who mounts frontal attacks upon a patient's characterological defenses. Can the same therapist make "homework assignments," require patients to keep diaries of behavioral events, and so on? I do not pretend to know the answer, but I wonder whether therapists are not at their therapeutic best if they follow a technical approach that is maximally congenial to their own personality style. I do not wish to be misunderstood as advocating that the therapist should, without training or extensive clinical knowledge, do "what comes naturally," but it does seem that there should be a harmonious marriage between the therapist's personality makeup and the techniques he or she uses. Furthermore, interpretations must be anchored in, and emerge from, the therapist as a total human being rather than a therapeutic machine.

Person–Technique Blend

The foregoing considerations have important implications for the practice of time-limited dynamic psychotherapy. In light of the preceding exposition, I wish to advance the hypothesis that the time-limited therapists whose writing are currently in vogue are largely and perhaps predominantly successful not so much because of the particular kinds of interpretations they use (and consider uniquely effective), but rather because their particular personalities and the technique they have evolved constitute a special blend which works because these therapists are the kinds of people they are. Add to this the finding that the therapist's enthusiasm (plus, undoubtedly, his or her commitment) conduces to better results, and one arrives at the conclusion that the effects of therapy are a function not of the techniques per se, but rather of the unique constellation consisting of the therapist-as-a-person-in-conjunction-with-certain-techniques.

If this is so, we are faced with the thorny question concerning the extent to which particular techniques are teachable to others whose philosophy and personality makeup may be different from that of the originator of the system. The answer seems to be that just as certain patients benefit peculiarly from certain techniques, if the latter happen to coincide with what they need and find congenial, so particular therapists tend to gravitate toward certain therapeutic approaches for much the same reasons. Thus, there are distinct limitations with respect to the kinds and numbers of therapists who can be trained in a particular approach.

Having said this, I believe it is important to counteract the possible impression that technical developments in time-limited psychotherapy are foredoomed. This has been the problem of classical analysis. Because of the unfounded belief that the "classical model" was immutable, very little experimentation with technical alternatives occurred for many years, and

Alexander's (Alexander & French, 1946) attempts in this direction were greeted with a fair degree of hostility. Although there appear to be clear limits to what interpretations (and other techniques) may accomplish, it does not follow that *no* technical developments should occur, nor does it follow that therapists should allow themselves the luxury—society no longer does!—of waiting for the "right" patient to come along, that is, one who fits a rigid technical model.

Progress in technique development has also been retarded because many therapists have adopted a totally open-ended stance, which seemed to say that sooner or later, something of therapeutic value may transpire without the therapist doing much to hasten its occurrence. It is in this area that time-limited therapists have made significant contributions that merit further development. Such efforts will produce a sharper delineation of which patients can be helped by particular therapists who have been trained along particular lines. In the concluding section, therefore, I attempt to spell out, as clearly as possible, the directions in which the field must move for progress to occur.

FUTURE DIRECTIONS

In order to clarify my points, I would like to introduce a schematic presentation which, needless to say, should not be taken literally. Figure 1, parts A and B, summarizes major results of the research literature presented in the preceding section:

A1: Patient's Ego Resources Strong—Resistances Relatively Weak. Provided the patient possesses strong ego resources (including successful adaptation to life, high motivation for therapy, ability to become engaged in a collaborative relationship with a psychodynamically oriented therapist) and character resistances and distortions that are not too severe, the therapeutic outcome will generally be good. The diagram is designed to suggest that in this case, the therapist's human qualities (empathy, commitment, warmth, etc.), as well as specific technical skills, play a relatively minor role, as long as certain minimal requirements are met and the therapist is generally constructive and not psychonoxious. One qualification may be noted: therapists functioning at a high level, that is, those who are able to bring to bear an optimal combination of human qualities and therapeutic skills, achieve particularly impressive results with such patients. In this case, the therapist's skills seem to exert a synergistic effect. This is the

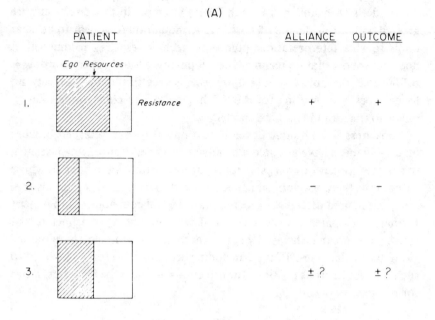

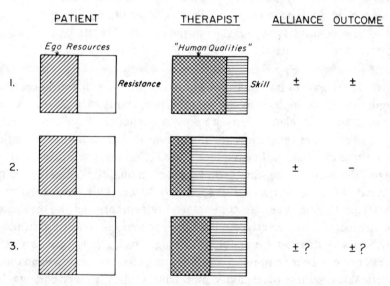

FIGURE 1. *Major determinants of outcome in time-limited psychotherapy.*

select group of patients who do well in short-term dynamic therapy of the kind advocated, for example, by Sifneos (1972, 1979).

A2: Patient's Ego Resources Weak—Resistances Strong. Based on adverse childhood experiences with significant adults (Strupp, 1972), such patients have difficulty in forming a productive therapeutic alliance, regardless of the therapist's human qualities and technical skills, and the outcome will generally be poor. These are not promising candidates for time-limited dynamic therapy. The reason is that unfortunate life-experiences have exerted a severe crippling effect on the character structure of such patients, and impressive short-term results are not to be expected. Falling into this category are schizoid characters, borderline conditions, and the wide range of patients suffering from problems in the area of impulse control. While one may expect that some of these patients can benefit from long-term, intensive psychotherapy, the available empirical evidence does not justify strong conclusions.

A3: Patient's Ego Resources Moderate—Resistances Moderate. From the standpoint of the clinician and researcher, these are the most challenging patients, who incidentally make up a sizable proportion of the patient pool. They represent a largely understudied and underresearched population, and in my view, this is where future clinical and research efforts should be concentrated.

Consequently, Figure 1, part B, presents an elaboration of the research possibilities suggested by this patient group. It will be noted that the patient characteristics remain constant, and the outcome is determined by factors relating to the therapist and the therapeutic alliance.

B1: Therapist's Human Qualities High—Technical Skill Low. These therapists are well exemplified by the college professors participating in the Vanderbilt Psychotherapy Project. With patients presenting moderate characterological disturbances and having relatively unimpressive ego resources, these therapists achieved only modest therapeutic results. Nonetheless, the outcomes were no worse than those obtained by highly experienced and skilled professional psychotherapists. Relative beginners (e.g., residents, graduate students in clinical psychology) might be expected to do equally well with such patients. What these therapists may lack in formal training may be compensated for by commitment to the patient and enthusiasm (Malan, 1963).

B2: Therapist's Human Qualities Low—Technical Skill High. This combination results in poor therapeutic results and may present the greatest risks for negative (psychonoxious) effects. It is exemplified by a sizable group of therapists who have undergone through training but who, for various reasons, are unable to invest significantly of themselves in the therapeutic task. They may actively dislike the patient, consider therapy routine or a "business," adhere slavishly to a set of techniques, and be insufficiently sensitive and responsive to the patient's psychological needs. (For other examples, see Hadley & Strupp, 1976.)

B3: Therapist's Human Qualities Moderate—Technical Skill Moderate. This combination represents probably the most common situation in clinical practice. A therapist of average professional competence and average "human qualities" is confronted with patients who fall short of optimal suitability for time-limited forms of psychotherapy. Paradoxically, while these individuals are in the greatest need of professional services, they are also the ones who have been most neglected by mental health professionals (Rabkin, 1977). This judgment applies with particular force to time-limited dynamic psychotherapy, which has traditionally focused on the selection and treatment of the most promising candidates (Butcher & Koss, 1978). It is noteworthy in this regard that the extensive contemporary literature dealing with borderline conditions and narcissistic personality disorders is almost entirely devoted to long-term intensive therapy (e.g., Giovacchini, 1979; Kernberg, 1975; Kohut, 1971). An exception is Malan, who has attempted to treat more "difficult" patients in time-limited dynamic psychotherapy.

It should be clear from the foregoing discussion that the most important challenge facing time-limited dynamic psychotherapy entails systematic exploration of the extent to which patients of greater than average difficulty (i.e., individuals with moderately severe resistances and characterological distortions) can be treated by time-limited methods. In these instances, the outcome depends, to a very significant degree, on the therapist—his or her human qualities and skills in achieving particular therapeutic objectives. Accordingly, attention must focus on the therapist, and we must examine what measures might be taken to forge a more potent therapeutic instrument, by which I always mean the therapist's personality in combination with his or her techniques. Based on accumulating research evidence and clinical experience, the following avenues, in combination, appear to be the most promising:

- Techniques should be optimally geared to the achievement of reasonably specific therapeutic objectives identified early in the course of treatment.

- The therapeutic situation should be designed to meet the unique needs of the individual patient, as opposed to the tacit assumption that the patient conform to the therapist's notions of an "ideal" therapeutic framework. Techniques should be applied flexibly, sensitively, and in ways maximally meaningful to the patient.
- Steps should be taken to foster a good therapeutic relationship (working alliance) from the beginning of therapy, thus enhancing the patient's active participation and creating a sense of collaboration and partnership.
- Negative transference reactions should be actively confronted at the earliest possible time.
- Concerted efforts should be made to help therapists deal with negative personal reactions, which are characteristically engendered by patients manifesting hostility, anger, negativism, rigidity, and similar resistance.
- While time-limited psychotherapy poses particular challenges to all therapists (especially demands for greater activity and directiveness), they should resist the temptation to persuade the patient to accept a particular "solution," impose their values, and in other respects diminish the patient's strivings for freedom and autonomy.
- Rather than viewing psychotherapy predominantly as a set of "technical operations" applied in a vacuum, therapists must be sensitive to the importance of the human elements in all therapeutic encounters. In other words, unless the therapist takes an interest in the patient as a person and succeeds in communicating this interest and commitment, psychotherapy becomes a caricature of a good human relationship (the ultimate negative effect!).
- Closely related to the foregoing, therapists should keep in mind that all good therapeutic experiences lead to increments in the patient's self-acceptance and self-respect; consequently, continual care must be taken to promote such experiences and to guard against interventions that might have opposite effects.

My proposal is to implement a specialized training program for professional psychotherapists (i.e., individuals who have already acquired a reasonable level of expertise), in which the foregoing points will receive systematic attention. In developing this program, I am proceeding from the hypothesis (which I plan to test empirically) that in therapeutic work with particular patients, a competent therapist, who possesses appropriate personal qualities and has mastered the principles and techniques outlined above, will achieve better treatment results than a comparable person without such specialized training. In advancing this hypothesis, I am not asserting that either a set of techniques described in the abstract or a patient population defined largely in terms of a presenting symptom (e.g., phobias) is superior to a "general" therapeutic approach: this line of research has proved disappointing (Parloff, 1979). Instead, I propose that a relatively specific treatment approach, one which is aimed at a stringently defined target population and takes careful account of technical problems that arise in the patient–therapist interaction (Burke, White, & Havens, 1979), holds considerable promise. In broader terms, I believe that the future of psychotherapy rests with the growing refinement of clinical practice. Conversely, I judge that the relatively meager evidence for the effectiveness of psychotherapy as a generic treatment modality is largely a function of poor alignment (matching) between important patient and therapist characteristics, the lack of clearly formulated treatment objectives, and the more or less indiscriminate application of diverse techniques (Bergin & Lambert, 1978; Strupp, 1978).

The proposed treatment approach comprises a series of integrated elements which are schematically presented in Table 1. These elements have been distilled from (1) the findings of the Vanderbilt Psychotherapy Research Project, (2) the literature on short-term dynamic psychotherapy, and (3) contemporary trends in psychotherapy research and practice. I believe that the uniqueness of the proposed approach lies in the integration of principles and techniques that offer the greatest promise at the present state of knowledge.

In conclusion, I propose to explore the frontiers of time-limited dynamic psychotherapy with the view toward examining its potential and limitations. It is my contention that we have not gone far enough in this endeavor, nor has the research been nearly as systematic as it might have been. When all is said and done, I believe we shall find that there are definite limits to what time-limited dynamic psychotherapy (or, for that matter, any form of psychotherapy) can accomplish, and that outcomes depend importantly on patient selection, the goals to which the therapist (and the patient) aspire, and the nature of the therapeutic changes the therapist is able to engender. With regard to the latter, I reject the notion of the therapist as an "influencing machine," nor have I much faith that "treatment manuals" will significantly further our objectives. Rather, I view therapeutic change as a process that usually proceeds at a relatively

TABLE 1. *Salient Features of Proposed Treatment Approach*

	Element	Comment
Patient population	Specific, replicable patient population; psychiatric condition with presumably homogeneous dynamic basis (avoidant personality disorder)	Usually not specified in short-term dynamic therapy
Patient selection	Careful selection and assessment; patient must have good adaptive resources and capacities, yet need not be "ideal" candidate for short-term dynamic therapy; recognition that most patients have "character" problems and that isolated neurotic conflicts in a largely "healthy" personality are very rare; patient must have reasonable motivation for therapy (range of suitability specified)	Usually a narrow band of "ideal" candidates is selected
Link between assessment and therapy	Definition of dynamic focus and formulation of therapeutic goals; therapy geared to specified goals (therapeutic plan)	Advocated by Alexander and French (1946), Malan (1976a), and Sifneos (1972)
Goals	Symptomatic as well as characterological change	Usual emphasis is on symptomatic improvement
Pretraining	Enhancement of patient's motivation and preparation for therapy through role induction	Not usually done in a systematic way; considered promising (Strupp & Bloxom, 1973)
Contract	Based on formulation of goals, contract is negotiated with patient (dynamic focus, however, is not necessarily shared with patient)	Not usually done; considered promising
Time limits	Up to 40 hours to permit more intensive therapeutic effort aimed at character change	Advocated by Malan (1976a)
Technique Therapist activity	Fairly active; insight through "here and now" interpretations; enhancement of patient's autonomy; firm control and guidance of therapy without frontal attack on defenses; systematic emphasis on quality of patient-therapist interaction	Deemphasis on therapist's "charismatic qualities"

(continued)

TABLE 1. *(continued)*

	Element	Comment
Therapeutic alliance	Early formation crucial; stress on therapist's empathy	Systematic emphasis considered highly promising
Management of transference	Crucial, particularly confrontation of negative elements; stress on early attention to problem	Not usually done
Consultation	Periodic review of therapeutic progress, focus, and specific problems by therapist in consultations with a group of experienced clinicians	Not usually done
Deemphasis of specific techniques	Main techniques consist of questioning, clarification, interpretation, yet no claims made that single techniques are uniquely effective (see below)	Most approaches unduly emphasize specific techniques
Curative factors (Marmor, 1976; Frank, 1971; Strupp, 1976)	1. Patient–therapist relationship (alliance) 2. Corrective emotional experience 3. Cognitive learning (interpretation) 4. Suggestion and persuasion 5. Identification with therapist 6. Mastery and competence through success experience	See preceding comment. In my view, therapeutic learning occurs on a broad front in which common factors are important; therefore, efforts should be made to enhance the effect of these influences.

slow pace. This is because therapeutic change coincides with the patient's personal maturation, which cannot be significantly hastened, and which follows laws whose basic characteristics are, as yet, poorly understood. If we, as therapists, approach our task with the proper humility and respect for another human being, however, if we can listen and fathom the meanings of the patient's latent schemata, if we can be good role models of maturity ourselves, if we can successfully deal with our own shortcomings and conflicts, and if—a big if!— we can mesh the foregoing requirements with broad clinical knowledge and experience, we will have gone as far as is humanly possible in helping our patients. That, I submit, will be no trivial accomplishment.

REFERENCES

Alexander, F., & French, T. M. *Psychoanalytic therapy: Principles and applications.* New York: Ronald Press, 1946.

Bachrach, H. M., & Leaff, L. A. Analyzability: A systematic review of the clinical and quantitative literature. *Journal of the American Psychoanalytic Association,* 1978, *26,* 881–920.

Beck, A. T. *Cognitive therapy and the emotional disorders.* New York: International Universities Press, 1976.

Bergin, A. E., & Lambert, M. J. The evaluation of therapeutic outcomes. In S. L. Garfield & A. E. Bergin (Eds.), *Handbook of psychotherapy and behavior change* (2nd ed.). New York: Wiley, 1978.

Burke, J. D., White, H. S., & Havens, L. L. Which short-term therapy? Matching patient and method. *Archives of General Psychiatry,* 1979, *36,* 177–186.

Butcher, J. N., & Koss, M. P. Research on brief and crisis oriented therapies. In S. L. Garfield & A. E. Bergin (Eds.), *Handbook of psychotherapy and behavior change* (2nd ed.). New York: Wiley, 1978.

Davanloo, H. (Ed.). *Basic principles and techniques in short-term dynamic psychotherapy.* New York: Spectrum Press, 1978.

Frank, J. D. Therapeutic factors in psychotherapy. *American Journal of Psychotherapy,* 1971, *25,* 350–361.

Frank, J. D. The present status of outcome studies. *Journal of Consulting and Clinical Psychology,* 1979, *47,* 310–316.

Freud, S. On psychotherapy. In J. Strachey (Ed.), *Standard edition of the complete psychological works of Sigmund Freud* (Vol. 7). London: Hogarth Press, 1953. (Originally published, 1905.)

Freud, S. On beginning the treatment. In J. Strachey (Ed.), *Standard edition of the complete psychological works of Sigmund Freud* (Vol. 12). London: Hogarth Press, 1958. (Originally published, 1913.)

Freud, S. Papers on technique. In J. Strachey (Ed.), *Standard edition of the complete psychological works of Sigmund Freud* (Vol. 12). London: Hogarth Press, 1958. (Originally published, 1911–1915.)

Freud, S. Transference. In J. Strachey (Ed.), *Standard edition of the complete psychological works of Sigmund Freud* (Vol. 16). London: Hogarth Press, 1958. (Originally published, 1917.)

Freud, S. Analysis terminable and interminable. In J. Strachey (Ed.), *Standard edition of the complete psychological works of Sigmund Freud* (Vol. 23). London: Hogarth Press, 1964. (Originally published, 1937.)

Giovacchini, P. *Treatment of primitive mental states.* New York: Jason Aronson, 1979.

Gomes-Schwartz, B. Effective ingredients in psychotherapy: Prediction of outcome from process variables. *Journal of Consulting and Clinical Psychology,* 1978, *46,* 1023–1035.

Greenson, R. R. *The technique and practice of psychoanalysis* (Vol. 1). New York: International Universities Press, 1967.

Hadley, S. W., & Strupp, H. H. Contemporary views of negative effects in psychotherapy: An integrated account. *Archives of General Psychiatry,* 1976, *33,* 1291–1302.

Keithly, L. H., Samples, S. J., & Strupp, H. H. Patient motivation as a predictor of process and outcome in psychotherapy. *Psychotherapy and Psychosomatics,* 1980, *33,* 87–97.

Kernberg, O. F. *Borderline conditions and pathological narcissism.* New York: Jason Aronson, 1975.

Kernberg, O. F., Burstein, E. D., Coyne, L., Appelbaum, A., Horwitz, L., & Voth, H. *Psychotherapy and psychoanalysis: Final report of the Menninger Foundation's psychotherapy research project*. Topeka: Menninger Foundation, 1972.

Kohut, H. *The analysis of the self*. New York: International Universities Press, 1971.

Luborsky, L. Measuring a pervasive psychic structure in psychotherapy: The core conflictual relationship theme. In N. Freedman (Ed.), *Communication structures and psychic structures*. New York: Plenum Press, 1977.

Malan, D. H. *The study of brief psychotherapy*. New York: Plenum Press, 1963.

Malan, D. H. *The frontier of brief psychotherapy*. New York: Plenum Press, 1976. (a)

Malan, D. H. *Toward the validation of dynamic psychotherapy*. New York: Plenum Press, 1976. (b)

Malan, D. H. *Individual psychotherapy and the science of psychodynamics*. Woburn, Mass.: Butterworths, 1979.

Mann, J. *Time-limited psychotherapy*. Cambridge: Harvard University Press, 1973.

Marmor, J. Common operational factors in diverse approaches to behavior change. In A. Burton (Ed.), *What makes behavior change possible?* New York: Brunner/Mazel, 1976.

Parloff, M. B. Can psychotherapy research guide the policy maker? A little knowledge may be a dangerous thing. *American Psychologist*, 1979, *34*, 296-306.

Rabkin, J. G. Therapists' attitudes toward mental illness and health. In A. S. Gurman & A. R. Razin (Eds.), *Effective psychotherapy: A handbook of research*. New York: Pergamon Press, 1977.

Sifneos, P. E. *Short-term psychotherapy and emotional crisis*. Cambridge: Harvard University Press, 1972.

Sifneos, P. E. *Short-term psychotherapy: Evaluation and technique*. New York: Plenum Press, 1979.

Sloane, R. B., Staples, F. R., Cristol, A. H., Yorkston, N. J., & Whipple, K. *Psychotherapy versus behavior therapy*. Cambridge: Harvard University Press, 1975.

Strupp, H. H. On the technology of psychotherapy. *Archives of General Psychiatry*, 1972, *26*, 270-278.

Strupp, H. H. The nature of the therapeutic influence and its basic ingredients. In A. Burton (Ed.), *What makes behavior change possible?* New York: Brunner/Mazel, 1976.

Strupp, H. H. Psychotherapy research and practice: An overview. In S. L. Garfield & A. E. Bergin (Eds.), *Handbook of psychotherapy and behavior change: An empirical analysis* (2nd ed.). New York: Wiley, 1978.

Strupp, H. H. Success and failure in time-limited psychotherapy: A systematic comparison of two cases. *Archives of General Psychiatry*, 1980, *37*, 595-603.

Strupp, H. H., & Bloxom, A. L. Preparing lower-class patients for group psychotherapy: Development and evaluation of a role-induction film. *Journal of Consulting and Clinical Psychology*, 1973, *41*, 373-384.

Strupp, H. H., & Hadley, S. W. Specific versus nonspecific factors in psychotherapy: A controlled study of outcome. *Archives of General Psychiatry*, 1979, *36*, 1125-1136.

CHAPTER 9
CHOOSING A METHOD OF SHORT-TERM THERAPY: A DEVELOPMENTAL APPROACH

Henry S. White
Jack D. Burke, Jr.
Leston L. Havens

INTRODUCTION

In recent years, a number of methods of short-term, individual dynamic psychotherapy have been introduced. These methods differ significantly in their techniques and in the types of problems or conflicts which are used as the foci of the therapy. They include the interpretive method, based on vigorous interpretation of Oedipal conflicts, the empathic method, based on a brief, empathic encounter with the patient around the experience of loss, and the corrective method, based on the therapist's use of suggestion and transference management.

Because of the important technical differences among the methods, we suggest there may be types of patients for whom a particular method would be especially useful. Such a schema for matching method and patient would permit a therapist to take full advantage of the technical distinctions.

Furthermore, we suggest that a schema based on adult developmental stages integrates these schools of short-term work and provides a way of testing and determining their areas of application. We have chosen a developmental schema (rather than, for example, a diagnostic one), because

HENRY S. WHITE. Department of Psychiatry, Harvard Medical School at the Massachusetts Mental Health Center, Boston, Massachusetts.

JACK D. BURKE, JR. Applied Biometrics Research Branch, Division of Biometry and Epidemiology, National Institute of Mental Health, Bethesda, Maryland.

LESTON L. HAVENS. Department of Psychiatry, Harvard Medical School at the Massachusetts Mental Health Center, Boston, Massachusetts.

many of the methods of short-term dynamic psychotherapy easily formulate themselves in these terms: there is a striking congruence between the foci of the different methods and the developmental tasks of the different stages of adult life. In addition, the effectiveness of short-term work can best be seen, perhaps, as helping patients over developmental impasses rather than "curing" individuals or producing profound character changes, unless such changes are a function of development.

Without a way to choose among the different short-term schools, a therapist may try to fit the patient to the method rather than the method to the patient. A therapist following this procedure runs the risk of committing what we have called the "fallacy of misplaced objectivity" (Burke, White, & Havens, 1979). That is, the therapist might assume that the patient's apparent pathology exists independently, as an objective fact, and might assume that the therapist's perception of the patient is not influenced by preconceptions or expectations the therapist has. In this way, the therapist who preselects the method might find the patient suitable to a certain chosen method only by the process of finding in the patient what is expected or wished for. With a broader horizon and an orderly way to choose among many different methods based on a prior assessment of the patient, a more appropriate match between patient and method may be possible.

We begin the chapter with a description of three different methods of short-term dynamic psychotherapy, emphasizing their differences in technique and choice of focus. In the second part, we present the principal features of the currently hypothesized developmental stages of adult life, stressing those aspects which appear to have clinical relevance. Finally, we indicate the method of short-term work which appears to fit best with the developmental stage.

APPROACHES TO SHORT-TERM DYNAMIC PSYCHOTHERAPY

Writers approaching short-term therapy from a psychoanalytic background have generally assumed that they need to narrow the scope of work for therapy. Typically, they have done this by focusing on a characteristic problem which they find in some patients and which they assume is due to a particular underlying conflict. This effort to set an agenda is sometimes done explicitly with the patient and at other times is only implicit. In either case, it represents a noticeable departure from the open-ended approach of long-term psychoanalytic psychotherapy.

Focusing therapeutic attention on a characteristic problem has a possible consequence which we want to consider. If the problem to be addressed has an association with a particular type of unresolved conflict, it seems reasonable to expect that there is a particular therapeutic technique suited to dealing with the problem. In fact, we believe that each of the short-term methods does rely on a characteristic technique. In this section, we will examine the methods of therapy developed by major writers, describing the problems they treat and the characteristic modification of psychoanalytic technique which they make to sharpen their approach to that problem. The following summary represents a condensation of our previous work (Burke *et al.*, 1979) describing the differences between the methods.

The interpretive approach, as described by Sifneos (1973, 1979), is used in high-functioning patients. The characteristic problem addressed by this method is the patient's frustration in attaining satisfactory intimacy and companionship in a heterosexual relationship. The goal of therapy is to have the patient understand the connection between this current problem and the underlying Oedipal fantasies and conflicts. To provide this understanding, the therapist relies on vigorous interpretive techniques as an "unemotionally involved teacher."

We shall describe two forms of the empathic approach. According to Mann (1973), the characteristic problem is the patient's passive wish to hold on, a wish that keeps the patient stuck in inappropriately dependent behaviors. The aim of therapy is to foster the patient's ability to separate from the sustaining figures by overcoming separation anxiety and by developing more positive, less ambivalent, internal representations of the important figures. The therapist provides an empathic encounter within the rigid framework of a time-limited therapy, acting as an "empathic helper" who can stay with the patient's feelings, both positive and negative. The other variant of the empathic approach, described by Goldberg (1973), is addressed to patients who have suffered narcissistic injuries. The characteristic technique is to tolerate, share, and ultimately interpret the patient's grandiosity and hurt feelings, with a goal of restoring a narcissistic equilibrium.

The third principal approach is the corrective approach. In the variant described by Alexander and French (1946), the method is directed at previously high-functioning patients who experience a failure of performance, which is caused by a combination of inhibitions due to past experiences and current demands for new responsibilities. The aim is to have the patient overcome the obstacles either by "transference management" in the therapeutic relationship or by achieving success in a series of prescribed actions designed to show that success is, in fact, possible.

In the variant of the corrective approach described by Beck (1967, 1970), the characteristic problem is the patient's self-critical thoughts based on past experiences. The characteristic techniques are clarification, reality testing, and suggestion.

It is easier to appreciate how these writers have modified the more typical psychoanalytic approach through their focus on a characteristic problem by considering the alternative: an open-ended, short-term method without any narrowing of the scope of work. Schafer (1979) described such an effort conducted at the Yale University Student Health Services, where limits of time and resources demanded the use of brief therapy.

By maintaining the "analytic attitude," the therapist attempts no predefinition of the patient's problem but waits to see what issues come up in the course of treatment. The focus of work, then, is not a characteristic problem or the associated underlying conflict, but the resistances and transference fantasies related to the still hidden content. Schafer feels that sooner or later, after the resistances have been considered and resolved, the repressed content is introduced into therapy. This approach follows the "basic technical rule" of Greenson (1967):

> These rules of technique are basic: analyze resistance before content, ego before id, and start with surface. Working with content may be more interesting, more scintillating; working with resistances is more plodding. . . . The basic technical rule means that content interpretation will not become effective until the significant resistances have been analyzed sufficiently. (p. 143)

Although the distinction should not be made too rigidly, and the analysis of content and resistance becomes an interactive, progressive process, this difference between the "basic" approach and the one adopted by the short-term therapists, which we shall describe, is helpful in understanding the various methods. For example, Sifneos (1979) emphasized this difference in discussing his short-term, anxiety-provoking psychotherapy: "Contrary to the classical psychoanalytic technique of dealing with the defenses first, this approach tends to focus more on the drive or the impulse behind the patient's defense mechanism" (p. 95).

We suggest that each of the major writers on short-term therapy takes a similar approach, choosing patients with a characteristic problem and a particular underlying conflict assumed to be associated with the presenting problem.

THE INTERPRETIVE APPROACH: SIFNEOS

Working mainly with young adults, whose symptoms or complaints seem related to frustration of their desire to achieve satisfying heterosexual relationships, Sifneos (1979) has developed a vigorous interpretive method aimed at producing insight by quickly exposing the presumed underlying conflict:

> The underlying psychological conflicts which are usually involved in the therapeutic foci of (these) patients have to do with Oedipal–genital or triangular–interpersonal interactions. . . . The . . . therapist . . . can afford to be selective and can concentrate on areas in which, in his opinion, most of the patient's conflicts exist—the Oedipal focus. (pp. 42, 95)

Classical psychoanalytic technique emphasizes slowly overcoming resistance. In contrast, Sifneos (1973) proposed a direct interpretive approach as an "unemotionally involved teacher" (p. 117). The aim is to recover the forgotten and forbidden memories and expose the repressed content as efficiently as possible. Although this technique runs the danger of increasing the patient's resistance, Sifneos contended that vigorous uncovering of repressed Oedipal issues arouses enough anxiety that patients cannot avoid learning something profound about the nature of their problems and the source of their frustration in their relationships. The educational experience must be guided by an active, didactic therapist who can maximize the impact of this self-discovery, if the latter is to be effective:

> DOCTOR: Well, it is interesting, because the image you had when masturbating, about that boy who is built like a girl, and was wearing . . .
> PATIENT *(Interrupting)*: Oh, my God! Oh, no!
> DOCTOR: Yes.
> PATIENT: I never thought of it this way all the time. You read about all that stuff in magazines; but sex with my mother in that way! It is horrible! (Sifneos, 1973, p. 190)

The interpretive technique which Sifneos used relies on clarifications, confrontations, and summaries; much less attention is directed to the patient's affects or resistances. Although the patient's transference feelings are noted and sometimes emphasized, the transference is used mainly as a springboard for a quick lesson, not as an opportunity to explore the patient's associations. When the transference is less directly related to the central Oedipal issue, which Sifneos seeks to expose, he dismisses it more readily, not allowing any interference in his effort to learn the forbidden secret:

> PATIENT: This is hard. Why do you make me do this?
>
> DOCTOR: I don't make you do anything. I just think there is something else that bothers you. Why were you feeling guilty?
>
> PATIENT: Because I chose my husband over my mother.
>
> DOCTOR: That was a matter of choice. Maybe it was the wrong choice. But why guilty? Guilty implies a crime—one pleads guilty or not guilty to a crime. What was the crime, Mrs. R.? (Sifneos, 1973, p. 156)

The purpose of this single-minded effort to uncover the hidden content is to have the patient understand and learn the truth about himself. Once the secret is exposed, the need to hide the disconnected parts is gone, if the resistances have been sufficiently broken, as indicated by the patient's intense anxiety. With patients who are as motivated and intelligent as Sifneos recommended they should be for this method, the discrepancy between how much they want from a mature relationship and what little they have managed to obtain is mystifying to them. By informing them that there is a reason, one which can easily be found and which is understandable, Sifneos motivates them to lift the cover from the mystery. Patients may then respond to the therapist's promise that the truth, once known, will set them free:

> DOCTOR: Do you think that maybe your mother's death had something to do with your wanting to be a wife to your father?
>
> PATIENT (*Pauses for a long time and then says*): God forbid, not in *that* way. I never thought of it. (*Seeming to be very upset; finally.*) I don't want to think about it.
>
> DOCTOR: It's time you thought about it, if you want to understand yourself. . . .
>
> DOCTOR: Do you have to choose someone who is so different just to avoid thinking of your father in this way?
>
> PATIENT: It's so horrible.
>
> DOCTOR: There is nothing horrible about it if it's the truth. . . . (Sifneos, 1973, pp. 160 ff.)

Besides this faith that understanding is the key to relief, which the therapist conveys to the patient, there are other reasons this technique of vigorous interpretation of an unconscious conflict may be beneficial to these patients. Having a persistent, conscientious tutor may be especially useful with patients whose cognitive style, especially when thinking about themselves, is generally diffuse and global (Shapiro, 1965). Being able to talk with and hopefully internalize a calm, nonthreatening, matter-of-fact therapist also provides a reassuring experience for patients whose repressed fantasies involve fears of retaliation or condemnation.

In contrast to other methods we shall discuss, termination is relatively less important in this method. Sifneos (1979) suggested that resolution of the Oedipal conflict usually entails less mourning than other types of separation or loss.

THE EMPATHIC APPROACH: MANN

Mann's (1973) approach to brief therapy is aimed at a central issue he considered so basic as to be universal: the unresolved conflict about the "recurring life crisis of separation–individuation" (p. 24). The patients he selected demonstrated their acute distress about this problem by their dependent, passive natures, their fantasies of union with nurturant figures, and their childish expectations of unlimited time in relationships. It is this fantasy that a perfect, eternal relationship is possible, Mann said, that keeps the patient from facing life's challenges and fosters a dependent, passive holding on instead of a mature engagement with the demands of adult life. Mann believed this type of conflict is uniquely suited to a time-limited approach, because the certainty of termination in a deliberately brief relationship reflects the passage of time and the necessity of separation.

Although the therapist operates within a framework of psychoanalytic knowledge, Mann did not formulate "psychodynamic hypotheses" about underlying conflicts and repressed memories that need to be exposed to the patient by vigorous interpretive work. Instead, he addressed himself to the patient's feelings. The goal of this method is neither to provoke anxiety by teaching the patient a particularly hard set of facts about his or her life nor to uncover a painfully difficult lesson. It is, rather, to share the patient's anxiety about separation, so it can be mastered in a more positive relationship. At the outset of treatment, the patient's "present and chronically endured pain" is acknowledged by a statement which "immediately brings the patient closer to the therapist out of his feeling that he is in the presence of an empathic helper" (Mann, 1973, p. 18).

This opening move by the therapist engages the patient on the basis of unrealistic fantasies about being perfectly understood, of a magical, long-sought union with a sustaining figure. The next move by the therapist is to point in the direction the therapy will proceed, from the patient's fantasy to the strict and unyielding reality which the therapist will come to represent: he sets a termination date. By doing this, concretely marking the date on the calendar, the therapist makes the inevitable separation as real as possible. These two opening moves by the therapist, setting up an empathic bond for which the patient has yearned and then announcing that it will be terminated, build a structure for the therapy that will continue throughout its course, with the oscillation between magical fantasies and harsh reality. "Union and separation become the major poles of treatment, thereby diminishing . . . all other phase-specific conflicts" (Mann, 1973, p. 33).

Mann advised therapists to accept the patient's wish for a perfect bond without interpreting or avoiding it. By the therapist truly accepting the patient's wish and thereby establishing an empathic bond at the beginning with the patient's unrealistic wishes, both therapist and patient will be prepared for the therapist's continued empathy later, at termination, when the sharing of feelings of disappointment and loss becomes so important.

> The specific limitation of time and the framework of the treatment agreement create in this kind of treatment a clearly demarcated beginning, a distint middle, and an unavoidable end. The beginning restores to the patient the golden glow of unity with mother, preseparation in endless time. The middle brings with it the disappointment that a relationship once wholly unambivalent will once more become ambivalent. And the end introduces the unavoidable harsh reality that what was lost must be given up. (Mann, 1973, p. 28)

At termination, the patient's disappointment and sense of loss threaten to overcome the treatment. Rather than teaching the patient an anxiety-provoking lesson, as would be done in the interpretive technique, the therapist is expected to help the patient tolerate the difficult feelings being experienced. The therapeutic benefit comes not from increased understanding, but from experiencing the negative feelings aroused by termination without withdrawing prematurely from the relationship. If the therapist can stay with the patient's "sadness, grief, anger, and guilt," the empathic relationship will be sustained, even through termination. This separation, more successful than others in the patient's life, because it engenders feelings of closeness even in disappointment, "will allow the patient to internalize the therapist as a replacement or substitute for the earlier ambivalent object. *This time the internalization will be more positive . . . less anger-laden, and less guilt-laden, thereby making separation a genuine maturational event"* (Mann, 1973, p. 36).

THE EMPATHIC APPROACH: GOLDBERG

Arnold Goldberg (1973) described another empathic approach to short-term therapy, which relies on Heinz Kohut's (1971) formulation of a psychology of the self. Goldberg suggested that a therapist's empathic stance can help patients recover from acute narcissistic injuries, that is, damaged self-esteem. This method uses the basic techniques developed in the psychoanalysis of narcissistic problems, particularly the self-object transference, but does not attempt to achieve character restructuring through the interpretive work that would become the mutative process in the longer therapy. According to Goldberg, restoring equilibrium to the narcissistic portion of the self is an adequate goal for brief therapy.

For example, in the case of a 35-year-old professional who became depressed and irritable after a lecture had been criticized by students, Goldberg provided an empathic "mirroring" relationship to reflect and strengthen the patient's injured self-esteem. When the hurt feelings were repaired, the patient was able to function without the need for an admiring therapist.

THE CORRECTIVE APPROACH: ALEXANDER

More than the other writers we have discussed, Alexander and his colleagues (Alexander & French, 1946) focused on the patient's current life problem, instead of on a presumed underlying conflict, as the proper target for therapeutic action. The therapist is expected to bring psychoanalytic understanding to the formulation of a "grand strategy" for helping the patient consider the interaction between his or her powers of adaptation and "latent neurotic tendencies." The aim, however, should never be shifted from the current life problem: "the patient must never be allowed to forget that he came to the physician not for an academic understanding of the etiology of his condition, but for help in solving his actual life problems (p. 34).

This stress on the patient's current ability to perform was a natural consequence of the psychiatric experience with traumatic neuroses in World War II. To correct the patient's failing performance, in war or in

private life, the authors recommended a managerial position whereby, after assessing the obstacles which keep the patient from action, the therapist can move against either the internal conflicts or the external situation.

Alexander and French (1946) recommended that if the restraints on
the necessary performance derive from earlier, unresolved conflicts, the
therapist should use the transference relationship to provide a "corrective
emotional experience." They advised the therapist to manage the transference by acting in a way which is markedly different from the way the
earlier authoritarian figures in the patient's life acted. With a 42-year-old
businessman, for example, who was having trouble with his job, his marriage, his children, and his health, Alexander and his colleagues reported
that

> the analyst made every effort to counteract (the patient's tendency to see him
> as an authoritarian father) by leaning over backward in an attempt to avoid
> the role into which the patient instinctively tried to inveigle him. Had the ther-
> apist followed rigid rules of technique, he would have remained passive, al-
> lowing the patient to make him the father of his childhood; he decided, how-
> ever, to take just the opposite attitude in the hope of breaking up the patient's
> pattern of behavior more quickly (p. 57)

Role playing of this sort, according to Alexander, liberated the patient from "the protracted effects of paternal intimidation," leaving him
free to perform his own duties as worker, husband, and father.

If the obstacles to the patient's performance lie in the present, however, they recommended even more direct management of the situation.
The therapist should explicitly supervise the patient's performance, either
by using suggestion or by giving direct advice and "should encourage the
patient (or even require him) to do those things which he avoided in the
past" (p. 41). One unfortunate side effect of this new, more gratifying relationship with a helpful, managerial figure might be to increase the patient's dependence on the therapist. But this problem can be handled like
any other current problem, that is, by telling the patient to change his behavior—in this case, requiring "as radical a reduction of interviews as is at
all tolerable for the patient" (p. 35). Termination is a natural consequence
of the patient's ability to perform on his own, without direction by the
therapist.

Alexander's approach to therapy utilizes a comprehensive assessment
of both historical and current problems in a patient's life, with an emphasis on current and future ability to perform. Understanding of past
conflicts and mastery of deep-seated anxieties are not as important as the

achievement of a new integration of past experience with a commitment to undertake new responsibilities.

THE CORRECTIVE APPROACH: BECK

Another form of corrective therapy was developed by Aaron Beck (1970). In contrast to Alexander, who focused on the patient's actions, Beck focuses on the patient's thoughts. In his therapeutic approach, the patient monitors any self-critical thoughts and "replays" them with the therapist. With a process of "logical analysis and empirical testing," therapist and patient can correct any misinterpretations of reality and work to substitute more appropriate beliefs in the patient's thinking. This process also relies on trial runs, with "homework assignments" to help the patient master the old "insuperable" problems.

MATCHING METHOD AND PATIENT

In this section, we propose a way of integrating the various approaches to short-term psychotherapy by using a schema based on the developmental stages of adult life. It seems to us that the kinds of problems or conflicts addressed by the different methods are very similar to the central issues and tasks of the various developmental stages. Therefore, we hypothesize that a developmental schema provides a way of matching method and patient—or, in different words, that determining the developmental stage of a patient (i.e., making a developmental diagnosis) indicates the most appropriate method of short-term therapy. Such a matching would be similar to the way an internist identifies the type of bacteria causing an infection in order to choose the most appropriate antibiotic, rather than using one or two favorite antibiotics on all patients.

In order to create a developmental context, we have drawn upon the theories and descriptions of adulthood that have recently appeared. We have relied heavily on the work of Levinson (1978), Vaillant (1977), Neugarten (1968), Gould (1978), and Erikson (1963). The focus of this empirical work has been predominantly the lives of middle-class males, and conclusions, therefore, should be applied with caution to other population groups.

One of the problems in reviewing this literature is the confusing plethora of terms used to describe the various life stages. We have adopted the following nomenclature, which has the benefit of being relatively jar-gon-free: late adolescence, early adulthood, settling down, midlife, ma-ture adulthood, and old age.

We have organized our discussion by developmental stages, pointing out the salient themes and issues that seem to characterize the stage and help to identify patients who are in the midst of it. Each stage has at least two aspects: one new, one old. At each stage, there are new tasks, skills, roles, and relationships that must be mastered. Simultaneously, there ap-pear to be a rekindling and a consequent reworking of certain childhood developmental issues. It is as if certain of the childhood developmental stages resonate with particular adult developmental stages. For example, a young adult's struggle to form intimate, heterosexual relationships may stir up unresolved Oedipal conflicts.

We then attempt to demonstrate how the method of short-term ther-apy that fits best with the developmental stage can be used to help patients who are having difficulty with the developmental challenge.

LATE ADOLESCENCE

Throughout the life cycle, the complementary issues of separation and in-dividuation surface again and again. Late adolescence is one of the periods in which these issues come to the fore. An adolescent faces the task of separating from home and parents in order to transform his or her rela-tionship with the world from a childhood to an adult pattern. Part of this process requires the capacity to tolerate a physical separation in order to take on a role and lifestyle frequently different from that left at home, thus forming the nucleus of the adult self.

A psychological separation also takes place. Peter Blos (1968) sug-gested that "the developmental task . . . lies in the disengagement of . . . cathexes from the internalized infantile objects" (p. 252). Such a disen-gagement allows a reworking and integration of these childhood identifi-cations into the ego. Functioning almost like transitional objects during this period are peer groups and certain social institutions, such as college and army, which support a nascent adult's shaky sense of identity while serving as counterweights to the regressive pull toward home.

Occurring simultaneously with this separation process is identity for-mation. Perhaps most critical to identity formation is the accomplishment of a stability and independence of ego functioning, leading to a sense of ego identity (Erikson, 1963). With this maturation of the ego, the adolescent begins articulating childhood fantasies and wishes into more clearly defined options and making the first tentative choices of adult roles (Levinson, 1978).

We want to emphasize the mutuality of the separation and the identity formation processes. As in childhood, separation and "disengagement of cathexes" lead to the internalization of the object relations and their integration into the ego; the growth of the ego and the formation of a stable character make the individual more independent and help maintain the separation. Thus, a modest intervention (such as a course of short-term psychotherapy) in support of a youth who is having trouble separating could have far-reaching effects.

Failure to negotiate this phase leads to role confusion, doubts about sexual identity, failure to make even a tentative occupational choice, a codification of dependent traits into character, and perhaps the lack of a coherent sense of self. Vaillant (1977) described several of his subjects who never completed adolescence. He termed them "perpetual boys": they remained closely tied to their mothers, friendless; if they married, "they assumed a feminine role in a rather distant marriage"; they never committed themselves to a career.

It would seem that the empathic approach of time-limited psychotherapy described by Mann (1973) would be most useful for the conflicts of a late adolescence. Because of its emphasis on termination, this method offers an opportunity for mastery of conflict around separation–individuation. In fact, the goal of this treatment, as stated by Mann (1973), is to help the patient tolerate and live through and resolve a separation *"from the meaningful, ambivalently experienced person"* (p. 34). This is precisely the maturational task of late adolescence—to tolerate separation and to internalize significant relationships from childhood.

Mann (1973) speaks to the use of his technique with the late adolescent:

> There is a very large group of patients for whom the twelve hour treatment plan is admirably suited, even indicated. Young men and women, roughly in middle or late adolescence, mostly college students, who present themselves with any of a multitude of psychological and somatic complaints make up the majority of this group. . . . The particular pressures and strains of college life, with its attendant problems related to career, independence, identity and so forth confront each student with almost daily challenges to his growth and development. (p. 76)

This method succeeds in providing such a growth experience because of its use of empathy as one of the primary therapeutic techniques.

Through the empathic sharing of the patient's "chronic and presently endured pain," the therapist can get close enough to the patient to stimulate the patient's fantasies of union and merger, so that the experience of separation at termination becomes affectively meaningful. The empathic approach thus provides the late adolescent with an experience in the therapy of a "model" separation in which he or she can work through the dependent longings, conflicts about being autonomous, and ambivalent internalizations that may be blocking the development of ego identity.

We illustrate this matching with one of Mann's cases, a graduate student from a fundamentalist family, who presented with conflicts about leaving home and moving to an apartment of his own. Such a conflict is typical of late adolescence. His difficulty leaving was a result of conflictual identifications: to be a man was either to be destructive and vengeful like his brother or weak and ineffectual like his father. During the early part of the treatment, the patient retreated into passive longings to remain at home or to be nurtured by the therapist. By reexperiencing and resolving his ambivalence toward his important male introjects, however, the patient was able to internalize their positive aspects. In addition, he internalized the tolerant though realistic therapist, who supported his strivings to be independent. His ability to master his dependent longings carried over to the rest of his life, imparting a sense of independence and increased self-esteem. Thus, the patient used the separation from the therapist as a way of working out, in the transference, his conflicts about separating from his parents.

EARLY ADULTHOOD

The task of this phase can be summarized as learning how to make commitments to love and to work. The previous phase was marked by a turning inward; here, the newly won sense of identity is applied. "Having disengaged itself from the past, the newly hatched butterfly must reestablish viable links between itself and the outside world" (Vaillant, 1977, p. 215). These links are the intimate relationships with others and the preliminary choice of an occupation. "The young adult, emerging from a search for and insistence on identity, is eager and willing to fuse his intimacy with that of others . . . to commit himself to concrete affiliations" (Erikson, 1963, p. 263). This period is characterized by a trial-and-error process in forming relationships and by an occupational identity as the young adult searches for a compatible niche.

There are really two contradictory tasks that must be undertaken during this period: making tentative choices in order to explore possibilities and opportunities, while putting off making final commitments that would stunt or stifle this search (Levinson, 1978). Conflict around commitment becomes a central theme of the period. "The focal issue for young adults is the issue of social role, of the *individual's relationship to the structures of the established society.* . . . The task of youth is to find or create some congruence, in a broad sense, between individual and existing institutions" (Keniston, 1968, p. 269).

During this period, childhood attachments to parents persist in fantasy. These may take the form of believing that emulating one's parents will automatically bring success, or that one's parents will always be available to rescue one from painful situations (Gould, 1978). Such fantasies may determine occupational choice or, conversely, lead to internal prohibitions against certain choices. They are played out in object relations. Marriages formed during this period may be reenactments of the family romance, or they may be "conspiracies" in which the partners share the unconscious wish that the other will make up for deficits, as parents had so recently done, or they may aid in the avoidance of adult responsibilities.

In this phase of life, an individual moves toward what Erikson (1963) called "true genitality." This may stir up unresolved conflicts from earlier psychosexual phases. In particular, unresolved Oedipal attachments and conflicts become problematic as the young adult begins to form intimate, heterosexual relationships. Given the developmental thrust toward genitality during this period, a course of short-term psychotherapy directed at resolving these conflicts may be effective, whereas the same treatment at another developmental stage would not have succeeded.

In the sphere of work, similar kinds of Oedipal conflict may surface. Faced with the necessity of occupational choice, many young people reexamine their relationships with their parents and their parents' occupational choices. Conflicts about occupational success or competitive strivings interfere with this process and may block the assumption of adult roles, as manifested, for example, in a graduate student's inability to complete his thesis.

The consequence of failure at this stage is isolation, a fear of intimacy, and consequent self-absorption. Keniston (1968) framed this in sociological terms as "a kind of alienation either from self or society—a denial of the reality or importance of . . . social reality" (p. 270). A person who has failed to traverse young adulthood remains in limbo, caught between the world of childhood and the world of adulthood.

In summary, the phase of young adulthood continues the process of identity formation. The completion of adolescence imparts a sense of personal identity, while the completion of young adulthood leads to the formation of a social identity.

We suggest that the interpretive method appears to fit best with patients having difficulty with the developmental task of young adulthood. The use of Oedipal issues as a focus is particularly relevant to the developmental tasks of this life stage. In fact, the patients that Sifneos (1979) felt respond best to the interpretive method are "patients who linger . . . too long in their attachment to the parent of the opposite sex, tending to procrastinate in choosing to abandon their wishes for and competition with their parents and in finding a suitable surrogate among their peers" (p. 50). In other words, these are patients without major pregenital fixations, who delay in taking the maturational step of young adulthood because of unresolved Oedipal attachments and conflicts.

In addition to the choice of focus, the technique of the therapist produces a maturational experience for these patients. We noted how the use of time limits and empathy produces an emotional experience of separation in the empathic method. In the interpretive method, the therapeutic experience partly depends on the elicitation of anxiety by confronting patients with their own repressed and highly conflictual emotions. Such an experience, if successfully mastered by a patient, can lead to a generalized increase in anxiety tolerance. This, in turn, may enhance the individual's ability to develop and maintain close relationships, with all of the tangled and conflictual emotions such relationships elicit. In other words, the patient has the opportunity to experience and work through, in the microcosm of the therapy, the conflicts and difficulties that block the achievement of intimacy. Perhaps one reason for the importance of making therapist–parent links in interpretations, as emphasized by Malan (1976) and Sifneos (1979), is that such links heighten the patient's experience of conflictual feelings toward the therapist.

Finally, there is the factor of identification with the therapist. In this form of therapy, the therapist offers him- or herself as an unemotionally involved problem solver, able to face but not act on highly charged, conflictual fantasies and impulses. If the patient is able to identify with the therapist, he or she emerges with a more positive attitude toward interpersonal relations, feeling a sense of competence in being able to sort out and understand emotional problems, rather than being bewildered or overwhelmed by them. Such an attitude is important as a factor in a young adult's willingness to enter into close relationships.

For an example of a patient in young adulthood for whom the interpretive method seems most apt, we mention one of the cases presented by Sifneos (1979), a 23-year-old woman whose chief complaint was, "I can't choose the right kind of guy. I'm attracted to men who treat me badly." In the absence of other areas of major dysfunction, a complaint of difficulty with intimate, heterosexual relationships locates the patient in a developmental arrest in the young adult phase. Sifneos focused the treatment on her Oedipal conflicts, allowing her to become more aware of her longings and contemptous feelings toward her father. These had been played out in her relationships with men: she would get involved in brief encounters, after which she would grow tired of and ultimately discard the lover. The result of treatment was an improvement in her capacity to tolerate close relationships with both men and women as well as a decrease in her masochism.

SETTLING DOWN

The settling-down period brings an end to the provisional, exploratory quality of the young adult phase; commitments that had been postponed now must be made. Externally, the theme that dominates this period is career consolidation. According to Vaillant (1977), individuals in this phase are like latency age children: "they were good at tasks, careful to follow the rules, anxious for promotion and willing to accept all aspects of the system" (p. 216). During settling down, the young adult makes a choice of career and works hard at establishing him- or herself in it. If not done previously, many establish marriages and begin the process of childbearing.

The intrapsychic correlate of the consolidation of careers and family life is the maturation of youthful narcissism. Childhood aspirations are rekindled and reworked. Faced with the reality of the occupational world, the patient realizes that the grandiosity of childhood and adolescence must be relinquished. Levinson (1978) described two aspects of this process. The first is the formation of a dream, "a sense of self-in-adult-world. It has the quality of a vision, an imagined possibility that generates excitement and vitality" (p. 91). The dream can be thought of as a derivative of the childhood ego ideal now being gradually modified so as to be consonant with the life situation of the adult. While the dream needs to reflect the realities of the chosen life, it is likewise important that the life integrate and contain possibilities for the living out of the dream.

The other aspect of this maturational process is the creation of a relationship with a mentor. A mentor is a person who is part parent and part peer, who has the "qualities of character, expertise and understanding that the younger person admires and wants to make part of himself" (Levinson, 1978, p. 100). The mentor serves a transitional developmental function, helping the individual consolidate an identity as a full-fledged adult. The mentor can be conceptualized as a self-object (Kohut, 1971), one who supports and admires the person while the latter's narcissism is being tempered by the demands of reality, an idealized role model that the person internalizes during the process of forming an occupational identity.

The settling-down period is a crucial way-station along the line of narcissistic development, during which youthful idealism and grandiosity are channeled, modified, and transformed to become congruent with the actual opportunities and limitations of the person's life. This period is the conclusion of the youthful phase of adult life and the process of identity formation; an occupational identity is added to the personal and social identities formed during previous life stages. Definite lasting commitments and obligations are formed. "The future becomes less open and the individual establishes a more-or-less enduring mode of relationship to his society—be he critic or executive, revolutionary or yeoman, radical or apologist, apathetic or indignant" (Keniston, 1968, p. 271).

Failure of the settling-down process leaves an individual with an inadequate sense of an adult self, without a secure occupational identity. A vulnerability to narcissistic injury results from failing to transform childhood grandiosity into adult dreams.

During the settling-down period, there appear major differences between the developmental sequence of men and that of women. For example, while career consolidation may be straightforward for men, it can involve major role conflict for women who choose to both raise children and have careers (Notman, 1978). Women who have chosen to remain childless until their 30s may experience difficulties as they face the decison of how or whether to combine career and child rearing. This confrontation with limitations of time and mutually exclusive options can be thought of as the female equivalent of a man's need to make a more lasting commitment to a choice of career during this phase.

Because narcissistic issues come to the fore during this period, it appears that the method of short-term psychotherapy developed by Goldberg (1973), a variant of the empathic approach, would be particularly indicated for people at this developmental stage. This method is directed at the rapid resolution of narcissistic injuries. As mentioned above, such psychotherapy "aims to reestablish the narcissistic equilibrium with the therapist as the available narcissistic object and hopefully (but not necessarily) to uncover a screen for the childhood fantasy" (Goldberg, 1973, p. 724).

We illustrate the use of this method during the settling-down period with one of Goldberg's (1973) case reports mentioned earlier, a 35-year-old professional man who presented with depression and increased irritability. The narcissistic injury appeared to be the negative reaction of a group of students to a lecture he had given; in the discussion afterward, they had called him pompous. In therapy, the patient soon appeared to be "a grandiose although overbearing little boy who wanted admiration and/or reflection but who was likewise quite vulnerable to attack or rejection" (p. 724). Conceptualizing this man's problem in developmental terms, it appears that he had difficulty with the maturational tasks of the settling-down period, that is, modification of the childhood narcissism into a more mature, reality-based form. Unable to form a secure, stable occupational identity, he remained highly dependent on his students' admiration and had the constant need to prove he was cleverer than his associates. Rather than confront the developmental failure (i.e., confront directly the patient's grandiosity), Goldberg adopted an empathic stance and shared "the patient's wish to be great and really impress his audience and the bitter disappointment at rejection" (p. 726) and his use of the therapist as a narcissistic object. Kohut (1971) has described two forms of narcissistic transference: the mirror transference, in which the patient wishes to be admired by the therapist, and the idealizing transference, in which the patient idealizes the therapist. These transference relationships, which are used in this approach to short-term work, are very similar to the functions of the mentor, as described by Levinson (1978):

> He fosters the young adult's development by believing in him, sharing the youthful Dream and giving it his blessing, helping to define newly emerging self.... [The mentor has] qualities of character, expertise, and understanding that the younger admires or wants to make part of himself. (pp. 99, 100)

Thus, in this form of short-term psychotherapy, which appears particularly helpful during the settling-down period, the therapist functions as surrogate mentor, maintaining the narcissistic balance while helping the individual develop a more realistic view of himself.

MIDLIFE

Settling down is dominated by the business of climbing occupational hierarchies and establishing families. In midlife, concern shifts from outer reality to the inner life. Prompted by realization that the time left to live is less than time lived, that one's children are entering adolescence, that parents are sick or have died, an individual undertakes a major reappraisal of his life. One of the central tasks of this phase is to take a clear and hard look at the realities of life, to acknowledge and bear parts of the self that were, until now, denied or repressed. In various descriptions of the period, there is a striking commonality of theme:

> As he attempts to reappraise his life a man discovers how much it has been based on illusions and he is faced with the task of deillusionment. . . . The process of . . . reducing illusions involves diverse feelings—disappointment, joy, relief, bitterness, grief, wonder, freedom—and has diverse outcomes. . . The major task is to reappraise the life structure of the Settling Down period, within the broader perspective of early adulthood as a whole. (Levinson, 1978, p. 192-193)

> [In the midlife a person must relinquish the fantasies that] "there is no evil or death in the world," "death can't happen to me or my loved ones." The sense of timelessness in our early thirties is giving way to an awareness of the pressure of time in our forties. . . . To enjoy full access to our innermost self, we can no longer deny the ugly, demonic side of life, which our immature mind tried to protect against by enslaving itself to false illusions that absolute safety was possible. (Gould, 1978, pp. 217-219)

> Late adolescent and early adult idealism and optimism accompanied by split-off and projected hate, are given up and supplanted by a more contemplative pessimism. . . . This early adult idealism is built upon the use of unconscious denial and manic defenses . . . against two fundamental features of human life —the inevitableness of eventual death and the existence of hate and destructive impulses inside each person. . . . The explicit recognition of these two features, and the bringing of them in focus is the quintessence of successful weathering of the mid-life crisis. (Jaques, 1965, p. 504-505)

> In middle adulthood one becomes impressed that one will indeed die. It becomes apparent that the limitation of physiology and life span will not permit the full accomplishment of all one's projects. (Lifton, 1976, pp. 39-40)

> The middle years of life . . . represent an important turning point, with the restructuring of time and the formulation of new perceptions of self, time and death. It is in this period of the life line that introspection seems to increase noticeably and contemplation and reflection and self-evaluation become characteristic forms of mental life. (Neugarten, 1968, p. 140)

The sharpening awareness of death and of time and the limitations of the self dominate this period. These themes differentiate midlife from young adulthood and, in themselves, may precipitate a depression. If midlife issues are negotiated successfully, however, the outcome is a sense of generativity, "a concern in establishing and guiding the next generation" (Erikson, 1963, p. 267). To become generative can represent a way of dealing with the depressing realities of midlife: though one cannot have personal immortality, involvement with the next generation can bring a sense of symbolic immortality. Vaillant (1977) noted that "in middle life, the men's career patterns suddenly diverged and broadened" (p. 227), and there was "a wish to be of more service to those around them" (p. 222).

The sequence and timing of developmental stages in women may be more complex than in men. Notman (1978) a student of female adult development, conceived of developmental stages in women as "an interweaving of those experiences related to childbirth, parenting and family development with those of establishment of personal identity—separation and autonomy, intellectual growth and the relationship to work" (p. 16). In particular, midlife issues in women are strongly influenced by changes within the family. "Women, but not men, tend to define their age status in terms of timing of events within the family cycle. For married women, middle age is closely tied to the launching of children into the adult world" (Neugarten, 1968, p. 95). Women who have invested very heavily in child rearing may experience significant depression at menopause, whereas women who are in the advantaged position of having career options other than parent may greet with enthusiasm the growing independence of children, which signifies liberation rather than loss (Notman, 1978).

Failure to negotiate midlife successfully can take many forms: a sense of stagnation, a chronic depression, a flight into a second adolescence, perhaps a serious illness. We would expect, then, that of the multiple types of clinical issues that might emerge at this point, two would predominate. The first is a generalized sense of depression at the enormity of the reassessments to be performed, the losses that must be mourned. The second is conflict around generativity—in particular, unresolved conflict associated with one's internalized parents that comes to the fore in the process of assuming responsibility for the next generation and in facing the aging or death of one's parents. While becoming generative (e.g., a parent, mentor, teacher), a person is confronted with the relationship with one's own parents, because in assuming parental roles, one becomes more aware of the identification with one's parents. If the relationship with the parents was conflictual, and there remains intense ambivalence toward their internalization, serious problems may occur in assuming generative roles in midlife.

The corrective approaches of Alexander and French (1946) and Beck (1967, 1970) would seem to have particular usefulness at this developmental stage. These methods are well suited for treating the kind of depression often experienced in midlife. Rather than giving the patient an empathic encounter, which would turn him away from the tasks at hand, or confronting him with his maladaptive solutions, which may exacerbate the depression, these methods aim at restoring the patient's level of functioning by giving him an experience of mastery. This goal of treatment is stated explicitly by Alexander and French (1946): "The chief therapeutic value of the transference situation lies in the fact that it allows the patient to experience this feeling of success in rehearsal, a rehearsal which must then be followed by actual performance" (p. 40).

Likewise, in Beck's method, the goal of treatment is to control and detoxify the depressive cognitions, not to gain insight into their origins. The emphasis is on giving patients a feeling of mastery over their feeling states.

Such therapies speak to the needs of the demoralized person in midlife. They aim at restoring a sense of optimism and competence, so that the patient can deal with the developmental tasks at hand.

For example, Beck (1967) described a depressed, 40-year-old woman who presented with a complaint frequently heard in midlife: "What's the use of living. I've got to die sometime anyhow." In this case, the woman was overwhelmed by the awareness of her own mortality. While such an awareness is typical of midlife, it was intensified in this woman because her mother, a diabetic, had become ill at age 40. Beck told her that her depression was due to an identification with the mother: "You believe that you are following in your mother's footsteps. You got the notion when she was dying that when you reached her age (40 years) you would start to have strokes and go to pieces. The truth of the matter is that all our tests have shown that your physical health is perfect" (p. 138). Though not addressing himself to the developmental issues involved, the therapist gave the patient a rational explanation for her symptoms and with it a sense of control over her affective state and thinking process.

This case example, in which the identification with parents plays a central role, brings us to the second reason for matching the corrective method with patients facing midlife issues: to help a patient alter internalizations in order to become more generative. An example of this is the case mentioned earlier, a 42-year-old, domineering businessman, who heavily identified with his own tyrannical father (Alexander & French, 1946). This man expected the therapist to be as authoritarian as his father had been. In the face of the therapist's determined tolerance, however, the patient became increasingly confused by his own hostile, competitive behavior. This led him to be aware of his identification with his father and his excessive need to appear important and strong. The patient seemed to replace his identification with his father with an identification with the benign, accepting therapist, which allowed him to be more generative. The authors reported that

> the conditions in the home improved markedly. This started by his assuming a paternal attitude toward his son, with whom he had been competing as with a younger brother. . . . He himself recognized that he could now act as a father toward his son because he had at last found in the treatment what he had always wanted—understanding and support from a person in authority. (p. 59)

MATURE ADULTHOOD

The period of mature adulthood represents a second settling down. There is "a sense of having completed something, a sense that we are whoever we are going to be" (Gould, 1978). Erikson called this acceptance "ego integity." Levinson (1978) saw the time after the midlife transition as a period of rebuilding, in which a person must once again commit him- or herself to a particular life structure. Neugarten (1968), one of the principal investigators of this period, described the characteristic changes she observed:

> It is in this period of the life line that introspection seems to increase noticeably and contemplation and reflection and self-evaluation become the characteristic forms of mental life. . . . Men become more receptive to nurturant and affiliative promptings; women more responsive toward . . . their aggressive or competitive strivings. . . . In both sexes, older people become more egocentric . . . and attend increasingly to their personal needs. (p. 140)

Failure to develop a stable life structure and sense of ego integrity leads to a bitter, fear-filled old age, dominated by a sense of time running out and of despair.

OLD AGE

Old age brings with it another set of developmental challenges. Limits of space prevent our discussing the substantial literature of the problems and challenges of late life.

The use of short-term therapy in these developmental stages remains an important area for further investigation. We mention a recent case report (Hoyt, 1979) of the use of a time-limited approach with a 69-year-old widow, with the focus on her unresolved mourning for her husband. Such an approach may be well suited to these patients, given their realistic perception of the limitation of time and of their own lives. In contrast, Small (1979) appears to advocate a supportive orientation to the short-term treatment of this population.

CONCLUSION

A therapist using this developmental schema faces the question of how to make a developmental diagnosis as a prerequisite to knowing which short-term method to use. Such a diagnosis must be based on consideration of multiple factors, including the patient's chronological age, his presenting problems (e.g., a complaint of difficulty leaving home would seem to imply late adolescent issues, even if the patient were chronologically older), a broad review of the type of developmental tasks the individual is currently facing, and the patient's current level of psychosocial functioning. Much work is needed in order to develop a valid and reliable method for making such diagnoses. Loevinger's (1966) scale of ego development represented the first step toward such a developmental assessment of adults.

We note that each of the developmental stages in adult life seems to activate a particular childhood developmental issue (Colarusso & Nemiroff, 1979). For example, the tasks of late adolescence stir up old conflicts around dependence–independence and separation–individuation; the tasks of early adulthood stir up Oedipal issues; the tasks of settling down bring to the fore childhood narcissistic concerns. We therefore wonder if the kind of underlying conflict seen at a particular time might be used as a clue to the adult developmental stage.

In summary, we have presented a developmental framework for matching method and patient. This approach appears to have a firm theoretical basis, and we look forward to its clinical application and testing.

ACKNOWLEDGMENT

The opinions expressed herein are those of the authors and do not necessarily reflect the opinions of the United States Public Health Service.

REFERENCES

Alexander, F., & French, T. *Psychoanalytic therapy: Principles and applications.* New York: Ronald Press, 1946.

Beck, A. T. *The diagnosis and management of depression.* Philadelphia: University of Pennsylvania Press, 1967.

Beck, A. T. Cognitive therapy: Nature and relationship to behavior therapy. *Behaviour Research and Therapy,* 1970, *1,* 184–200.

Blos, P. Character formation in adolescence. *Psychoanalytic Study of the Child,* 1968, *23,* 245–263.

Burke, J. D., White, H. S., & Havens, L. L. Which short-term psychotherapy? *Archives of General Psychiatry,* 1979, *36,* 177–186.

Colarusso, C. A., & Nemiroff, R. A. Some observations and hypotheses about the psychoanalytic theory of adult development. *International Journal of Psychoanalysis,* 1979, *60,* 59–71.

Erikson, E. *Childhood and society.* New York: Norton, 1963.

Goldberg, A. Psychotherapy of narcissistic injuries. *Archives of General Psychiatry,* 1973, *28,* 722–726.

Gould, R. L. *Transformations.* New York: Simon & Schuster, 1978.

Greenson, R. R. *The technique and practice of psychoanalysis* (Vol. I). New York: International Universities Press, 1967.

Hoyt, M. F. Aspects of termination in a time-limited brief psychotherapy. *Psychiatry,* 1979, *42,* 208–219.

Jaques, E. Death and the mid-life crisis. *International Journal of Psychoanalysis,* 1965, *46,* 502–514.

Keniston, K. *Young radicals.* New York: Harcourt, Brace & World, 1968.

Kohut, H. *The analysis of the self.* New York: International Universities Press, 1971.

Levinson, D. J. *The seasons of a man's life.* New York: Knopf, 1978.

Lifton, R. J., *The life of the self.* New York: Simon & Schuster, 1976.

Loevinger, J. The meaning and measurement of ego development. *American Psychologist,* 1966, *21,* 195–206.

Mann, J. *Time-limited psychotherapy.* Cambridge: Harvard University Press, 1973.

Malan, D. H. *The frontier of brief psychotherapy.* New York: Plenum Press, 1976.

Neugarten, B. L. (Ed.). *Middle age and aging.* Chicago: University of Chicago Press, 1968.

Notman, M. T. Women and mid-life: A different perspective. *Psychiatric Opinion,* 1978, *15,* 15–25.

Schafer, R. *Brief analytic psychotherapy.* Lecture presented at Massachusetts General Hospital, Boston, April 24, 1979.

Shapiro, D. *Neurotic styles.* New York: Basic Books, 1965.

Sifneos, P. E. *Short-term psychotherapy and emotional crisis.* Cambridge: Harvard University Press, 1973.

Sifneos, R. E. *Short-term dynamic psychotherapy.* New York: Plenum Press, 1979.

Small, L. *The brief psychotherapies.* New York: Brunner/Mazel, 1979.

Vaillant, G. E. *Adaptation to life.* Boston: Little, Brown, 1977.

SECTION IV
PLANNED SHORT-TERM
GROUP THERAPY

CHAPTER 10
SHORT-TERM GROUP PSYCHOTHERAPY: HISTORICAL ANTECEDENTS

James E. Sabin

INTRODUCTION

Short-term group psychotherapy is a new and relatively unfamiliar form of treatment to clinicians who are not associated with the Harvard Community Health Plan (HCHP). To be candid, it is not an inherently plausible mode of psychotherapy to practitioners with a psychodynamic perspective. While it is not difficult to understand how an inspirational group can act rapidly, it is far from obvious how meaningful psychotherapy can be done in 15 group sessions. I am assuming that most readers of this volume will be dubious about short-term groups. But in actuality, however dubious you may be, there are probably more good reasons to be skeptical about short-term group psychotherapy than you have thought of.

To begin with, serious group psychotherapy has, to date, been virtually exclusively long term. Irvin Yalom (1975b), the best clinical thinker about group psychotherapy, conceptualized the group healing process as an enterprise of at least one to three years. Psychodynamically based group psychotherapy, as we currently understand it, is almost, by definition, medium to long term. According to Yalom (1975a):

> Group therapy is less a bargain than it seems. . . . [It] offers no substantial temporal advantages in that the total length of treatment in group therapy is no less than individual therapy. Although there are some therapists who have attempted brief group therapy on a crisis-intervention model, they have not demonstrated its efficacy and, for the most part, group therapy remains relatively long term therapy. (p. 708)

JAMES E. SABIN. Harvard Community Health Plan, Wellesley, Massachusetts, and Department of Psychiatry, Harvard Medical School, Boston, Massachusetts.

This was published in 1975. In the view of my colleagues at the HCHP, it no longer applies. But Yalom spoke with real authority—not simply for himself but for a broadly shared perspective on the essential nature of group psychotherapy, so the reader should peruse our material with a critical spirit.

The fact that we, as clinicians at a health maintenance organization (HMO), have a vested interest in developing and using low-cost forms of therapy provides the second major reason for readers to approach our work with skepticism. Whereas the private practitioner earns his or her income piece by piece, with income increasing as the amount of treatment provided increases, an HMO, in effect, receives its income on the first of the month, spending it thereafter in providing services. In private practice, more treatment means more income. Conversely, in HMO practice, more treatment means less income (for the organization).

Clearly, short-term groups *do* cost less than comparable individual psychotherapy. If eight HCHP members are treated by James Mann's (1973) 12-session technique, 96 hours of therapist time are required. If the same eight members have 3 evaluation sessions and then 15 1½-hour group sessions in the type of group describe by Budman, Bennett, and Wisneski (Chapter 12, this volume) slightly less than half the 96 hours are necessary. Having done outcome studies (Budman, Demby, & Randall, 1980; Budman, Randall, & Demby, submitted), we are convinced that short-term group psychotherapy is an effective mode of treatment. But while its effectiveness is a necessary condition for using it, it is not a sufficient one. The reason we actually use it in preference to other modes of treatment of potentially equal effectiveness is that in addition to being effective, short-term group psychotherapy is relatively cheap. Especially given that many critics of the health system believe that fee-for-service financing encourages *over*treatment, logic and fairness demand that you approach our program with an equal but reversed suspicion and ask whether we, at an HMO, have a tendency to *under*treat. As befits mental health professionals, you should question our motives and ask yourselves if our clinical endorsement of short-term groups is unwittingly motivated by thrift.

Short-term group psychotherapy did not spring full-blown from the frugal bosom of an HMO. Although intellectual history has a deceptively rational way of making one event or movement seem to flow from another with a kind of translucent inevitability, there *is*, in fact, a clear line of development in psychology and social science that eventuates in this particular treatment mode.

In the sections that follow, I delineate the major antecedents of short-term group psychotherapy. My method of historical explanation may be described as a building block or "lego" theory. Short-term group therapy is not a radically new clinical technique. The development of short-term group treatment is more a process of practical construction, evaluation, and refinement than a new vision of psychotherapy or human psychology. But while all the pieces from which short-term group psychotherapy was constructed were available by the mid-1960s, these pieces did not come together by dialectical necessity. The cost containment emphasis of the HMO provided us with a motive for recognizing the possibility of assembling the short-term group mode from its constituent parts.

KURT LEWIN

The parent figure of T-groups and the encounter movement, and thereby of short-term group psychotherapy, is Kurt Lewin, a German-born experimental and applied social psychologist (Marrow, 1969). Lewin never practiced as a clinician. He was associated with the Gestalt psychologists at the University of Berlin until he came to the United States in 1932. In America he was a professor at Cornell and Iowa until 1945, when he established the Research Center for Group Dynamics at MIT. Lewin had been dreaming of and planning this center for years, but he was not able to fulfill his ambitions. He died in 1947 at the age of 56. The center itself was transplanted to the University of Michigan, where it continued to evolve and flourish.

Lewin was educated in the very individual-centered or atomistic tradition of psychology prevalent at the turn of the century. But the great discoveries made by the Gestaltists, who demonstrated that perceptions are shaped by the structure of the perceptual field and not simply by the individual units in it, helped Lewin to come to see human motivation and behavior as likewise the product of a field of forces. This approach to human psychology, known as "field theory," is more important as a view of psychological reality and an analytical method than as a body of specific findings. Lewin (1951) defined his "principle of contemporaneity" as follows: "any behavior or any other change in a psychological field depends only upon the psychological field *at that time* [italics in original]"

(p. 45). This proved to be especially important for its subsequent implications for therapeutic practice. In contrast to the historical "there and then" emphasis of the psychoanalytic movement, the clinical methodologies that ultimately evolved out of Lewinian psychology were much more attuned to forces for change residing in the "here and now."

Although his theoretical writings are Germanic and, to the clinician, obscure, Lewin was a master of pithy phrases which capture basic attitudes. He taught that to understand a person we must study his "life space"—in current argot, something like "the space a person is coming from." The life space is conditioned by the person's way of perceiving his internal and external world. Whatever the world is really like, we live our lives in terms of our understanding and expectations of it. The most powerful determinants of the life spaces we are in are the people and groups of our world—those we are actually part of and those we carry within. Gordon Allport summarized the "unifying theme" of Lewin's work as follows: "The group to which an individual belongs is the ground for his perceptions, his feelings and his actions . . . it is the ground of the social group that gives to the individual his figured character" (Introduction to Lewin, 1948, p. vii).

Like so many who lived through the 1930s, Lewin's basic view of human nature was profoundly shaped by the Nazi movement. Hitler's power to transform groups into mobs demonstrated the malignant potential of group forces. If the life space can bring about such destructive changes, presumably there are equivalently creative forces available to be unleashed. Lewin devoted the last 15 years of his life to studying how the field of forces created by groups and our total life space can be altered to strengthen democratic institutions and make us better people.

The crucial opportunity to develop and test ideas about the power of group process initially came to Lewin in an unpromising form—a consultation request from a pajama factory! The Harwood Manufacturing Company had opened a plant in rural Virginia. To compete, the company had to train 300 inexperienced workers to meet standards of productivity set in industrialized areas of the north. Although the workers were eager, they were demoralized by what they experienced as unrealistically high expectations, and their output was poor. Older workers, who were potentially a source of needed skills, could not be integrated effectively, because supervisors had what amounted to fixed negative stereotypes of the elderly. Furthermore, necessary and realistically achievable changes in job content and on-the-job behavior evoked fear, anger, and resistance. Looked at generically, these issues arising in the factory—demoralization, self-defeating stereotypes, and resistance to adaptive change—represent the core issues addressed in psychotherapy as well. In each work situation, Lewin found that people could change themselves and adapt to external demands if they faced the change as part of a group that was actively guiding the change process. The best technique for achieving successful change was to engage a small group in studying how to bring about the changes to which each individual was committed. Although the setting was a pajama factory in rural Virginia, the processes are essentially those we currently use in group psychotherapy. Parenthetically, it is interesting and, in retrospect, prophetic that some of Lewin's industrial work was first reported in 1944 at a conference on short-term psychotherapy: the Second Brief Psychotherapy Council of the Chicago Institute of Psychoanalysis (Lewin, 1948)!

EMERGENCE OF THE NATIONAL TRAINING LABORATORIES

History has a way of assuming mythic form, and if Kurt Lewin is the spiritual father of short-term group psychotherapy, the summer of 1946 represents the first tentative step by which the word became flesh (Benne, 1964). The Connecticut State Interracial Commission had asked Lewin and the Research Center for Group Dynamics to train community leaders in more effective techniques for combating racial and religious prejudice. For Lewin, this invitation presented a splendid opportunity to carry out what he called "action research" (Lewin, 1948). The leaders would be trained in a group setting, and then they would apply their newly refined skills as change agents in back-home groups. Perhaps most important, the two-week workshop, which took place in June 1946 at the State Teacher's College in New Britain, Connecticut, could itself be a laboratory for study of the group methods that Lewin and his colleagues were developing. Forty-one community leaders and agency workers participated; one-quarter were black, one-quarter Jewish, and one-half what was then called "other."

The participants were divided into three groups, each of which took problems from the home community as their focus. By current standards, the group techniques were relatively conservative—free group discussion or brainstorming, decision-making exercises, and some role playing. What was special was that research observers sat in on the groups and at evening staff meetings presented their observations. Most of the participants commuted to the conference, but one evening, three who were staying on campus asked to attend the staff's discussion. Some of the staff were edgy about this, but Lewin, who was always on the lookout for new methods and new data, agreed.

The results of this casual evening venture were electrifying. Hearing one's own group behavior discussed objectively had thunderbolt force. It is difficult for mental health professionals accustomed to extensive comment and even unasked-for psychoanalytic speculation about our behavior, to project backward an understanding of how astonishingly fresh an experience like this was. In 1946, encountering objective, compassionate, probing responses to one's public self had the excitement of newly discovering wine or romance; and that first evening session at New Britain had the further excitement of a primal scene—a hidden truth was revealed by observing the ordinarily cloistered parents.

The workshop at New Britain demonstrated that what came to be called "feedback" was a technology with great power. Drawing on the success of the workshop, the staff planned a three-week session for the summer of 1947, which was held at a boarding school, Gould Academy, in Bethel, Maine. Until Esalen emerged 15 years later, Bethel was *the* symbol of the new group movement. Given the subsequent turn toward social radicalism taken by the encounter movement, it is interesting to know that one of the sponsors of the initial Bethel venture was the United States Navy's Department of Research.

The group format used at Bethel in 1947 and then again in 1948 was the Basic Skills Training Group, or BST. The BST was designed to help the members learn how group process evolves and how they could catalyze effective group function. Personal change in the participants was not the objective. The group was aided by a researcher who observed the meetings and then took the role of a Greek chorus, feeding his observations back into the group. In this early format, feedback was largely the function of the researcher. Accurate and useful feedback was regarded as a skill, not just a spontaneous effusion of reactivity.

Although the BST groups were designed to teach about group process and not to explore the self, they quickly became very personal, and trainers had difficulty holding on to the back-home focus. Even after the first workshop, which so clearly aimed at developing skills for changing organizations, some participants were so moved by the experience that they proclaimed themselves to be human relations trainers. From its inception, the laboratory movement has generated enthusiasts and zealots. It has had an extraordinary magnetism for participants.

FROM T-GROUPS TO THE ENCOUNTER MOVEMENT

At the third annual Bethel workshop in 1949, the training staff was expanded to include several clinicians of both Rogerian and Freudian approach. The original leaders of the BST groups, who stood for the emphasis on skill training and organizational change, were deposed from overseeing the groups. The groups were renamed T, or training, groups, and while they still aimed at developing skills, the focus of learning shifted in a much more personal direction (Benne, 1964).

Structurally, what the National Training Laboratory (NTL) was trying to do in 1949 was akin to what my colleagues and I at the HCHP found ourselves doing 25 years later. The T-group was supposed to join the practical, problem-solving objectives and techniques of the BST with a more personal, therapeutic focus derived largely from individual psychotherapy. Blending the skills of psychotherapists with those of group problem solvers could have led to the kind of brief, problem-solving therapeutic groups described by Budman, Bennett, and Wisneski (Chapter 12, this volume).

But the time was not right, and this did not happen. Neither long-term dynamic group psychotherapy nor focused short-term individual psychotherapy of the sort described by Mann and Sifneos (Chapters 3 and 4, respectively, this volume) had been developed sufficiently to provide a context for conceptualizing short-term group therapy. In the absence of a context that could help tap this aspect of its creative potential, the T-group movement proved too highly charged to hold together, and like an unstable atomic nucleus, it underwent fission.

On one side, the NTL founders argued that participants contracted to learn about groups and organizations, not to undergo therapy, and that even if they wanted therapy, the brief span of a Bethel conference was too short a time for any meaningful therapy to occur. Thus, even in the late 1940s, the issue of whether short-term groups could be therapeutic was a focus of controversy, much as it is today. Over the years, this group of trainers moved away from therapeutic use of the T-group into organizational development and management training. For health and mental health workers, this field is especially useful for purposes of team development (Blake & Mouton, 1975). But since management training, organizational development, and team building are not the subjects of this volume, I will say no more about the NTL and its subsequent evolution.

Not surprisingly, the other main fragment produced by the fission of the T-group spun out to California. In the early 1950s, the UCLA School of Industrial Management had a program derived from the BST group at Bethel, called "skill practice in supervision." Over a period of ten years, skill practice was transmuted into what was initially called "sensitivity training." Below is an excerpt from the manifesto of the UCLA group, called "The Self in Process," published in 1962.

> Our discussions in early training groups often dealt, at a rather superficial level, with there-and-then matters; but as time has passed there has been increasing involvement in "gut-level" here-and-now events. Whereas before, much effort was devoted to working on the specific, immediate on-the-job problems of participants, now only minor emphasis on such matters remains. Much greater attention is centered on broader, pervasive concerns of the group members, such as their central life values and their rarely faced feelings about themselves and others. . . . For us . . . sensitivity training is no longer primarily a technique for the improvement of group functioning, the development of interpersonal skills, the intellectual discussion of human relations problems, or the more surface discussion of neurotic manifestations. . . . Rather, sensitivity training is now pointed in the direction of the total enhancement of the individual. (Weschler, Massarik, & Tannenbaum, 1962, p. 34)

Sensitivity training, like the T-group, could have evolved rather directly into short-term group therapy. In fact, the UCLA faculty thought of sensitivity training as "therapy for normals." But what actually happened to the sensitivity techniques developed at UCLA was California and the 1960s. I am sure we are all familiar with the greening of the sensitivity movement into touchy–feely groups, nude groups, and all the other modes that blossomed with the flower children of the 1960s and early 1970s. The blossoming was profoundly antiintellectual, anticlinical, and especially antipsychiatric. Sickness resided in society. The therapeutic maxims were "turn on, tune in, drop out" and "you have to go out of your mind to come to your senses." Sensitivity groups were seen not as treatment of sick individuals, but as liberation from a sick and destructive society. Participants were not patients, but people seeking to enhance their growth.

FROM ENCOUNTER GROUPS TO
SHORT-TERM GROUP PSYCHOTHERAPY

What came to be called encounter groups were clearly very powerful and engaging, and among a broad range of clinicians, there has been a general sense that encounter experiences were sometimes very beneficial for participants. In an effort to discern some underlying order in the jumble of different approaches and to see what merit could be found in the extravagant claims often made for encounter groups, Lieberman, Yalom, and Miles did an extensive study at Stanford University, which was reported in 1973 in *Encounter Groups: First Facts.* They studied 18 encounter groups representing 10 different methods or schools. Although the format varied between a few massed or marathon sessions and shorter sessions done at intervals, the total "treatment" time was 30 hours for each method.

For our purposes, the important aspect of their work is the demonstration that a leader's ideology does not correlate with his or her actual conduct in the group or with outcome as defined by a wide variety of outcome measures. What they were able to do was to define a constellation of leader activities that do correlate with outcome. Specifically, leaders who offer a great deal of warmth and positive support, who provide a rich cognitive framework within which group members can make sense of their experience, and who monitor the group process vigilantly to prevent scapegoating and to ensure broad participation had, by far, the best results.

For us at HCHP, these findings were extremely valuable. From practice, we were familiar with focused, short-term individual psychotherapy as described by Mann (1973), Sifneos (1972), and Malan (1976), among others. Many of us had extensive experience with long-term group psychotherapy, generally carried out in accord with Yalom's (1975b) formulations of technique. The demonstration that 30 hours of encounter group experience could have a modest but significant positive outcome encouraged us to consider the possibility that short-term dynamic group psychotherapy (utilizing modified forms of techniques we were already using in brief individual psychotherapy and longer term group psychotherapy) might be an effective and efficient addition to our treatment program.

Although we did not adhere to the encounter philosophy of change epitomized by spatial and kinetic metaphors, such as "getting *behind* facades" or *"breaking* through blocks," nor certainly, to the antiintellectual and anticlinical bias, we did subscribe, rather unknowingly, to the basic encounter optimism about the powerful therapeutic potential of a short-term group experience. For us, this readiness to believe that short-term group psychotherapy could be effective proved to be the crucial legacy of the encounter movement. Frankly, given the mental set that short-term group therapy is a plausible model of therapy, it was not a hard step to bring together concepts and techniques already well developed and readily available.

Since my job is to present history, not fiction, I will not pretend that our short-term group program emerged from a highly self-conscious study of Kurt Lewin, the NTL and its offshoots, and other forebears I have not even mentioned. In actual fact, and this will be no surprise to readers who have started clinical programs, our group program developed by a series of pragmatic decisions and trial-and-error efforts. It is only in retrospect that the origins of what we have been doing becomes so clear.

The clientele we have been working with in short-term groups present with a variety of neurotic, characterological, or situational problems, often with prominent emotional and physiological symptoms and dysfunction in major areas of their lives. Unlike encounter-group users, they are not simply seeking optional growth experiences. Nor did we, as clinicians, define the groups we began to offer in terms of the prototypic encounter belief that change is essentially the function of a single dimension, be it relinquishing facades, breaking through blocks, or getting in touch with the body.

Here, to summarize and conclude, I shall shift from historical to culinary terms. We want this volume to be useful to you in your practice, so in that spirit, I offer you a simple, basic recipe for preparing short-term groups.

From the encounter movement, take a good measure of optimism about the efficacy of brief group experience, so that the therapeutic power or placebo effect of the therapist's belief in the treatment will be maximized (Frank, 1973).

From short-term individual psychotherapy, take a sophisticated ability to develop a sharply defined treatment focus, which will be explored intensively within the confines of brief, concentrated work (Malan, 1976; Mann, 1973; Sifneos, 1972).

From long-term dynamic group psychotherapy, take skill at formulating psychological issues and treatment goals in the kind of interpersonal terms that allow both patient and therapist to understand how the group process may work (Yalom, 1975a).

Finally, from research, draw on such studies as *Encounter Groups: First Facts* and work of the kind presented by Strupp (Chapter 8, this volume) for a picture of the broad types of therapist activities common to effective therapies.

As described by my colleagues in subsequent chapters, we at HCHP have accumulated extensive clinical experience in the use of short-term group psychotherapy, and we continue to evaluate the efficacy of these groups. This brief foray into history indicates that a new and potentially controversial mode of psychotherapy actually emerged by a gradual process spanning more than 35 years. The fact that short-term groups were implemented at an HMO is not a coincidence or accident of the historical process—the *setting* of clinical practice has more influence on the forms of practice than is generally recognized (Sabin, 1978). This particular kind of setting, a group practice which attends to a large and definable population, and which emphasizes considerations of cost effectiveness, encouraged techniques and attitudes potentially available for many years to be brought together in a fiscally practical, clinically powerful way.

REFERENCES

Benne, K. D. History of the T group in the laboratory setting. In L. P. Bradford, J. R. Gibb, & K. D. Benne (Eds.), *T-group theory and laboratory method*. New York: Wiley, 1964.

Blake, R. B., & Mouton, J. S. Group and organizational team building: A theoretical model for intervening. In C. L. Cooper (Ed.), *Theories of group processes*. London: Wiley, 1975.

Budman, S. H., Demby, A., & Randall, M. Short-term group psychotherapy: Who succeeds and who fails? *Group*, 1980, *4*, 3–16.

Budman, S. H., Randall, M., & Demby, A. *Outcome in short-term group psychotherapy*. Manuscript submitted for publication.

Frank, J. D. *Persuasion and healing* (Rev.ed.). Baltimore: Johns Hopkins University Press, 1973.

Lewin, K. *Resolving social conflicts: Selected papers on group dynamics*. New York: Harper & Bros., 1948.

Lewin, K. *Field theory in social science: Selected theoretical papers*. New York: Harper & Bros., 1951.

Lieberman, M. A., Yalom, I. D., & Miles, M. D. *Encounter groups: First facts*. New York: Basic Books, 1973.

Malan, D. H. *The frontier of brief psychotherapy*. New York: Plenum Press, 1976.

Mann, J. *Time-limited psychotherapy*. Cambridge: Harvard University Press, 1973.

Marrow, A. J. *The practical theorist: The life and work of Kurt Lewin*. New York: Basic Books, 1969.

Sabin, J. E. The therapeutic relationship in neighborhood psychiatry: Impact of clinical setting on clinical practice. *Psychiatry,* 1978, *41,* 24–32.

Sifneos, P. E. *Short-term therapy and emotional crises.* Cambridge: Harvard University Press, 1972.

Weschler, I. R., Massarik, F., & Tannenbaum, R. The self in process: A sensitivity training emphasis. In I. R. Weschler & E. H. Schein (Eds.), *Issues in human relations training.* Washington, D. C.: National Training Laboratories, 1962.

Yalom, I. D. New directions in group therapy. In D. X. Freedman & J. E. Dyrud (Eds.), *American handbook of psychiatry* (Vol. 5, 2nd ed.). New York: Basic Books, 1975. (a)

Yalom, I. D. *The theory and practice of group psychotherapy* (2nd ed.). New York: Basic Books, 1975. (b)

CHAPTER 11
THE CRISIS GROUP:
ITS RATIONALE, FORMAT,
AND OUTCOME

James M. Donovan
Michael J. Bennett
Christine M. McElroy

This chapter describes the development of a short-term, crisis-oriented psychotherapy group begun in 1971 at the Harvard Community Health Plan (HCHP) in Boston. We report on it from a number of viewpoints. First, we describe how the crisis group evolved within our setting; then we explain the rationale, the format, and the clinical management of the group. We analyze outcome data from a sample of 43 patients who participated, and we include case studies of 2 of these to lend experiential illustration to the statistical data. Finally, we discuss the significance of these outcome findings and the curative factors within the group. We suggest ways in which this modality might be adapted to other settings.

The crisis group is a generic mode of treatment which might be utilized in one form or another within a range of settings, although, so far, this has not happened. The form of the group would probably vary according to the constraints within the mental health unit in question. For this reason, we describe our own department at some length to demonstrate how the group naturally evolved for us. The HCHP is a complete, multispecialty health maintenance organization (HMO). Its primary treatment units are two ambulatory care centers, one in Boston and one in Cambridge, which are affiliated with particular Harvard teaching hospi-

JAMES M. DONOVAN and MICHAEL J. BENNETT. Harvard Community Health Plan and Department of Psychiatry, Harvard Medical School, Boston Massachusetts.
CHRISTINE M. MCELROY. Department of Mental Health, Harvard Community Health Plan, Boston, Massachusetts.

tals. Some 90,000 prepaid patients receive most of their medical care at the HCHP or its affiliated hospitals.

HCHP, which began in 1969, offers broad mental health benefits. By 1971, the number of requests for mental health services was substantial. We often observed that fundamentally healthy people with a realistic life crisis, such as a divorce, were being referred. These individuals needed to be treated quickly, usually with brief, straightforward therapy. We decided to begin a group to treat such patients in cooperation with the triage nursing staff. Triage is the walk-in, acute-care medical area from which most of the acute mental health referrals emanate. Another objective of including triage staff was to teach the nurses about the diagnosis and treatment of psychological crisis.

In sum, we had within our setting a large number of relatively socially advantaged but troubled patients with realistic life crises, and we had a limited mental health staff to treat this population; we were integrated within a medical setting in which mental health care was accepted as a shared responsibility of the mental health and other medical departments. We hypothesized that a timely, realistic intervention could rapidly and effectively ameliorate the symptoms of the crisis. Furthermore, we hypothesized that the professional therapist did not have to be the only agent of change. Other medical personnel and fellow patients could participate within a system which treated the individual patient. We believed that rapid access to this sytem, rapid assessment of the problem, and feedback to the patient were at a premium in treating their difficulties. Given this outlook, and given the parameters of our setting, the development of the crisis group seems a predictable phenomenon. Indeed, by 1971, only two years after our center opened, the crisis group was fully formed and actively functioning and has thrived ever since.

THE FORMAT AND MANAGEMENT OF THE GROUP

Although it would be accepted practice at this point to review the literature in the area of short-term, crisis-oriented psychotherapy groups, this would be meaningless without first describing the specifics of our own group. For that reason, we delay the literature review.

According to the format of our group, the patient in psychological or medical distress, like all our referrals, is directed to us by a medical department, usually the triage area which, in our setting, handles those people in acute distress. The referral might also come from a primary care medical area. The crisis group candidate is someone who has experienced the acute onset of significant symptoms (e.g., sleeplessness, inability to work) in connection with a definable precipitating event or stress. This patient is not psychotic, homicidal, or suicidal, and he or she is willing to attend eight twice-weekly sessions over a four-week period.

The group is led jointly by a triage nurse and a mental health professional (a psychiatrist, psychologist, or psychiatric nurse). In the crisis group intake, performed by one of the two cotherapists, the patient and therapist examine the patient's crisis and its symptoms. The therapist develops a psychological formulation of the crisis and relates the symptomatic picture to that formulation. This evaluation is shared with the patient in an attempt to establish a working alliance and a common viewpoint. The therapist describes the group and suggests that the patient join. If the invitation is accepted, they agree upon workable goals for the treatment.

The group of six to eight members meets in the health center twice weekly for 1½-hour sessions, usually on Monday and Friday mornings from 9:00 to 10:30. The patient agrees to a therapeutic contract of eight consecutive sessions. Therapists rotate with all the adult mental health staff and five to six triage nursing personnel involved. Termination of therapists is overlapped, so that one of the two therapists terminates and is replaced each four sessions.

The group focuses on the present, especially the problem that provoked the individual's crisis reaction. Unlike other therapy groups, there is only secondary emphasis on group process. Each patient takes a turn telling his or her story, sometimes at great length, and perhaps like a Greek chorus, the other members listen, occasionally commenting. At the story's end, fellow patients and the therapist question, clarify, advise. Often there is a spirited debate in the group about the patient's problems and what he or she can do to improve the situation. In each subsequent session, the patient is queried about further progress and the diminution of symptoms. When one patient has finished his or her story in a particular session, the group turns to another. The tone of the group is invariable warm, supportive, and task oriented. The implicit purpose of the group is to help each member with the particular focused problem, such as whether or not to get a divorce, how to resolve grief over a parent's death, and the like.

The therapists are active and directive and take the lead in clarifying and explaining the patient's feelings and behavior to him or her. They interpret neurotic patterns quickly ("You're hanging onto this man who has been continually unfaithful. How come?''). They allude to the group process ("What does this long silence in the group mean when this woman tells us she will be terminating the group early?''). Group issues are important and are used therapeutically, but the core of the treatment is for the group to concentrate on individual patients serially. The changing cast of the group often makes group issues less important. The therapist presents him- or herself as a model of an alert, insightful group member from whom the other members are able to learn to question, interpret, prod, and confront. When the group has learned these skills, the therapist recedes and allows the group to do its work with its individual members.

The deepening of transference to the therapist is not seen as helpful in the treatment and is discouraged through rapid clarification of reality. We are trying to promote ego-oriented problem solving, not regression. Extra group meetings with either therapist alone are granted reluctantly, and the use of medication is avoided whenever possible. Patients are continually asked, explicitly and implicitly, what they can do to help themselves. This often includes reaching out to friends and family who have not yet been used for support.

Over the course of the group, there may be extensive, informal contact among members. Once the formal session ends, the whole group will often repair to a local restaurant to continue the session without the therapist. We do not criticize this; we feel that group cohesion is the medium of treatment, and the group is of such short duration that extensive clinging is unlikely to occur. In our outcome evaluation data, we concretely substantiate what was already obvious to us, specifically, that the therapist is not the key person in the treatment. It is the support and feedback from the other group members which has the most power.

Nearly all the patients terminate the group within the allotted eight sessions. After termination, a few group members maintain supportive relationships with one another for a few months and occasionally longer. About half the patients in our outcome studies sought further treatment, either in our setting or privately. This treatment was often group therapy. Beyond designing an active, short-term, crisis-oriented group with a specific number of sessions, we did little to plan the development of this group culture; it was a serendipitous evolution. Our outcome data demonstrate that when such a temporary society is to the patient's liking, and he or she remains within it, substantial benefit is almost always received. We shall elaborate on this point below and speculate on the exact nature of this benefit and the specific curative factors within the crisis group.

REVIEW OF THE LITERATURE

Apart from encounter and classroom laboratory groups, it is almost impossible to find literature on short-term psychotherapy groups employed as defined clinical interventions. Since our group has been so helpful to us and our patients, we are mystified by this phenomenon. There are probably at least two reasons for it. First, short-term groups may be in frequent use in a range of settings but are not so designated. For example, almost all inpatient milieu programs use group therapy, and since hospitalizations are often brief (15–30 days), these groups are probably, in effect, crisis groups focusing on the reason for hospitalization and on the patient's progress toward rehabilitation. Various psychoeducational groups within the community are, in fact, to a degree short-term focused therapy groups (e.g., Seminars for the Separated and Smoke-Enders).

The second reason may be that group therapy is usually seen as a long-term modality, its most notable proponents often state that good results can be expected only after one or two years of treatment (Yalom, 1975). Maybe there remains some sensitivity about group therapy as an inferior mode of treatment, so that practitioners are loathe to experiment with or to mention experiments that they have already done where they offer a brief group treatment. It is as if group treatment is enough of an embarrassment, and it is too much to make it brief. After all, short-term individual treatment has gained respectability only very recently, probably only in the last five to ten years. Probably to our credit, when we in the mental health field endeavor to treat the emotional problems of our fellow human beings, we feel that unless we offer them unassailably humanitarian and substantial treatment, we are being callous. In other areas of medicine, this would not obtain. A brief, cost-effective surgical procedure in place of a more extensive one would probably be readily accepted if positive outcome data were available.

When we search the literature, we find almost no reference to short-term groups which in any way resemble our own, and we find few attempts at outcome evaluation. The one startling exception is the work of Allgeyer and her associates in Los Angeles (Allgeyer, 1970, 1973; Strickler & Allgeyer, 1967). Since 1967, these practitioners have been using a model nearly identical to ours. When we started our group, we had no knowledge of Allgeyer's work, which is so similar, but which, oddly, is the only remotely parallel format mentioned in publication.

Strickler and Allgeyer (1967) rated 25 of 30 patients as "improved," and a majority of those as "maximally improved," after the crisis group. There was no follow-up, however, to ascertain if these effects lasted. The Allgeyer groups consisted of five to six members who met for six two-hour sessions. The therapy was focused, directive, and supportive on the part of both the leader and the patients. The group was continuous, but each person participated for only six sessions, so there was a constant turnover from experienced patients to novices. The Allgeyer groups were conducted in a similar way to our own; the positive reactions of both the patients and the therapists are consistent with our experience, as is the general positive clinical outcome.

In one setting, Allgeyer (1970) used a group with patients of lower socioeconomic class, some of whom had major mental illness. Again, the group was effective. Our patients were predominantly middle class, and those with major mental illness were screened out. Allgeyer's experience indicated that the crisis group need not be restricted to advantaged populations, socioeconomically or psychiatrically. We shall discuss below patient selection for a crisis group and the breadth of population that might be served. The range of applicability of the crisis group is one of the most important questions about it.

We mention other citations in the literature to show where the crisis group fits in the spectrum of clinical interventions and how others have developed somewhat similar procedures.

Trakos and Lloyd (1971) described a crisis group at the Illinois State Psychiatric Institute, which seemed to be designed to treat those who could not wait for or tolerate other forms of therapy. Therapist activity, the early formation of goals, and rapid admission to the group were all significant aspects of the treatment. Unlike our group, involvement with the family and outside agencies was stressed, and medication was used frequently. Outcome evaluation was attempted: 83% were reported improved.

Sadock, Newman, and Normand (1971) used a crisis group that was similar to ours, except that it was comprised of socially deprived patients. The group served as an intake procedure as well as a treatment mode; there appeared to be little previous screening of the patients. The group was apparently used primarily to deal with unreliable, possibly frightened, or poorly motivated patients. No specific clinical population was defined. There was no outcome evaluation or follow-up.

Allgeyer's work aside, the crisis group seems generally to have been used either as a measure of last resort for patients who would otherwise receive no treatment or as an intake group modality to quickly absorb

large numbers of patients in a clinical system which lacks sufficient therapists. The crisis group format has usually not been seen as an individuated,
legitimate form of treatment in itself. We are proposing that it be construed in just this way.

OUR OUTCOME STUDY

As we worked with the crisis group, we became struck with how helpful it
was to patients and how underutilized it might be in other settings. We designed a study to substantiate or refute the positive effects of the crisis
group. Such a study necessitated a longitudinal design. The first criticism
of any short-term method or treatment is that its effects are only short-
term. In our design, we studied a sample of 43 patients, large enough to
control for individual variation, and we provided for patient assessment at
three data points—just before entrance to the group, on termination of the
group, and one year following termination. We present the results of this
outcome study and then two case studies to lend vitality to the statistics.

METHOD

In our outcome study, we included patients who had participated in the
group at some time from November 1972 to January 1975. During this
time, 141 patients had been in the group, but 40 were withdrawn from the
study because they had attended fewer than four times, and 15 were excluded because they had failed to adequately complete our initial evaluation forms. Thus, we sent out 86 one-year follow-up forms and received 43
back.

Each subject contributed the following data: a pretreatment questionnaire asking for a description of his or her difficulties and expectations
of the treatment, a posttreatment questionnaire asking, through direct
questions, how successful the group had been, and a one-year follow-up
questionnaire assessing, again through direct questions, how many of the
treatment effects seemed to have persisted.

The patients also completed the Zuckerman and Lubin (1965) Multiple Affect Adjective Checklist and the Barron (1963) Ego Strength Scale
before beginning the group, just after the group, and again at one-year
follow-up. The Zuckerman test measures a person's subjective feelings of
anxiety, depression, and hostility at the time the test is taken. It has been

validated with a variety of groups, both in normal state and under hypnotic suggestion. The Barron test purports to measure ego strength, which, as defined by Barron, is the ability to gain from psychotherapy, to be spontaneous, to have vitality of feeling, and to have high self-esteem. It is negatively correlated with defensiveness, rigidity, and hypochondriasis. The Barron test, derived from the MMPI, is composed of 68 true-or-false questions that have been empirically related to ego strength by Barron and his colleagues.

We analysed the score changes on the Zuckerman scales (anxiety, depression, and hostility) and on the Barron scale, using one-way analysis of variance. Our hypothesis was that if the crisis group were clinically effective, the Zuckerman scores would decrease, and the Barron scores increase, from pregroup to postgroup, and that this change would be maintained for the subsequent year. Finally, the therapists were asked to complete pre- and posttreatment questionnaires on each patient, assessing the patient's clinical status on entering and leaving the group.

RESULTS

The sample of 43 patients appeared to be representative of the HCHP population: they were predominantly young (74% were between 18 and 35 years old), white, middle class, and highly educated (89% had graduated from high school, 53% from college); and 79% were women. The patients came for help in a focal, acute, interpersonal crisis; 75% entered the group because of a troubled relationship, usually a marital problem or a broken romance.

From both the patients' and the therapists' viewpoint on direct and indirect measures, we considered treatment an outstanding success. At the close of the group, 91% felt the group was "helpful," and 95% "liked" the group. The therapists rated 26% of the patients "maximally improved" and another 49% "improved." Although the treatment was brief, the subjective effects seemed stable over time. At one-year follow-up, when the patients were asked a number of direct questions about the efficacy of the group, they were again highly positive.

The changes in the three affective dimension scores on the Zuckerman tests were submitted to one-way analysis of variance. Both the anxiety and depression scores shifted downward from before the group until just after it; this change was maintained and augmented through the follow-up period. These differences met statistical significance. (Hostility scores decreased only slightly from pre- to postgroup and from postgroup to follow-up.) The Barron ego strength scores describe a similar pattern. One-way analysis of variance showed a statistically significant increase of ego strength through the three data collection points.

Finally, on postgroup evaluation and on follow-up, the patients gave reasons why the crisis group had been helpful. (One individual could give any number of responses, so the following percentages total to greater than 100.) The answers pointed to the importance of group support and cohesion. In the postgroup evaluation, 47% felt that the group support was helpful; 44% mentioned that it was helpful to know that others had the same problems; 42% felt that the chance to ventilate feelings was productive; but only 7% mentioned that the therapist was helpful. The perception of the functioning of the group was similar at one-year follow-up.

Participation in the crisis group may be a prelude to further psychotherapy, particularly group psychotherapy. In the year following the group, 44% of the sample received further psychiatric treatment. This was distributed evenly among individual and group psychotherapy and did not seem to relate to positive or negative outcome measured at one-year follow-up. Since less than 25% of patients in our department were in group therapy during that period, it appears that group psychotherapy is differentially chosen as a mode of treatment by the ex-crisis-group patient.

Two case studies of quite typical crisis group patients follow.

CASE STUDY NO. 1

This 31-year-old, white, single man entered the group in November 1974. He presented to triage with depressive symptoms and fleeting thoughts of suicide. The object of his sadness was a long-term girlfriend, who was repeatedly unfaithful. He played the long-suffering, stable, understanding partner, but as the pattern repeated over several years, he became increasingly symptomatic and agitated, though not overtly angry. Bright and intellectual, this man attended only two years of college and worked at a somewhat stimulating but low-paying position with little chance for challenge or advancement. No stranger to psychotherapy, he had perhaps 50 sessions of treatment prior to joining HCHP and 4 sessions with a staff psychiatrist before entering the group. He could not stand up for himself when abused by his girlfriend, and he did not pursue education and career with much ambition. Previous psychotherapy had been helpful but evidently not sufficient.

This man had a very positive course in the group. He liked the staff psychiatrist who referred him, and in the four pregroup sessions, he was already experiencing symptomatic relief. The psychiatrist liked him and felt that his prognosis in the group would be

> good for resolution of the crisis and for growth. At the moment, I do not anticipate the need for follow-up therapy. He must come to some decision about the relationship with his girlfriend. This will require some ability to tolerate his emotional reaction to the way he is apparently being treated and to experience some of the support of the group in order to do this.

Upon entering the group, the patient had a view of his central problem and his personality difficulties that was identical to that of the psychiatrist.

QUESTION: Describe the problem for which you are now seeking help.

ANSWER: Inability to sever unsupportive relationship after four-year duration. Inability to determine if relationship has potential or if I've been projecting value into it.

QUESTION: Describe the things you expect or hope will happen in the therapy group.

ANSWER: Feedback! Help in reevaluating certain values. Reaffirming certain self attitudes. Getting the active/passive into better perspective. Gaining some insight into the feelings of others, especially women. Hope to learn—remember—everyone's name in the group.

At the start of the crisis group, a positive two-way bond with the referring therapist and with the idea of the referral was obviously in place. This man had a clear idea of the external and internal difficulties that necessitated treatment and of his goals in it. His attitude toward group therapy was positive. He wanted to learn everyone's name and to receive feedback. He wanted to be involved, to be part of the group. His remarks indicated an ability and a motivation to speak and feel in the language of psychotherapy and a realistic knowledge of what issues were appropriate for therapy and what therapy could and could not offer.

This man's career in the group was highly positive. He improved a great deal symptomatically and appeared to grow internally. On termination, his reaction was enthusiastic: "warmth, feedback, input, a taste of reality, communality, varying perspective, good shit." His group therapist concurred:

> Excellent course. Very active participant in group. Still seeing old girlfriend but is less involved and has begun a new relationship with another woman.

Seems to have a better awareness of how he sets himself up in a relationship to be father/therapist, etc., and how this keeps him from getting what he wants.

At one-year follow-up, the group retained a positive glow, and, as predicted further treatment had not been necessary. He felt that participation in the group definitely did help him with his specific and general difficulties:

I had an opportunity to see others in their relationships. This helped me gain a better perspective on my own. I also met some very fine, caring people in the group. It permitted me to relax enough to get back in the swing of my job and personal interests. I had an opportunity to compare and contrast myself to others. It allowed me to reaffirm my self-evaluation and esteem. It helped me realize that I was a good, valuable person even though my relationship was ending.

QUESTION: Have you had similar difficulties in the past year to those that brought you to the group and how did you deal with those?
ANSWER: Varied, new acquaintances viewed more realistically so as not to set up old situations.

This man's Barron scores were 43, 51, and 48, respectively, at pregroup, postgroup, and one-year follow-up, indicating an increase in ego strength, although the high level at termination was not quite maintained. His Zuckerman scores followed a similar pattern, with anxiety and depression decreasing over the three data points.

This patient was in acute pain when he came to the group, could formulate his problem accurately, and could view treatment as a realistic and positive opportunity. He had resources in himself that the group could reaffirm; in the group, he reached out to others and appreciated them. Thereafter, he experienced himself with more approval, and his symptoms declined as his self-esteem rose appropriately. His treatment helped him with his focused problem and somewhat with his personality difficulties in general. More work perhaps needed to be done, and in subsequent years, he has returned, on occasions to his original therapist in the department, asking for specific help in one or two sessions but each time also reporting a better life for himself. He appears to be doing some of this work on his own.

CASE STUDY NO. 2

This 49-year-old, white, married woman, mother of four, was a member of a group of 43 people who did not return the one-year follow-up questionnaire but did participate fully in the group. She was contacted later by phone. Her experience paralleled that of the group on which we have full test data. The problem for which she sought help was that her husband could not finish his dissertation after many years of temporizing. His job was in jeopardy, and the family had been continually on edge as he struggled with this project. Her first husband had not adequately supported the family, and she had, with great anquish, divorced him some 12 years before. She had had a three-year course of individual psychotherapy in another town four years before entering the group and had found it helpful.

She attended all eight sessions of the crisis group and reported that it definitely helped her with her difficulties ("I was really upset; they did a lot.").

QUESTION: What was helpful?

ANSWER: It made me realize the feelings I was having were not unique. Behavior under stress is similar for everyone. Having a common experience is reassuring.

QUESTION: Would you participate in the group again under similar circumstances?

ANSWER: Oh yes.

QUESTION: Have the changes you experienced in the group been maintained under the present?

ANSWER: I think some. I can't separate the effects of individual treatment, in the year after the group. *[The patient had had 12 sessions of individual therapy.]* I still have some ups and downs but I talk about them. I do handle things better. My relationship and my job have improved. I have come to the conclusion that when other people in the family get upset, I don't need to go into therapy, they do.

Although this woman retained psychological difficulties ("ups and downs") and remained within a difficult marriage, the crisis group clearly helped her with her fury and helplessness over her husband's dissertation work and, in a general way, with subsequent upsetting circumstances. She came to the group with a defined problem. She was used to the procedure of psychotherapy, which she viewed positively, and she participated a great deal within the group. She appreciated the other members of the group and found the universality and cohesiveness of the crisis group of great personal importance. Over a year later, she remembered it very positively, particularly the input of the others in the group. She seemed to have gained the perspective that she did not need to be ashamed about her emotional reactions to problems, and that she did not need to take responsibility for the difficulties of every family member. Her husband did finish the dissertation, but one wonders if he would have, had his wife not sought treatment and subsequently separated herself from his writing difficulties.

DISCUSSION

The 43 patients studied here appear to have benefited significantly in terms of symptom change, that is, feeling that the group had helped or feeling less anxious or depressed by the group's end. They may also have made more profound developmental gains through the experience. Many reported changes that indicate greater general maturity: "I do handle things better." The pattern of the Zuckerman anxiety and depression scores and the Barron ego strength scores over the follow-up period corroborates such changes. Interestingly, the benefit to the patients seemed to come from the group culture, not specifically from the therapist. If they learned to look to peers more, and to parent figures less, for support and advice, this no doubt stood them in good stead after treatment and contributed to their favorable adjustment.

There are many potential criticisms of the outcome study. One criticism might be directed at the large number of those who participated in four or more group sessions but did not return the questionnaires one year later. We contacted as many of these patients by phone as possible, however, and they did not seem to differ appreciably from the research sample in their positive assessment of the treatment experience or their postgroup adjustment.

What can be said of the 40 patients who withdrew from the group before completing four sessions? It is possible that help could be had in one, two, or three sessions of a crisis group. Patients whom we later see in individual treatment often report that, but it is more likely that many of these withdrawals, some 28% of the participants in the group during the research period, were not helped significantly in the few times they attended. We assume that for them, the curative principles—universality and group cohesiveness—were, for whatever reason, inapplicable. These hypotheses speak to people who probably did not have a positive treatment experience; nor, to our knowledge, were they overtly harmed by it, unless one defines *harm* as the differential between this and some preferable treatment they might theoretically have received.

We know of only one instance of an apparent casualty among the 141 patients. A 26-year-old woman whose mother was dying of a lingering cancer became increasingly depressed in the group, did not respond what-

ever to the confrontation and support of the group culture, and finally had
to be removed from the group and treated individually with long-term psychotherapy and chemotherapy. This woman's capacity to regress and her
incapacity to respond to this psychological intervention was missed entirely by the original evaluators. This negative outcome of the case was utterly
unforeseen and might easily have occurred were individual therapy or no
therapy the disposition. This case was the only instance of a possible
"casualty" among a large number of patients. The crisis group may not be
applicable to everybody, but it does not appear to be a dangerous form of
treatment.

Those patients who dropped from the group should have been pursued and encouraged to return or offered alternative treatment, if appropriate. This is the policy of our department. We have no record of how
often it was actually followed or with what result, but our guess is that
there was further contact with many of these patients who left prematurely. No one form of treatment fits everyone. Dropouts from group therapy
are rather common, particularly at the beginning of the treatment. The
usual figure for dropouts from group therapy is 20–30%, just as it is here.
More thorough group preparation and a more careful screening of patients could reduce the number of withdrawals and should be done, but we
have to accept a certain percentage of disaffected patients, particularly
among acutely upset people who do not feel very confident about themselves and are perhaps fearful of group interaction. The discussion of withdrawal from treatment leads directly to a consideration of patient selection and group composition. These are discussed later.

Another potential criticism of the outcome study and of the efficacy
of the crisis group is that our patients were so advantaged educationally,
economically, and psychologically that almost any kind of treatment or no
therapy would have worked for them. It is important to note, however,
that all these patients were symptomatically impaired enough to seek referral; for that reason, no therapy was obviously not an alternative. The
symptoms usually improved rapidly at the time of treatment, and this trend
continued through the following year. It was our impression that this
change was caused by the treatment experience and would not have occurred as readily without it. The patients shared this view.

These conclusions about the efficacy of treatment might be studied
further, possibly by in-depth interviews of the patients and by the use of a
matched, untreated, or differentially treated control group. Such
strategies were impossible in our setting because of both financial and
ethical restraints.

THE CURATIVE PARAMETERS OF THE GROUP

The above qualifications considered, the crisis group appears surprisingly effective despite its brevity. Two specific curative factors—the cohesiveness of the group culture and the knowledge that others are in similar difficulties and want to help—seem the key to the treatment. It is important here to recall how insignificant the patients felt the therapists to be as change agents, in comparison to fellow patients. Interested and involved group members seem to replace the lost or disappointing person who has abandoned the patient and precipitated the crisis. Fellow group members, who often represent a broad age range, may also stand for family members to whom the patients might have turned in younger years. The presence of people who are terminating therapy, having solved many of their problems, and who can realistically advice and encourage newer patients is, no doubt, important. They socialize new patients into the group culture. The timeliness and intensity of the intervention, which comes at the height of the crisis, when the feelings are strongest, and which occurs twice weekly for 1½ hours per session, probably are also important. The facts that the patients have received all their medical care in the building where they attend the group, and that one therapist is always a medical nurse, may subconsciously make it a particularly safe haven.

However timely the group is, the patient knows it will also be brief. Most new members feel vulnerable and are open to seeking care from others, realizing they will have to receive it quickly, if at all. The feelings communicated in the group tend to be very positive (although much anger may be vented on outside people in abstentia). Perhaps there is a sense that there is no time to work through negative feelings. The patients feel they have found a place where others have the same problems and are accepting and highly supportive. They want to contribute to that atmosphere, helping others as they themselves have been helped.

The therapists capitalize on the positive atmosphere of the group. Regression is discouraged. Transference tends not to build because of the rotating therapists and the small number of sessions. Its use in the treatment is minimal, although the therapist's expectations that the patient will improve are a very important part of the treatment; in this way, transference is an unspoken presence. Negative transference regression is particularly discouraged. Insight by patients and therapists is used much less to further elucidate underlying conflict than to historically define the situation that is overwhelming the patient and to encourage a resolution. "You chose a man who would ignore you the way your father did and now you can't stand it, but you won't leave, either." When the patient can add to such formulations, and when the insight and support of the group begin to diminish the patient's feelings of worthlessness and pain, he or she gains a sense of greater mastery and self-esteem. This person can then often help someone else in a similar fashion.

When termination comes, the patient leaves with praise for getting better, warm encouragement for the future, and a feeling that he or she has graduated. For many, the separation becomes a corrective emotional experience and a first test of newly regained competence. Unlike the loss that brought them to the crisis group, it has a positive quality which authenticates, not denigrates, the self. The crisis group is not primarily insight oriented, but rather is aimed at problem solving and helping the patient return to independent living. The group culture, abetted by the therapist, communicates the expectation that the patient will present his or her problem, gain support, advice, and insight, confront the problem, take steps to resolve it, and improve symptomatically, and leave.

These are the curative parameters that we have been able to observe in the life of the group. We disclaim conscious responsibility for the development of much of this powerful group culture. We wished to undertake crisis intervention in a group, primarily because of the time pressure and training need. We speculated that group support would be helpful to the patients. We did not know that it would be this helpful nor that the process of the group would follow this particular format—a development that takes place week by week, year in and year out, regardless of different patients and different therapists. We certainly did not realize that the primary instrument of the treatment would be the group culture, not the therapists' activities.

As part of this powerful group experience, it is predictable that the patient will improve symptomatically within the group, but why does this improvement remain or even increase throughout the year after? The reason is not that 44%, as mentioned, received more treatment in the following year. Those who did tended to be slightly more symptomatic on follow-up testing. Alternatively, perhaps the crisis was a psychiatric low point in the person's life history. With the help of the group, he or she simply returned to a normal level over a year's time. A second possibility is that the positive experience in the group helped resolve some facets of a neurosis (probably by decreasing interpersonal inhibition and reliance on parental figures). This increased inner freedom may, in turn, have led to further psychological change after treatment. Wolberg (1965), for one.

believes that a brief, powerful intervention, such as a crisis group, can ease conflicts and allow the personality its own growth process. Those whose test scores improved from pre- to postgroup and even more markedly from postgroup to follow-up seem to fit Wolberg's schema. In the telephone follow-up and on the questionnnaires, many reported what appeared to be a global increase in psychological well-being and problem-solving ability following the group experience. These data, however subjective and certainly not applicable to all the group patients, imply that the crisis group does enhance personal development in a number of the participants and does not simply return them to a premorbid adaptational level.

Both these models of the effect of the crisis group may be accurate. Some individuals simply gain support at a difficult time and return to their previous style of functioning. For others, it is a generally liberating experience that induces further development when treatment is over. Reason dictates that still another group gains relatively little, although our outcome data indicate that this is not a prominent group, unless it is represented by those who drop out after fewer than four sessions. Therefore, those who stay within the group often receive lasting benefit from it, but a significant percentage leave precipitously. For that reason, patient selection and the overall technical management of the group become all important factors in its efficacy or inadequacy for a given patient. Specific technical skills or personality traits of one therapist versus another are less important factors in our format, since so many therapists are involved that individual differences erode in significance. We are describing a method here, not the individual attributes of therapists.

For what settings is the crisis group appropriate, who should be in it, and how should the group be managed? The crisis group could be appropriate in almost any clinical setting where patients have definable psychological crises. The daily group meeting that is invariably held on short-term inpatient wards focuses on exploring the internal and external situations which precipitated the hospitalization and on rehabilitating the patient to the community. In their fundamentals, these groups clearly parallel the crisis group, although they are labeled differently. These groups often have no name whatever; they are rarely referred to in the literature, or they disappear under the rubric of "milieu treatment." A good deal of staff time is often allotted to these groups, and our guess is that they are highly effective modes of treatment. In other words, a crisis-group-like intervention may already be a customary part of many inpatient settings and may have broad applicability as a treatment to hasten the

rehabilitation and discharge of patients undergoing short-term hospitalization.

The crisis group has even wider potential as a variation of outpatient
treatment. Patients need not be so socially advantaged as those in our setting in order to benefit from it. It is not a "rich man's treatment." Allgeyer (1970) used an identical technique with socially disadvantaged patients and obtained the same positive results. A state institution in the
Boston area is experimenting with the crisis group as a primary treatment
for some of its outpatients, many of whom have or have had major mental
illness and a history of multiple hospitalizations. Since the group helps the
patient rapidly solve a disquieting crisis, it seems an ideal modality for
preventing hospitalizations in a high-risk population. It also seems an
ideal form of treatment for specific subgroups, such as the recently separated or the recently unemployed.

The major precaution in applying the crisis group in a particular setting with particular patients is that one must be ever mindful of what the
central curative parameters of the group really are, that is, universality
and group cohesiveness. If the patients in the group differ too widely from
one another and do not overlap in experience, life situation, or outlook,
the group will probably lose its potency. Those prone to major mental illness will no doubt mix badly with those who have primarily reactive depression and are far from any psychotic state. Impoverished people whose
complaints are related to economic insufficiencies will not strike a chord
of universality in a group of highly employable, professional people. A
volatile, borderline person who rages about the room will only be disruptive among more sedate patients. The hypomanic, homicidal, or suicidal
person will be equally at odds with the thinking and behavioral universality of most groups. The seriously character-disordered person will have
such different values and superego functioning than the mainstream of patients that he or she will also be seen as deviant, undermining group cohesiveness. Those with this type of extreme psychopathology, which excludes them from a regular crisis group, could, of course, be put together
in some sort of short-term group with people similar to themselves. AA
groups, though usually not short term, are one example.

A subjective definition of universality is very relevant here. Some
people, for reasons of inhibition, embarrassment, guilt, narcissistic en-
titlement, or simply realistic personal preference, do not want to talk
about their intimate problems in a group. Our guess is that many of those
who dropped early from our crisis group fall into this category. They may
have been coaxed into the group in the first place, or once there, they may

have disliked it. For those who do not wish it, the group does not have universal appeal, and these patients do not experience or contribute to the cohesiveness of the group. They should not be forced toward it, and alternative treatment should be provided, if needed.

The therapist should also behave to foster universality and group cohesiveness. He or she should be active, inquiring, and optimistic, encouraging the patients to rapidly confront their problems and one another. The therapist should directly exhort the group members to interact: "What did you think of what she said? Your problems seem similar. Mr. _____, you haven't talked much today, what is on your mind?" Again, enunciating the principles of universality, the therapist should remind the patients that they came to the group with a central goal, that is, to resolve a crisis, and should not allow the group to regress into a complaint session. The therapist should also be open and accepting enough for the group to feel that he or she is with them and not interacting with them from above. The former stance will increase cohesiveness and decrease problematic transference reactions. The therapist should consistently articulate the central goal of the group, namely, that the patients want to feel more independent and to have a better self-esteem and, conversely, to feel less controlled by symptomatology and other people. This behavior by the therapist contributes to the air of universality and group cohesiveness. Perhaps most importantly, the therapist should embody the confidence that difficult feelings can be examined, and conflicted human relations can be resolved to a degree.

These guidelines translate into a therapeutic style which is active, open, friendly, perceptive, often confrontative, but supportive; it is not a remote, blank-screen style, but rather a style which encourages patients to use their own resources (and those of the group, friends, and family) and not to look toward the therapist or conventional authority figures for all their solace. If the therapist can help the patient accept him- or herself and recognize the need to work on problems in a context with others, then the therapist is truly fostering a sense of universality and cohesiveness, which will enable the patient to gain from the group treatment and carry increased self-reliance and self-esteem from it.

CONCLUSION: LIMITATIONS AND STRENGTHS OF THE GROUP

The limitations of the crisis group as a treatment should be reemphasized. Although it probably can free people internally so that they can develop to higher levels than previously, the crisis group almost certainly cannot bring about major characterological change, since it is so brief. In our outcome study described above, nearly half the patients received further treatment in the year after the study, and approximately one-fourth of the patients referred to the group dropped from it; thus, the crisis group is often not a final form of treatment, and it is not applicable to everyone.

As mentioned earlier, an additional limitation is that the patients in the group probably must have a great deal in common in order for the group to work smoothly. Those with major mental illness will not mix with well-compensated but acutely upset neurotics. Patient selection is crucial. Since the group session should be in excess of an hour in length and be offered twice each week, and since each patient needs an individual evaluation before the group, staff time is probably not greatly saved by using this model. Frankly, we feel that it is usually a superior mode of treatment to individual crisis intervention, since it fosters feelings of independence and relatedness in the patient, but in terms of conservation of resources, it is not a dramatically economical mode of service delivery. This is particularly true if the cotherapist model is used. This is not obligatory, but the fast-paced, acute nature of the difficulties and the large number of patients lend preference to the cotherapy arrangement.

Such a model also allows the crisis group to be a training instrument, and here it probably has few equals. The experienced therapist can give on-the-spot supervision to the inexperienced. The number of patients who rotate through the group and through all phases of the treatment, however brief, can teach the newer practitioner a great deal about individual psychopathology and symptom formation and about the course of treatment. Group dynamics and crisis intervention principles are also there in abundance, ready to be learned by the novice and to be pointed out *in vivo,* by the lead therapist after each session.

Although it is neither a new nor miraculous form of treatment in terms of cost or efficacy, and although not every patient in every setting can use it, the crisis group can be a crucial part of an integrated clinical program. With a limited investment of staff resources, the group offers a surprising amount to a large number of people at a time when they need it and in a form in which they can use it. The cotherapy model is ideal for training purposes or for building cohesion among seasoned staff as they work in pairs.

REFERENCES

Allgeyer, J. M. The crisis group: Its unique usefulness to the disadvantaged. *International Journal of Group Psychotherapy,* 1970, *20,* 235–239.

Allgeyer, J. M. Using groups in a crisis-oriented setting. *International Journal of Group Psychotherapy,* 1973, *23,* 217–222.

Barron, F. Ego strength and the power to rally from setback. In F. Barron (Ed.), *Creativity and personality freedom.* Princeton: Van Nostrand, 1963.

Sadock, B., Newman, L., & Normand, W. D. Short term group psychotherapy in a psychiatric walk-in clinic. In L. Barten (Ed.), *Brief therapies.* New York: Behavioral Publications, 1971.

Strickler, M., & Allgeyer, J. M. The crisis group: A new application of crisis theory. *Social Work,* 1967, *12,* 28–32.

Trakos, D. A., & Lloyd, G. Emergency management in a short term open group. *Comparative Psychiatry,* 1971, *12,* 170–175.

Wolberg, L. R. The technique of short-term psychotherapy. In L. R. Wolberg (Ed.), *Short-term psychotherapy.* New York: Grune & Stratton, 1965.

Yalom, I. D. *The theory and practice of group psychotherapy* (2nd ed.). New York: Basic Books, 1975.

Zuckerman, M., & Lubin, B. *Manual for the Multiple Affect Adjective Checklist.* San Diego: Educational & Industrial Testing Service, 1965.

CHAPTER 12
AN ADULT DEVELOPMENTAL MODEL OF SHORT-TERM GROUP PSYCHOTHERAPY

Simon H. Budman
Michael J. Bennett
M. J. Wisneski

At present, the thinking in psychodynamic group psychotherapy remains at about the point where the thinking in dynamic individual psychotherapy was prior to the great innovations of Balint, Malan, Sifneos, Mann, Wolberg, and others. That is, major theoreticians, such as Yalom (1975), consider group therapy a long-term treatment modality, with brief group approaches seen as providing inferior and palliative care. What Wolberg (1965) described as "prejudices of depth" dominate the group therapy literature.

The Harvard Community Health Plan (HCHP) short-term group therapy program grew out of a need to treat a large, psychologically oriented population in a high-quality, cost-effective manner. In 1976, when the Commonwealth mental health law went into effect, it required that all Massachusetts insurance carriers include coverage for chronic psychiatric conditions. As many of our resources at HCHP needed to be refocused on this population, it became necessary for us to consider new approaches for the healthier part of our membership. It should be explained that HCHP is a large, prepaid, group-practice-type health maintenance organization (HMO) with three centers located in the greater Boston area. The Kenmore (Boston) Center of HCHP and its mental health program as a whole are described in greater detail elsewhere (Budman, Feldman, & Bennett, 1979).

SIMON H. BUDMAN, MICHAEL J. BENNETT, and M. J. WISNESKI. Harvard Community Health Plan and Department of Psychiatry, Harvard Medical School, Boston, Massachusetts.

By 1976, we had had considerable experience with short-term individual treatment approaches and with the crisis group program. There had also been some less well developed experience with short-term groups for people in midlife and late midlife. Early in 1976, we began to direct more of our energies toward the implementation and clearer conceptualization of short-term group psychotherapy.

At first, the homogeneity of these groups, in terms of age of participants, was an administrative convenience; for example it was easier to keep track of the particular group to which a patient should be referred. Only gradually did we come to realize the theoretical and technical reasons that such divisions made sense. At that time, we were operating with very little guidance from the group therapy literature, since much of that literature rejected the idea of changes occurring quickly in group therapy.

A number of clinicians at HCHP formed a monthly, short-term group therapy workshop and began to meet regularly in order to understand more fully the process and theory of the short-term groups. Early in the history of these meetings, several things became clearer to us. For one, people of a similar age (and, we presumed, at a similar stage of adult development) had common issues and concerns and could quickly become a cohesive group. For another, the process of these groups at different age levels was not the same.

These two "discoveries" may not seem to be earthshaking, but both were quite important in helping us further clarify our thinking about, and refining our practice of, short-term group treatment. We realized that people of different ages had different needs. (These commonalities of issues among people at a given age level were most striking if the latter were not psychotic or too severely disturbed.) Nowhere in the group therapy literature was there discussion of these phenomena.

At that same time, we began to examine more closely the literature on adult development. Life history research, such as that by Vaillant (1977) and Levinson, Darrow, Klein, Levinson, and McKee (1978), did support our experiences and framed them within a conceptual system. Our short-term group patients began to teach us that for people at a given level of development, the great common areas of concern could cut across very different initial symptom pictures. It also became clear that beginning to work on these common areas of concern within the context of a short-term group could have great impact on a patient's life during and after the group. Thus, it appeared to us that people could have major difficulties negotiating one or another stage of adult development, and that a brief group intervention focused on these developmental issues or tasks could have an important impact in enabling patients to continue their growth.

The notion that group process differs according to level of adult development was also new. For the most part, it had been and continues to be asserted that the unfolding of group process within small groups is inexorable, occurring regardless of leader, patient, or situational exigencies. As we discussed our experiences, it became clearer to us that although the process of the short-term young adult groups closely paralleled the literature on group process and group development (presumably because most studies of group process had been done with this population), there were major differences in how the process evolved in early and later midlife groups.

We also learned a good deal from the literature on short-term individual psychotherapy. In particular, this literature addressed the importance of focality in brief treatment (Malan, 1963; Small, 1979; Ursano & Dressler, 1974; Wolberg, 1965), therapist activity level (Barten, 1971; Butcher & Koss, 1978), patient and therapist expectations of improvement (Butcher & Koss, 1978), patient selection factors (Hartley, 1979; Strupp, 1980), and the clear conviction supported by research (Sloane, Staples, Cristol, Yorkston, & Whipple, 1975) that significant change can, indeed, occur in brief treatment. Our experiences with short-term group treatment helped us develop a conceptual frame of reference. In turn, this theoretical understanding has helped us refine our techniques and approaches (Budman, Bennett, & Wisneski, 1980). At this point, we believe that important and generalizable therapeutic work can begin within the context of a relatively short-term group therapy experience by (1) helping group members focus upon, and grapple with, life-stage issues, (2) modifying technique and structure in the group to more closely match the particular life-stage issues being dealt with, and (3) keeping group members attuned to the brevity and time-limited nature of the treatment.

We shall describe the three types of short-term adult developmental model groups done at the Kenmore HCHP mental health department. These are (1) groups for young adults (early 20s to early 30s), (2) midlife groups (mid-30s to early 50s), and (3) later midlife groups (early 50s to early 70s). We shall discuss the central issues for members of these groups, patient selection factors, group processes, and issues of therapist activity. At this point, approximately 20% of our patient population is seen in such groups, and we have had experience with over 2000 patients in this treatment modality.

YOUNG ADULT GROUPS

Although there are many concerns for people going through young adulthood, we believe that the most common, unifying, and familiar ones center around problems of intimacy and closeness. The members of our young adult groups, who are usually in their early 20s to early 30s, are almost invariably dealing with problems in this area. We believe that most of these pati⌣nts are confronted with the issues which Erikson (1959) described as "intimacy versus distantiation and self-absorption," that is, the ability to be truly close and loving to another person rather than isolated, distant, and/or pseudointimate. Some of these patients make much use of what Elliot Jaques (1965), in his classic paper on death and the midlife crisis, called a "schizoid defense style." Vaillant (1977) stated that young adults tend to use "immature defenses," such as projection, hypochondriasis, withdrawal, acting out, and so on. He went on to say:

> Thus, psychiatrists who work exclusively with young adult (especially graduate student) populations discover that regardless of diagnosis, difficulties surrounding intimacy are the dominant motifs of their patients' complaints. The emotional disorders that selectively afflict young adults—schizophrenia, mania, impulsive delinquency, and suicidal inclinations—all reflect anguish about, or protest against, failures at intimacy. [Furthermore] to fail at intimacy . . . [is] to forfeit mastery in the next stages of the adult life cycle. (p. 215)

Clearly, a young adult who is unable to negotiate the establishment of intimate peer relationships is at risk.

Most individuals in our young adult groups are not devoid of skills in this area. For the most part, they were able to develop friendships in childhood and adolescence, and they have been able to gain some separation from their families of origin. They are having great difficulty, however, in being truly open, sharing, mutual, and committed in current relationships. These individuals can often relate reasonably well to others at work and in more formal interactions. They have great difficulty in closer relationships, however, and are, to some degree, lacking in the ability to be appropriately disclosing, supportive, assertive, and/or loving to significant peers.

As will be described, the format of the young adult groups and the leader's continual attention to the central issue of intimacy make this short-term group modality uniquely appropriate for those directly or indirectly dealing with young adult issues.

PATIENT SELECTION FACTORS

Patients referred for the young adult groups may be highly symptomatic and under great stress. It is critical, however, that they have a basic ability to relate to other people. Our research (Budman, Demby, & Randall, 1980; Budman, Randall, & Demby, submitted) has indicated that patients who are highly schizoid, with few if any friends, who are very suspicious of others, and who are relating most frequently to their family of origin rather than to their peers tend to do poorly. One needs a basic relatedness to other people in order to gain in short-term group therapy. We are in agreement with Grunebaum and Solomon (in prep.) when they write:

> We believe that an individual's behavior in group as well as in work settings and school depends on his/her ability to have ways of structuring peer relationships more than on his/her specific symptoms or past relationships with parent figures. (p. 2)

When screening patients for the short-term young adult groups, the therapist should, in particular, explore the patient's relationship history. Does the patient have friends? People to whom he or she relates? What has been the history of friendships? Did the patient ever have a best friend? Did the patient belong to groups, clubs, organizations as a child? If a patient lacks a history of at least some positive and productive interactions with peers, a group referral should be questioned.

The following case examples illustrate some background differences in two male members of the same young adult group. Although both entered treatment being highly symptomatic, Barry was far more able than Jack to "hook into" the group, and the group to him.

> Barry, a very anxious, 28-year-old administrator, was referred for a short-term young adult group because of increasingly severe phobic anxiety. He could not travel anywhere by public transportation and was forced to either drive or walk anywhere he went. His driving was also restricted, since he would quickly be overcome by anxiety, hyperventilation, and a dread that something terrible was about to happen to him.
>
> He reported a history of close childhood friendships with his siblings as well as with other children in his neighborhood. In high school and college, he had had several male friends and did some dating. In the group, Barry presented as a rather intellectualized but very humorous and engaging person. Although he was tense and stiff in early meetings and reported that several times he had considered running out of the room because he felt "trapped," he gradually started to open up. This process began around his being very soli-

citous of other members of the group. Especially during times of tension in a meeting, he would try to say something funny or supportive. The therapist and other group members began to point out to him that although he could be helpful and caring to others, it was quite difficult for him to reveal his own needs and issues. He began to experiment with talking more in the group about himself and his own problems. There followed several sessions where Barry spoke about a number of major family problems which he had previously discussed with no one, such as his mother's drinking and her severe depressive episodes. When these occurred, his father would call him for advice and solace.

Because of his willingness to relate in the group and to actively participate, Barry became a valued member. As he opened himself up for help and support, such caring from the group was forthcoming. Over the course of the 15 sessions, Barry changed his behavior in the group considerably. He went from someone who could be verbal and active regarding information, events, or someone else's problems to someone much more able to also discuss himself, his needs, and his concerns. By the end of the group, he had scheduled a vacation which would require a good deal of flying. At a three-year follow-up, he remained symptom free and still had fond memories of the group.

Jack, a 29-year-old insurance examiner, requested therapy for his difficulty in relating to women. He had never had an ongoing love relationship with a woman and, during high school and college, was isolated and withdrawn. Although he had some acquaintances, he tended to be without friends. The patient was born with a cleft palate and seemed to be quite self-conscious about this, although in no way did it overtly affect his functioning.

Two years before he sought therapy, his parents and divorced after a protracted separation. He was the oldest of four children, and he had decided to stay home with his father in order to "help Dad raise the others." This was in spite of the fact that his youngest sib was already in late adolescence when Jack's parents separated. He was extremely focused on the chaotic events at home and had never left home again after graduating from college.

Initially, Jack's attempts at relating within the group were generally contentious or ill timed. He would begin to dominate the conversation during early sessions with very specific and rigidly stated advice for any member or members who presented their concerns and problems. By the fifth meeting, his lecturing had become a source of irritation for several of the men and women in the group. In that session, it appeared that Jack might soon be scapegoated, as some members began to cut off his lectures or ignore him. The therapist tried to get Jack as well as the group to look at the responses which his pedantic behavior engendered. Jack could hear the leader's interventions only as critical and attacking. His position became, "If people don't like what I have to say, then I won't speak at all." From the fifth meeting to the end of the group, he was generally withdrawn, responding curtly to any invitation to speak. He ceased to actively participate and was left behind. At the end of treatment, he felt that he had made a few slight gains. Four months later, however, he was angry and disappointed and felt very defeated by the course of treatment.

Strupp (1980), in discussing psychotherapeutic outcome in time-limited individual psychotherapy, writes:

> The key determinants of a particular therapeutic outcome are traceable to characteristics of the *patient* . . . if the patient is a person who by virtue of his past life experience is capable of human *relatedness* and therefore amenable to learning mediated within that context, the outcome even though the individual may have suffered traumas, reverses, and other viscissitudes is, [*sic*] likely to be positive. . . . If on the other hand his early life experiences have been so destructive that human relatedness had failed to acquire a markedly positive valence and elaborate neurotic and characterological malformations have created massive barriers to intimacy (and therefore to 'therapeutic learning') chances are that psychotherapy either results in failure or at best in very modest gains. (p. 716)

The importance of this capacity for relatedness may even be greater in short-term group psychotherapy than in short-term individual therapy.

PREGROUP PREPARATION

It is quite clear to us that a major element of successful group therapy is adequate pregroup preparation. Effective pregroup preparation can function to more quickly enhance group cohesiveness and reduce the dropout rate (Budman, in press; Budman & Clifford, 1979; Budman, Clifford, Bader, & Bader, in press; Piper, Debbane, Garant, & Bienvenu, 1979).

In running a short-term therapy group, both these issues are of great importance. Both low cohesiveness and high dropout rate mitigate against a group quickly pulling together and becoming a working unit. For these reasons, and because we (and other researchers) have found the group dropout rate to be higher among younger patients (Budman, Demby, & Randall, 1980; Myers, 1975; Sethna & Harrington, 1971), we place a great deal of emphasis upon pregroup preparation for the young adult groups.

Prior to the start of a young adult group, patients are interviewed individually by the group therapist for a half-hour session. During this session, we attempt to clarify both the current issues and the goals for treatment, and we tell the patient something about the short-term group. In addition, this interview is used to give the group therapist a clearer idea about the patient's motivation and interest in group treatment and to screen out any patient who would appear to be obviously inappropriate (e.g., one who is psychotic, suicidal, or homicidal or does not wish short-term group therapy). During this interview, we also attempt to help the patient "reframe" his or her presenting problems into interpersonal forms. In particular, we focus on what a given symptom picture may mean about the patient's ability to be close to others.

Several days or weeks following this interview, we hold a pregroup preparatory workshop with all patients about to join a given short-term group. This workshop serves a dual purpose: it provides pregroup patient preparation, and it acts as a screening tool for the therapist. The best predictor of group behavior is group behavior (Bond & Lieberman, 1978). The workshop allows the therapist to see patients in group interaction, and it allows the patients to experience group interaction before they actually join. We see the workshop as particularly important in preparing young adult patients. Because the intimacy issue is so central, and because there is so much discomfort and anxiety in this area for our young adult population (which is not present in the same way for older adults), we do what is possible to reduce the threatening aspects of the group. In going through the pregroup workshop, a patient can decide before treatment begins whether or not he or she wishes to stay with it. Thus, the disruptive effects of dropouts are minimized. Within the context of our couples group program, a similar workshop structure reduced dropouts to below 1% (Budman & Clifford, 1979).

The workshop itself (which is described in greater detail in Budman, in press) has three components. In the first part of the workshop, patients meet one another under less tense, more structured conditions than might ordinarily occur in a therapy group. Patients are asked to pair off, introduce themselves to one another, and return after ten minutes to the larger group, where each introduces the person with whom he or she was speaking.

In the second part of the workshop, patients form small groups of four and are asked to describe an incident which they wished they had handled differently. As one person speaks, the other three listen and are then asked to role play with the person the way the situation actually occurred. The four then discuss alternative methods of handling the situation and role play these alternatives.

In the third component of the workshop, the group as a whole does a task. This task generally requires the participants to imagine themselves as part of a club or organization planning a dinner together.

Feedback regarding the workshop has been very positive. It allows patients to become more comfortable with one another under less stressful circumstances than generally exist at the beginning of a therapy group. We have screened patients out of the group at this point, if they appear to be an extremely poor fit with the rest of the group, or if they look very fragile or disturbed.

The following example illustrates how the pregroup workshop may be used for screening purposes:

Mark was a 21-year-old laboratory technician. He was intelligent and quite capable at his job but tended to be immature socially. He was small in physical stature and looked about five years younger than his stated age. Mark's problems were mainly in relationships with peers. He had a small group of male friends, all of whom were involved in chemistry as both a career and a hobby. He had distant relationships with women, which almost invariably ended in rejection if he tried to get close or start a dating relationship.

During the pregroup workshop, it became apparent that Mark did not fit well with the other prospective members of the group. In contrast to them, he appeared even younger and more immature in his concerns. He was the only group member still living at home and seemed unable to sympathize with the issues presented by others as problems. In the large group exercise, he was extremely anxious and concrete.

On the basis of the therapist's observations of Mark in the workshop, it was felt that he would do far better being the oldest member of a late adolescent group than the youngest member of a young adult group. The workshop allowed the therapist to make some clinical estimates of Mark's ability to fit into the group as well as gain a sense of the group. When the therapist discussed with Mark the possibility that he might not fit well with the group and proposed a group of younger persons, Mark seemed quite relieved and amenable to this.

THE GROUP PROCESS

Between one and two weeks after the pregroup workshop, the group itself begins. With young adults, we have closed, 15-session groups, in contrast to the midlife and later midlife groups, which have open, rotating memberships. We believe that the closed format highlights and enhances the intimacy issues within the group, whereas a rotating membership would work against the development of such closeness. Where we have tried a rotating membership with young adults, the group appeared to be far less successful than with the closed format.

Young adult groups are told that the primary goals are to help members get closer to one another and to examine their emotional responses to interpersonal interaction. For these reasons, there is an emphasis on here-and-now interaction, with there-and-now or historical materials woven in flexibly. Because intimacy and fears about intimacy are the central issues for young adults who are developmentally on track, the therapist must actively steer the members toward examining their interactions and affect within the group. We have found that there tends to be a great deal of passivity and dependency upon the leader, especially during the earliest and latest stages of group development. Therefore, the leader walks a fine line. If, on the one hand, he or she is too active, the group can easily become leader centered, with some members passively allowing the leader to run the show and/or others entering into a counterdependent power struggle with the leader. On the other hand, therapist inactivity often leads to much projection, anxiety, and struggle to get more from the leader.

The young adult groups, in order to stay with the task at hand, which is dealing more intimately, openly, and immediately with one another, must be group focused. In our view, the leader of these groups can and should actively help members stay task centered. This may be done by getting members' immediate reactions to events in the group, having members share feeling about one another, examining repetitive interactional patterns in the group, encouraging members to ask questions of one another rather than the leader, getting member feedback regarding other members, and so on. The following example illustrates the application of several of these techniques during the third meeting of a young adult group:

> The meeting began with some general discussion about how hard it is to talk to people and have them listen to you. Most members of the group (four men and four women) were in agreement that although they tended to be quite willing to take time out and listen to other people's problems, few of their friends were willing to do the same for them. Willy said that he was uncertain about opening up and then having the other person not respond or look at him as if he were "a total jerk." Ruth said that her friends would tell her that she was really strong, that they were sure she would handle things, and then pat her on the back and leave before she could say too much. She continued in a quiet voice, trembling with emotion, "If I were upset and felt lonely or afraid or that I couldn't handle things, there would be no one there for me." Almost immediately Greg intervened and told Ruth, "If people aren't listening to you, then they've got the problem, not you, so don't worry about it, forget it, you're fine." The therapist told Ruth that immediately before Greg's comments, she had looked very upset and near tears, and that afterward she again appeared strong, competent, and in control. He then asked her how she had

felt immediately before Greg's comments. She agreed that she was near crying but would have felt stupid if she had done so. The leader then asked each of the group members how they had felt when Ruth was so close to tears. Most had felt anxious or uneasy. Linda said that Ruth's tearfulness made her want to cry, and that she was terrified that if she (Linda) did indeed begin, it would be "hours before I get myself together." When Greg spoke, he again began to intellectualize and asked the group what was the best way to reassure someone who was upset. The leader gently but firmly told him that he was moving away from his feelings about Ruth's upset and asked him again how he had felt at the moment that she began to seem tearful. He was able to sit with the feelings for a few moments and then explained that a woman with whom he had lived for three years and had recently broken up with would "suddenly" become extremely upset, tearful, inconsolable, and suicidal. When he had seen tearfulness in a "strong person" like Ruth, he became frightened that she might become hysterical and "fall apart," too.

The incident above was quite productive for Ruth, Greg, and the other group members. In later discussion, it became clearer to Ruth how her fear of her own emotions made it difficult for others to give her support. She gave signals that what came out could be overwhelming to her, and that she was gladly deflected from pursuing her own concerns. For Greg there was the opportunity to see *in vivo* how he used intellectualization and how uncomfortable affect made him. For the group as a whole, the incident was of major importance, because they were dealing with feelings and with one another.

None of the interventions described in the above example is a patient–leader transference interpretation. We feel such interpretations are valuable if the progress of the group or of one or more members is being impeded by the transference to the leader. For the most part, however, the therapist's active interventions are intended to enhance intermember relatedness.

It has been our experience in training short-term group therapists that the tendency is for experienced (i.e., long-term) group therapists to be too passive in these groups. Sitting back and waiting for the process to evolve, not interrupting silences, and intervening infrequently are all aspects of treatment that can be acceptable in a long-term group, which may last indefinitely. Therapist inactivity or passivity is unacceptable in short-term group treatment for young adults. Group members have a limited period of time in which to work on their goals and need therapist support and active intervention to do so. The other tendency for neophyte young adult group therapists, especially those who have done much individual treatment, is to do individual therapy in a group. This may benefit a few members to some degree, but it defeats the goal of peer intimacy and defends against it.

The stages of group development in the short-term young adult groups closely parallel those described in other literature on process in small group interaction (Tuckman, 1965). The initial meetings of these groups are characterized by members directly or circuitously asking, "Who are the members of this group, and why are we here?" Initially, members share information about themselves and why they are in the group. From the beginning, young adult groups display much more passivity and dependence upon the leader than the midlife or later midlife groups. It is the leader's task to keep members dealing with one another and with their emotions. At no point should the leader deliberately attempt to frustrate members' dependency by silence or withdrawal but should actively attempt to communicate that "truth" does not reside in the leader alone. Regardless of how "giving" the therapist is, the groups reach a point in about the sixth session where there seems to be a group crisis. During the crisis, usually of one- or two-session duration, members are frustrated either by the leader's "ungiving" position or by the leader's overcontrolling stance. This frustration may be exemplified by an angry or depressive response from members and perhaps some questioning of what will be gained from the group.

The crisis will occur regardless of the therapist's level of activity. Its intensity and form, however, are very much related to the therapist's actions. A therapist who is relatively silent and outside of the group engenders a more extreme response than does an actively involved leader, in whose group the crisis may be quite limited. In the process of resolving the crisis, members realize that the leader does not have all the answers, and they turn to one another. The group becomes much more cohesive at this point, and one or another member often reveals his or her "real" reasons for being in the group.

The following example illustrates such a turning point in the seventh meeting of a short-term group:

> Although the group had gone quite well up to this point, it had been characterized by a great deal of inhibition among the four men and five women members. Meetings would generally begin slowly, with some presentation of problems which they had had in dealing with others during the past week. The leader would often attempt to pull the members back to examining their current interactions in the group. Although this refocusing would occur, it tended to be somewhat stilted and uncomfortable.
>
> In the sixth session, there had been some discussion about "where things

in the group are going," and some of the frustrations that members felt in the group were stated. For example, James, who had attended the meetings on a very irregular basis, had now missed two sessions in a row. Members expressed the concern that he hadn't gotten enough to keep him in the group, and a few said that, to a lesser degree, they shared some of those feelings. Shortly after this, the leader tried to draw Linda into the discussion. She was a very depressed, 26-year-old married woman, with a masters degree in rehabilitation counseling, who had for the past year worked as a clerk–typist because she was overwhelmed by anxiety, depression, and feelings of inadequacy whenever she attempted jobs requiring more responsibility. Linda, like James, had come late to several group meetings. She said that she often felt frightened about coming to sessions. She did not feel like "part of it" and was afraid that if she spoke, members would see her as odd and not fitting in.

The leader encouraged her to talk about why she felt "odd" and different. With the leader's support, she was able to describe a series of traumatic events in her family, which had occurred 1½ years previously. At that time, her parents, both of whom had long histories of severe depression, had died together in a suspicious automobile accident. Three months later, her younger brother, who had had a series of psychiatric hospitalizations, committed suicide. Linda's disclosure had a profound effect upon the group. Most members were very supportive and caring. Some spoke about painful losses which they had experienced. Linda's openness led to her becoming much more involved and committed to the group. Her courageous self-disclosure presented other members with a model for disclosure and asking others for help.

The disclosure may not be as dramatic as Linda's and may take the form of an admission of one's profound loneliness, sexual orientation, repeated rejections, and so on. Regardless of the specific form it takes, the increased openness and genuineness begins a period of active work for the group. This phase of the group is characterized by much sharing and mutual support and very little absence or irregularity of attendance. If a member has not dropped out by this point in the group, the likelihood of his or her becoming a dropout is practically nil. A short-term young adult group which continues to have uncertain attendance, low cohesiveness, and low support has not reached the working stage and is likely to be a low yield, poor outcome group.

During this central phase, the leader continues to encourage and actively support sharing and openness. If, for example, a member is talking about never really knowing how other people respond to her, the leader might intervene by asking if she would like feedback about this and then ask each member to talk about his or her reaction to that patient. If, on the other hand, a patient were to say that he can never express to people his reactions about them, he may be asked to describe his emotional responses to each group member. Group members, by this phase of the group, have often integrated the leader's interventions. Frequently they will raise a question and ask for feedback or will themselves talk about reactions to given events in the group. The focus of the treatment upon intimacy and openness can be accepted by the patients and worked on during this phase of group development. It requires constant vigilance on the part of the therapist, however, to stick with the goal and not let the group retreat from it.

During this period of the group, some patients, especially those who tend to be more quiet and withdrawn, can get lost in the shuffle. It is essential that the leader try to pull all members into the group each session. This can be done in a variety of ways. If all members have not participated to some degree during a given session, it would be useful to include those people in a "wrapping up" of the session by asking them how they felt about today's meeting.

As the group approaches the final three or four sessions, and thus the termination, there is, to some degree, a resurgence of the dependency and leader-centeredness characteristic of the earliest stage. Often there will be some recurrence of symptoms and anxiety about "what happens for me once the group ends." The role of the leader during this stage is to help members clarify their fears about ending, help them share their feelings of loss, and help them look at and specify the gains which they have made in the group. For members who have, indeed, modified their behavior over the course of the treatment, it is of the essence to help them look at what they are doing differently within the group and outside it. It is insufficient for a patient to merely say, "I'm talking more with people outside the group." In order for such a gain to be maintained and for the patient to feel as though he or she can, indeed, maintain it, the exact nature of the change should be clarified. The therapist might ask when, under what circumstances, and to whom the patient now talks more; or the leader can turn to the group and ask when and how the patient is now more open and able to speak in the group. The leader might also describe changes he or she has observed the patient make and the feelings that this has evoked. In any case, in order to reinforce changes and enhance the likelihood they will be maintained, they should be specified. This specificity keeps the patient attuned to the changes and continues his or her work on these issues after the group ends.

For some members who have not really made appreciable changes up until this point, the time-limited nature of the group can act as a catalyst in breaking free of a long-term pattern. For example:

Fred was a member of the same group as Linda (described earlier). He was a single, 28-year-old computer key punch operator, a job he had had for five years since graduating from college. Fred was supportive and well liked in the group but rather passive and shy when it came to speaking about himself or expressing his own needs within and outside the group. He had initially entered treatment because he felt that he could never follow through on things and could not be assertive at work, and because almost all the people who had begun working in his company at the same time and the same level had been able to leave to pursue their long-range career choices, while he had remained behind.

In the 12th session, the leader had asked members how they were feeling about the approaching termination and where they saw the problems with which they had begun the group. Fred said that he felt as stuck as he did before the group, and that now that the group was soon ending, he would again be "left behind" by everyone else making gains. He looked very sad and upset. Other group members began to explore with him why he was so frightened of making a move and pursuing a career. Members stated their own fears of failing at a career and of being "unable to compete."

This session proved to be very useful to Fred, and a year later he reported it to have been a turning point in freeing him to return to graduate school. It was only because of the specific time-limited nature of the group that such a session occurred. In open-ended group treatment, there is a timeless quality similar to that which Mann (Chapter 3, this volume) describes in long-term individual therapy. This timelessness allows members to postpone changes or postpone dealing with anxiety-provoking issues. In our short-term groups, members are constantly faced with the finitude of the group, which helps keep them focused on dealing with issues now, before it is too late.

In a short-term group, the leader should keep the members alert to the time issue. It is, in fact, rare that members are unaware that the ending is fast approaching, but it is essential for the leader to say regularly, "We'll be ending in x weeks on such-and-such a date." The fact of the approaching ending generates much feeling, which also becomes grist for the mill and can be examined and dealt with.

In the young adult groups, the leader also functions as a model for the expression of affect and openness toward group members. Such modeling and openness should not be mistaken as license for the leader to attack or be cruel to group members, nor is it the opportunity for the leader to receive therapy in the group. Rather, it permits the leader to look at his or her own emotional responses in the group and to use these feelings in a judicious and clinically responsible manner to help members, in turn, look at their own feelings and behaviors. A therapist who does this too frequently turns the group into a center for his or her own narcissistic gratification. If the leader rarely shares some of his or her own reactions, members feel that although the leader is advocating openness and intimacy, there is much hypocrisy in this stance.

In a service organization, such as HCHP, it is not possible for members ending a short-term young adult group to see this as an absolute termination of treatment. Consequently, we plan a reunion six months after the last session, and we let people know that they may recontact us for treatment again after the group. We do state, however, that the termination of a given group is very difficult, and that some of the feelings of anxiety and uncertainty will pass. We also make it clear that the group is only the beginning of a process. Much of the intent of the group is to help members start a process which they themselves may continue after termination. It is recommended that group members wait at least six weeks for "the dust to settle" before making plans for further treatment. Members almost invariably abide by this injunction. Although group members continue as HCHP members after termination of the group, and although we hold a reunion, the group termination is still a sad and uncomfortable time for most people. In many ways, members do experience the termination as final, because never again will their group exist as it did over the course of treatment.

MIDLIFE GROUPS

This is a 15-session group designed to serve patients aged 35 to 50. Normal people experience a period of reassessment and increased self-scrutiny at this point in life; this process is often turbulent but, for most people, does not lead to a crisis. Nevertheless, symptomatic distress sufficient to warrant medical or psychiatric attention is common. In our population, the most frequent presenting picture is that of depression, especially characterized by a sense of immobility or stagnation, a paralysis of the will. Why is the midlife individual prone to develop depression? The answer, suggested by the complaint of stagnation, is that this period of life is an active transitional period of psychosocial and psychodynamic evolution. Failure to evolve through the necessary tasks of midlife, because of conflicts or blocks emanating from the past, can produce a sense of immobility and a state of depression. The aim of treatment is to break the log jam and free up the normal forces of growth.

THEORIES OF MIDLIFE DEVELOPMENT

What are the psychosocial and psychodynamic issues? Jung (1971) spoke of "an important change in the human psyche," where suppressed aspects of the personality become manifest or even dominant. Recent theorists (Gutmann, 1975) have suggested an intrinsic pattern of change, across cultures, where men move in the second half of life from active to passive modes, while women tend to move in the opposite direction.

Most of the descriptive work on normal psychosocial development springs from the work of Erik Erikson (1959), who saw the task of midlife as achieving a state of concern about establishing and guiding the next generation, which he termed "generativity." Failure, according to Erikson, leads to self-absorption and a sense of stagnation. Levinson (1978) expanded the notion that individuals need to be needed as guides and mentors to the young, pointing out that the generative need complements the young adult's dependence on such guides for his or her own normal development.

George Vaillant (1977), studying Harvard graduates into their 40s and 50s, saw adult development as consisting of alternate periods of disruption and integration progressing along a developmental spiral, where success at one stage predisposes to success at the next. This is in contrast to the popular notion that adults choose alternative courses for themselves (e.g., career versus family). He sees midlife as a period of turbulent disruption, occurring usually in the 40s, with a quieter period of "career consolidation" preceding it and a quiet and integrative period succeeding it, which he termed "keepers of the meaning." Comparing midlife to adolescence as a time of new discovery, decreased instinctual barrier, and a redefinition of identity values, Vaillant described his normal subjects as "leaving the compulsive, unreflective busy work of their occupational apprenticeship to once more become explorers of the world within" (p. 220). He saw adult development as tending toward a greater social involvement and a maturing of adaptive (ego) defenses over time.

The psychodynamic issues of midlife were addressed by Elliot Jaques (1965). Drawing on the work of Melanie Klein (1935/1948), Jaques viewed the central task as the need to finally come to terms with depressive issues emanating from earliest infancy, avoided or only partly resolved in earlier stages of development. Klein theorized that in the second half of the first year of life, the infant experiences a quandary which forms the basis for its subsequent attitude toward life and death. Recognizing its mother, on whom it remains totally dependent for survival, as sometimes gratifying and sometimes frustrating, the infant must contend with its ambivalence toward her. Such ambivalence leads to a state of chaos, confusion, and depression termed by Klein "the depressive position": a separation anxiety stemming from the fear that mother will be hurt, destroyed, or driven away. This state is viewed as the core issue in neurosis, one which is reawakened throughout life by situations of loss and most intensely reawakened at midlife by the contemplation of one's own death, the ultimate and total separation and loss. Distinguishing between the conscious fear of death and the unconscious meaning of death stemming from the infantile depression, Jaques sees the midlife task as coming to terms with the limitations in one's love objects and the world as well as the imperfections—including hatred—in one's self. The successful resolution of the midlife depression, according to Jaques, is to achieve a state of resignation without despair. Having grieved for what will not and cannot be, the individual is free to make new choices which accept the limits in self and others.

TREATMENT AND THE RELEVANCE OF TIME

If the midlife individual is forced to come to terms with the limits and imperfections in self and in the world, it is the undesirable reality of time and its passage which forces the issue. Bernice Neugarten (1979) spoke of a new "time perspective," in which time is restructured into "time to live instead of time since birth," and the individual is challenged to decide "what is yet to be accomplished and what might best be abandoned" (p. 880).

The prod of time can be capitalized upon in the treatment of individuals with midlife problems, whose intense awareness of time has both real and symbolic value. Time-limited therapy, as described by Mann (1973), establishes a context which replays the separation paradigm of infancy and, in so doing, crystallizes the issue of ambivalence as a fundamental part of all important relationships. That is, the patient is invited to become dependent, but not for long, thus provoking but thwarting underlying infantile wishes for permanence, immortality, and perfection, which Mann views as core issues in neurosis. Such wishes are balanced by the healthy thrust toward separation–individuation, which Mann viewed as heightened at times of development or transition. Transition can be reinforced through effective brief treatment focusing on the ambivalence associated with the conflict between infantile and mature forces. The goal is to help the patient separate "without self-defeating anger or hatred or despair or guilt" (Mann, 1973, p. 28). This calls for an acceptance of inner feelings of anger and of one's destructive wishes, brought to the fore, in Mann's view, by the reality of time.

In our opinion, time-limited techniques are therefore most relevant in the treatment of the midlife individual, where we view the core issue as the need to come to terms with the impermanence and imperfections in the world (including one's love objects) and in one's self. The latter is especially relevant to the issue of self-esteem in midlife depression. The use of a group mode serves to reinforce the essential, normative, interactional and social nature of many of the issues of midlife as enumerated above, offering both support and peer pressure to do the work and move on.

THE MIDLIFE PATIENT

The prototypical presentation of the midlife patient within our setting is a man or woman in the 35 to 50 age range, who presents with symptomatic distress and/or functional impairment sufficient to warrant referral. Presentation is often prompted by a significant life change, especially a loss, although there may be a variety of symptoms, character types, and diagnoses. The patient is generally reassessing significant aspects of his or her life, feeling bogged down or stuck, feeling that options are limited, new choices must be made, life is passing quickly, and time is running out. Previous expectations and hopes may not have been achieved. Frequently, there is the sense that achievements are hollow and empty.

An important requirement for treatment is the patient's perception that it is he or she who must be changed in some fundamental way. This motivation to work on the inner issues which are seen as leading to the sense of stagnation does not mean that character change, per se, is the patient's goal. The patient sees that new life choices are being blocked from within. Often there is expressed concern with long-standing patterns of behavior which are now seen as obstacles to growth.

PATIENT SELECTION

Assuming the patient is sufficiently distressed to warrant treatment, is willing to work in a group, and accepts a brief treatment mode, certain criteria must be met:

1. There should be an absence of contraindications such as active psychosis, suicidal or homicidal intent, significant paranoid or schiz-

oid features, active alcohol or drug abuse problems, or major anti-social behavior.

2. The patient must view his or her problems as significantly internal; that is, patients who are preoccupied with external, situational causes to their distress, who are excessively hypochondriacal or preoccupied with symptoms, or who are in an actual state of crisis are considered poor candidates.

3. The patient must be able to communicate with others well enough to function in a group mode. This does not mean that social adeptness is required, but, as is true in the young adult groups, severe problems in relating to others or patterns of extreme social isolation would make group treatment a poor choice.

Candidates are interviewed by the group leader prior to being accepted. There is a frank discussion of the goals of treatment; the patient is told what to expect in the group and what will be expected of him or her. Questions are answered, and an attempt is made to help the patient view his or her problems in adult developmental terms—as normative, understandable, and capable of improvement. Every attempt is made to enlist the patient's active involvement in the process. He or she is told that the group will focus on two areas:

1. The commonalities among the members will be explored—common concerns such as aging, the fears of making new life choices, the problems of dying parents and growing children, and the like.

2. Since it is a group, there will be an opportunity to examine, first hand, patterns of relating to others in a social unit. Behavioral patterns, in turn, will be presented as reflecting self-perceptions and attitudes. Much of what will be worked on in the group, therefore, is couched in terms of self-esteem and identity issues.

THE GROUP PROCESS

The group is composed of eight to ten men and women ranging in age from 35 to 50 but tending to cluster in the early 40s. It meets weekly for 15 1½-hour sessions. Over the four years of its existence, it has been run, at times, as a closed group but, for the most part, as an open group, with new members being added when old members terminate. The group can be viewed both as time-limited treatment done in a group and as group psychotherapy done briefly.

Although many of the curative factors described by Yalom (1975) appear to operate, certain group phenomena do not occur to a significant degree in our midlife groups. For example, conflict with the leader and group crisis are rare, as are group conflicts around the issue of dominance. The "in or out" introductory phase tends to be brief, and actual dropouts are infrequent in this population (Budman, Demby, & Randall, 1980). Similar to other forms of brief treatment, and unlike extended group therapy, the working-through process is assumed to occur largely outside the group or after termination.

Much of the anxiety and the positive motivating force in the group seems to stem from the time limit, which is readily perceived by the group as replicating a major theme of the distress which brought them to treatment. Time and its passage operate to shift the group's attention from separate preoccupations to unifying concerns. The time limit ultimately forces, during the termination phase, a confrontation with universal, depressive issues: the inevitable disparity between what is wished for and what is possible, the fact that everything ends, and the need to come to grips with one's own anger and disappointment in order to make new, positive choices in the face of an imperfect self operating in an imperfect world.

Members are encouraged to use the group and take from it what they need. Despite this rather unstructured approach, most participants undergo a sequence which can be characterized and related to the psychosocial and psychodynamic issues described earlier. Since the midlife group has been run both in an open format, with new members added when old members terminate, and, at times, as a closed group, no clear correlation can be made between the course of the group as a whole and the treatment sequence for a given member. Thus, the closed group can be characterized as having a beginning, middle, and end phase, while no such phases can be clearly defined in the open group. Nevertheless, the treatment sequence appears to be similar. What follows is a characterization of a typical treatment sequence, using clinical examples to demonstrate how patients use the group to address and begin to confront both the psychosocial and psychodynamic challenges of the midlife issues which have brought them to treatment.

THE PROBLEM AND THE MYTH

Closed groups generally begin with a request that each group member state what has brought him or her to treatment and what he or she hopes to achieve. In open groups, new members are usually asked such questions by the group itself early in a first meeting. Characteristically, problems are presented in a tentative, brief, and conceptual manner, often couched in specific situational terms.

During the first two or three meetings, group response tends to be supportive and noncritical. Advice may be offered, other members may acknowledge similar problems or concerns, and there is a certain amount of questioning and factfinding. During this period, with the help of the leader and/or senior group members, there is a gradual shift from the specific problem to its antecedents, historical or biographical, and from the situational aspects to the member's role in bringing it about, perpetuating or sustaining it, or failing to resolve it. At this point, the problem comes to be viewed as an example of some chronic or repetitive pattern or propensity, and the latter is rationalized in the form of a personal or family mythology. This corresponds with Mann's (1973) statement that "for most patients, a crisis is generally an exacerbation of a lifelong conflict situation that may find what seems to be different avenues of discharge at different times" (p. 32). The following illustrates the beginning phase of treatment for a man in an open midlife group:

> Peter was a 42-year-old divorced engineer, who complained of being stuck in his life and of feeling empty and lonely. Several years following a divorce, he was contemplating making a commitment to the new woman in his life but was afraid to do so. He saw himself as a relative failure at work and as a man who had, all his life, "engineered failure": flunking out of college twice prior to graduating, doing passable work at his job but never living up to his own high expectations.
>
> Peter's problems with self-esteem were traceable to identification with a crippled and chronically depressed father, who, although living on his own father's income, had been autocratic and perfectionistic with the patient, pushing him to make up for father's failures. The Oedipal conflict was resolved by the patient's assumption of the myth, "I am an impotent man who can only function with a strong man by my side." He had had many years of psychotherapy, with little gain. He functioned in the group as an ancillary leader, able increasingly to challenge the therapist, whose response reinforced a picture of the patient as a knowledgeable and thoughtful grown-up who could run his own life.

THE ARGUMENT

At some point, usually by the third or fourth session, it becomes obvious that mutual support, acceptance, and well-meaning advice will not produce behavioral change. There is a sense of frustration, often shared by all in the closed-type group, and a pervasive sense that the group, like its members, is "stuck." Unlike the young adult groups, it is uncharacteristic for the midlife patients to blame the leader or to demand more from the leader at this point. Rather, there is an increased commitment to work harder and to be more critical and less accepting of themselves and of each other. This leads to the first serious questioning of facile explanations, rationalizations, and personal myths, which, in turn, increases resistance and leads to arguments between those tenaciously defending their need to be unsuccessful, depressed, or self-destructive in the face of alternative courses of action proposed to them but systematically ruled out. It is the recognition of character defenses and their role in protecting the mythology (and avoiding the anxieties which would follow from a loosening of such defenses) that allows for change beyond symptom reduction.

For the argument to be productive, a member must feel not only questioned but also supported by the group. It is important for the leader to identify the behavior or the attitude—not the patient—as being alien and, where necessary, to help the patient to view the group as being on his or her side. Given a state of cohesiveness, there is a strong incentive to modify the behavior or attitude for the group as well as for oneself.

> Sally, a 36-year-old, thrice-married artist presented originally with marital "boredom" and a general sense of stagnation in pursuing career goals. Heavily defended, only gradually did she make the extent of her depression and immobility apparent. In the group, she tended to intellectualize and monopolize group attention, but she was helpful to others. Halfway through treatment, still denying the extent of her unhappiness in her marriage, she entered into the following argument: She planned to return to the South to take care of her mother, while her father accompanied the patient's only sister to a hospital in another city, where the sister was to undergo surgery for presumed cancer. The patient made it clear that her mother, a harshly critical person who had made no secret of her preference for the sister over the patient, would fail to appreciate her sacrifice and would be both demanding and demeaning, as was her norm.
>
> The patient resisted all group efforts to find a less self-sacrificing alternative, insisting she "had no choice." When the therapist pointed out that she seemed determined to convince the group she had no alternative but self-sacrifice, she broke down in tears and began, for the first time, to examine her compulsive need to repeatedly seek to please her mother with the same, inevitably disappointing result. She was able to find a bearable alternative to the travel plan on her own, and in subsequent meetings, she began to examine her macochistic behavior in other areas of her life and ultimately in her marriage as well.
>
> Six months following her termination from the group, Sally had separat-

ed from her husband and was more actively taking risks in pursuing career goals. She was no longer bored or depressed but stated she was actively working on taking charge of her life, feeling less constrained by internal forces and less stuck.

THE CONFESSION

Once patients gain insight into the tenacity of character defenses in sustaining personal myths, they frequently identify factors or experiences in the past which are related. Early memories or experiences, frequently having to do with parental relationships, which reinforced a sense of shame, badness, or lack of worth, are most commonly brought up and shared; often, these memories have been kept secret and never shared, and they are presented in a tentative, confessional way. Such memories may or may not have direct relevance to the stated problem(s) leading to treatment. They are core depressive issues, which, in all cases, form an important part of the patient's self-image. With the sense of imperative to make internal changes and to come to terms with bad or unacceptable parts of the self, the patient is motivated to take the risk of sharing this aspect of him- or herself. Validation by the group is probably less important than abreaction and personal reevaluation, but it can be reinforcing of the patient's attempt to integrate a hitherto shameful part of him- or herself. Since it is the function of character defenses to keep such painful beliefs about the self at bay, some loosening of such defenses commonly follows.

> Joseph, a 45-year-old accountant, was referred because of anxiety and phobic symptoms stemming from conflict with a male superior at work. He had a history of mild recurrent depression associated with job instability and had entertained some recent suicidal fantasies.
>
> In the group, Joseph was obsessional and highly controlled. He tended to stay on the periphery of the group and repeatedly questioned its worth; nevertheless, he attended regularly and was helpful to others in an analytic, problem-solving fashion. As he came to recognize the group's importance to others, and as he started to feel better, Joseph began slowly to commit himself and share his profound sense of sadness. He was surprised at the group's acceptance and chose to share with them the fact that he had had a problem with soiling as a child. He had been known in his family as "the little shit." The empathic response of the group helped him connect his fear of losing control and his difficulties regarding assertion and free self-expression with his view of himself as a dirty, uncontrolled person. His aloofness in the group diminished, and he reported some lifting in his inhibitions at work. He was able to deal with the supervisor in an active, effective manner, and his anxieties diminished.

COMING UNSTUCK

As a group member starts to confront depressive issues, the group experience is beginning to draw to a close. It is usually around the tenth session that concerns about the end of the group begin to surface. At this point, the issue of time and its passage becomes focal. Although there may be anger expressed at the therapist, the organization, or the mental health department at this time, the limits and inevitable incompleteness and disappointment are much more likely to be viewed in an existential sense and to be seen as a manifestation of the reality that nothing goes on forever. The issue of time has a powerful effect on drawing the members of the group closer together in the shared experience of grieving their own death, both as a group and, to a greater or lesser extent, personally. Previous losses are discussed, and there is talk of aging, fear of illness, and fear of dying. Although a good deal of sadness may be shared, there is usually a renewed commitment to using the remaining time well, moving on, accepting the limits in a resigned but nondespairing way.

It is in this context that group members begin to plan for leaving the group, and there is some incentive to deal actively with the sense of being stuck and being unable to make life choices. This is a time when members are likely to experiment with new patterns of behavior and make decisions. Oftentimes, these actions reflect something more than resolution of the problem or situation which may have led to treatment, that is, a greater readiness to surrender old patterns of behavior and old myths.

Allan, a 37-year-old, divorced pharmacist, was referred with concerns that he was too emotionally constricted and unexpressive. Several years after a divorce, he was considering making a new commitment but was fearful of doing so. His ex-wife and children had recently moved from the area, and his aging parents, on whom he had been both emotionally and financially dependent, were in declining health. Recent somatic complaints were similar to those of his sick mother.

In the group, the patient was demanding of the therapist, whom he viewed as the expert with the answers. This mirrored his lifelong wish to be closer with his admired but ambivalently held father, seen as financially helpful but emotionally aloof. Assertiveness, independence, and self-expression were associated with the threat of loss of the care-taking object. Deprived of his day-to-day status as a parent, he had regressed and resumed his dependent relationship with his own parents, whom he now feared losing.

As other members of his open group terminated, Allan became senior. With the therapist's refusal to be the group mentor, Allan began tentatively to take that role, with good response from others, since he was a kind and genuinely helpful man. He was able to begin relating to the therapist more as a contemporary and less as a parent and, in the few sessions prior to termination, was able to share his fear of losing his parents. He also shared in the group his growing perception that in their old age, he must become a parent to them. He planned a testimonial dinner to his father and was its speaker. Termination from the group was uneventful.

Several months after termination, Allan remained independent of his parents, free of depression, and gave evidence of greater assertiveness in his dealings with others.

TERMINATION

The final phase of the group concerns saying good-bye and leaving with hope. As in any other form of short-term treatment, there is an assumption that the work will continue. Unlike the Mann (1973) model, the prepaid group practice setting does not permit a final good-bye, and members know they can return, if necessary. Despite this, considerable sadness and some anger are expressed. Old losses are recalled and experienced. Rarely do group members continue relationships with each other, and the end of treatment is usually accepted as a good-bye. For those who are especially sensitive to loss, this may be an extremely difficult but productive stage of the group.

Gladys, a 42-year-old, divorced florist, came to the group because of depression, with periods of tearfulness, and a sense of isolation and loneliness. These apparently were connected with a failing romance and the imminent departure of her last child from the home. Her history was of an illegitimate birth and infrequent contact with her mother during the early years of her life. She was raised in a series of foster homes until her adoption at age 14. She described always feeling on the outside of things, alien, and with unmet needs. These had been partially mitigated during child-rearing years.

In the group, Gladys functioned as an incisive, helpful person who held herself aloof, often keeping people at bay with her caustic wit. She initially attached herself to the therapist, being both dependent and seductive, but responded well to limit setting and became increasingly involved with the group. As termination drew near, she made phone calls to the therapist, seeking reassurance, and began to actively grieve old losses and to express fears of being alone and on her own. With group support, she was able to separate without bolting or denying the importance of the group, and she felt some pride in doing so.

When seen six months later, she was doing well. She had made an attachment to a man who sounded available and caring. She was also feeling better about her relationships and about her life in general. Gladys felt the group had been very helpful but still longed to go on in treatment in order to "wipe the slate clean" of old hurts. She responded well to reassurance and the offer of appointments if necessary in the future.

DISCUSSION

Throughout life, beginning in infancy, each individual must repeatedly contend with the disparity between what is desired and what is possible. This issue takes different forms at different times but finds its most intense expression in two areas: response to separation and loss, and self-esteem. The former can be traced to its earliest antecedents in infancy, while the latter is established gradually, over time, progressing as a precondition and consequence of successive steps in development.

In midlife, under the pressure of time and, in particular, the "shift in time-perspective" referred to by Neugarten (1979), both issues come sharply to the fore, and the individual is vulnerable to a state of depression characterized by a sense of stagnation and a paralysis of the will. This is brought about by a strong sense that options are limited, and both one's self and the world are less than one wished them to be.

The task of treatment is to help the patient face those aspects of self and the world which underlie the despair. The group offers both pressure and support, while the presence of time as an issue in the group underscores the imperative toward action. Because the patient tends to move, under such circumstances, to core conflicts and concerns, and because group members can be helped to recognize resistance to confrontation when it occurs, the group mode probably increases the anxiety at the same time it helps members to bear it through sharing the pain. The confrontation is with the impossible wishes: immortality, perfection in self and others, choices free of conflict or pains, complete security and fulfillment. The resolution involves coming to terms with shameful, angry, destructive parts of oneself as well as the limits in what one can expect from others. The regressive and infantile wishes are counteracted by the push to maturity characteristic at times of transition in adult life. This thrust is augmented by the pull of the group and the pressure of the reality of time.

There is an additional factor worth noting, one which correlates well with the psychosocial tasks of midlife. With "faith in the species," some measure of the old hope for permanence and perfection can be retained by reinvesting, not in oneself, but in the next generation. The shift in time sense involves not only a recognition that one's life will end, but also a shift from a narcissistic preoccupation (with the world as an extension of oneself and with one's own pleasures, success, and security as paramount) to a sense of one's self as a "bridge between the generations." This shift can often be seen in a limited way in the tendency of group members to move fluidly from a discussion of self to self-as-parent to self-as-child. It is also reflected in the wish of more experienced group members (especially in open groups) to share their wisdom with newcomers and to serve as guides and mentors. This spirit is reinforced, and the preoccupation with self as being alone is, in part, counteracted by the group mode.

In sum, the successful resolution of midlife depression requires both psychosocial and inner growth and a fundamental shift in emphasis. It requires confronting and coming to terms with certain painful realities which underlie character structure and which reappear in an intense form at midlife, causing turmoil but also permitting growth and resolution. Optimal resolution leads to a new view of one's self as a "good enough" self operating in a "good enough" world.

LATER MIDLIFE GROUPS

Consistent with Jaques's (1965) characterization of the midlife phase of adult development as beginning at about age 35 and reaching full maturity at about age 65, and considering the midlife group previously discussed, this particular group might best be described as the later midlife group, its members evolving in the developmental process toward "mature adulthood." This description deals with the short-term (20 sessions or less), open-ended group therapy of patients in the age range of, roughly, 50 to 70. In Erikson's (1959) view, people of this age are dealing with the conflicts of "ego integrity versus despair." This stage may be characterized by the acceptance of one's "own and only life cycle," by a sense of satisfaction with what one has done, with one's accumulated knowledge, experience, and so on, or by a deep despair that it is too late to start over, a despair represented by disgust, misanthropy, or displeasure, all of which are hiding a fear of death.

Vaillant (1977) saw the 50s as a quieter time of life than the 40s. Since the 50s are not a time of life when one can easily change careers, teaching what one knows or what one has already learned appears to be the only track open as a means of institutionalizing one's care of others. A transmission of knowledge and experience as well as an altruistic outlook tend to be characteristic of this period. Vaillant commented further:

> If the steps from infancy to childhood to adolescence lead in sequentially mastering our body, our reality, and our emotions, then from forty to senescence the steps lead in the reverse direction. *Thus if the forty-year-old struggles with feelings, the fifty-five-year-old struggles once more with reality.* [italics added] . . . Reality must replace the ideal, and we must accept that life's seesaw has tipped; that there are now more yesterdays than tomorrows. . . . The old person, like the infant, struggles with his body. At fifty-five, some men were slowly entering the last stage of the life cycle, where the task is to replace the indignities of physical decay with a sense of unshakeable self worth. (pp. 233–234)

Neugarten (1979), in discussing the strengths which older patients bring to psychotherapy, stated:

> An aging patient brings . . . a large repertoire of experience, long practice at working out solutions to problems, and much resources for recovery. Introspection and stocktaking are well-developed features of the mental life. The past lies close at hand, and the reliving and reworking of the past may come more readily than to a younger person. (p. 893)

Muslin and Epstein (1980), in an outstanding review article on the psychotherapy of the aged (those 50 to 60 or older!), summarize as follows:

> While differences in emphasis exist in the writers cited, all observers of the aged agree with certain manifest data: that the late years ordinarily accost people with major life crises in socioeconomic life style, outlets for achievement, and often changes in roles within the family. Most relate to the task of preparing for or denying the omnipresent specter of death. There is also a common emphasis on changes in the psyche of the elderly. These changes range from modification in the egodefenses and self-system to alterations in one's overview of the universe. (p. 6)

They go on to explain that is is essential for the older person to be able to come to terms with and accept his or her increased physical and psychic limitations without shame or a significant loss of narcissism or self-esteem.

Thus, for the patients in our later midlife groups, there is a greater need to deal with the realities of life than with feelings. There is also a need to deal with limitations, losses, and the knowledge that one's life is much more than half over. Patients in this group, however, also have significant strengths and coping skills which come from many years of living and survival and may contribute to the therapeutic process.

THE PATIENTS

Patients in this group are referred for evaluation for possible group treatment by other members of the mental health staff or by other health care providers at HCHP familiar with the later midlife group. All referrals are generally made in the context of a specific problem of later-life-phase mastery. Patients usually have a specific and immediate problem which precipitates the request for the consultation. These problems are generally manifested by symptoms of anxiety, depression, somatization, or aggravation of organic disease (e.g., high blood pressure, migraine, ileitis). Because many of these patients have had previous mental health treatment, and their educational level is generally high, they tend to be quite open to therapy, including group therapy.

STAGES OF GROUP DEVELOPMENT

After a patient is referred for an evaluation and possible acceptance into the group, one can look at the beginnings of group development as a function of attitudes toward HCHP itself and the relationship to primary care providers.

Although all forms of psychotherapy may, to a greater or lesser degree, depend on the institutional context to determine their effectiveness, this issue of context or institutional transference is probably particularly salient when treating older people. For example, Hoeper, Nyez, Regier, Goldberg, Jacobson, and Hankin (1980) ask:

> If such social supports are not available, and this is often especially true in the older population as social supports developed over a lifetime gradually disappear for a variety of reasons, does the health care system provide substitute social supports? (p. 210)

We believe the answer is affirmative. Many of the older patients in our later midlife group have strong bonds with the health plan as a whole. This bond or institutional transference further supports the group model proposed here.

Later midlife group patients appear to relate to the group leader differently from either young adult patients or midlife patients. The therapist is not idealized and seen as the one with all the answers (the case in the young adult groups, at least initially); nor is the leader seen as more or less a peer (as is often true in the midlife groups). Rather, the leader is seen as a physician who is willing to provide a setting where patients may try to help themselves and one another, but where the patient should not expect radical changes or miracles.

These older patients have had much life experience; some have had previous psychotherapy; most have formed significant intimate relationships during their lives and have experienced and tested them utilizing projected aggressive fantasies and impulses in the natural course of living. At this point in life, they are likely to have a sense of perspective, reality testing, and "object constancy" relative to human relationships and life in general, and they are most adept at "using" objects (human relationships, therapists, and therapy) in a more productively therapeutic manner and with less interference by projective defense mechanisms of identification (Winnicott, 1971) than is characteristic earlier in life. Because of those factors, people at this stage of adult development are perhaps best able to "use" therapy in a more direct and productive manner.

THE FORMAT

The structure of this group differs from either of the other two groups previously described, in that this group basically has a "revolving door" format. A member may attend the group for up to 20 sessions per year but basically uses the group as he or she, the group itself, and the therapist see as being most appropriate. There is a flexible use of sessions, with some patients attending weekly, others biweekly, and still others on a far more variable schedule.

Because of the looseness of structure in this group, it is made clear to patients that the setting, the time of meetings, the leader, and some of the members will remain constant. The group meets weekly for 1 ½ hours, and attendance may vary from two to ten members. (The average session has the leader and five members present.) The acceptance of this inconsistency may relate, in part, to the institutional transference mentioned previously and, in part, to the long life experience of these patients in adapting to new or stressful circumstances.

In general, most of the patients are fairly comfortable in attending the first session and subsequent sessions after the evaluation interview. Patients rapidly adjust to the group and, over the initial several meetings, quickly establish a relaxed relationship with the therapist and a few of the other group members. Because of the sometimes rapidly changing atmosphere from week to week, it seems that new patients try actively to establish a reassuring relationship with one or two other members of the group.

In the early sessions for a given patient, he or she will readily discuss the specific problems which brought him or her to the group. Patients are generally there-and-now oriented, with the focus being directed toward problem solving. In a group like this, where patients frequently discuss job or financial problems, family concerns, and difficulties with aging relatives or parents, the wealth of information and expertise of members who have had many years of life experience and wisdom is great. For example, one member who was in the group because of depression and sadness over an unwanted separation and divorce happened to be a very competent activities therapist in a geriatrics facility. She had extensive knowledge about most elderly resources in the area and was able to give expert advice and assistance with regard to such programs.

Economic problems are frequently discussed, as is job security. This is especially true in women who are in their late 50s or early 60s, and who may be extremely dissatisfied with their jobs but do not have many options and cannot move on. Job problems around intergenerational conflicts are also frequently discussed. This might relate to the difficulties that an older person who is preretirement is having with a younger supervisor, who is making the patient's job more stressful and perhaps even threatening the latter's job security. This generally activates a great deal of anxiety, mutual identification, and empathy in most group members and frequently begins discussion and a sharing of experience with regard to the universal experience of getting older.

Cohesiveness in the group develops rapidly and strongly. Despite the diversity and uniqueness of the individuals themselves, there is a remarkable incidence of commonly shared experiences. Since a number of the women are widowed or divorced, there is a great deal shared about how to combat loneliness and isolation. Most of these patients seem to be quite realistic about the possibilities of developing new heterosexual relationships at this point in their lives and frequently cite the statistic that women live longer than men, and that it will be unlikely that many will find another husband. There is a good deal of mutual sharing on how to utilize local community resources in terms of interests, activities, and social affairs to combat loneliness and isolation. Although members frequently express the fantasy and wish that they will make new friends in the group, relationships initiated between group members seem to be quite sporadic and tentative and generally do not develop into anything of a long-standing nature.

Members share fears about getting older, about developing physical illness, and about the general effects and deterioration of aging. Patients very infrequently discuss anxiety about their own personal death. But they are quite comfortable when the occasion arises to discuss and grieve deaths of significant others in their lives.

Those with severe or terminal disease do not do well in this group. On one occasion, a 62-year-old man with an early diagnosis of carcinoma of the pancreas was put into the group. After he mentioned his medical diagnosis, group members became covertly hostile and distant and denied his presence. After one session, he never returned. Another patient in his late 50s with severe pulmonary emphysema attended group sessions several times, ventilating his anxieties about his condition and his inability to quit smoking. In this case, the members were quite overtly hostile toward the man (who actually asked permission to smoke in the group), and he dropped out after a few sessions.

Generally, there are more women than men in the group. Moreover, females attend more meetings than males, and for a longer period of time. This is probably consistent with other, younger age group experiences, where women are more comfortable in discussing feelings and being open about themselves. When male patients come to the group, they usually come because of a relatively acute situation involving stress or problems on the job or difficulties with regard to career.

An important issue in this particular kind of group is that patients never really terminate. After resolving their acute problem or crisis, they leave the group with the understanding that they can return whenever they feel the need. This is done specifically with the thought in mind that in such a short-term group, the experiencing of feelings regarding termination might be too stressful and anxiety provoking.

The role of the therapist in the later midlife group is to help provide the group with a sense of "object constancy" and continuity. In addition, the leader can act as a facilitator and catalyst.

Since many patients in the group have had previous experience in therapy, they tend to be quite verbal and active in the treatment. It is not unusual, for example, for members themselves to set clear limits with patients who enter the group and are overly controlling or narcissitic. The leader may find it necessary to intervene, if the group beomes sidetracked or bogged down, or to draw out quieter and less active members. The patients themselves, however, are often able to relate easily to one another, quickly discuss their problems, and rapidly confront other members. The basic focus of the group is a practical, problem-solving, there-and-now orientation.

The following three clinical examples will give the reader some sense of the course of treatment for patients in this group and the types of issues dealt with.

Ralph was a 62-year-old, married, government worker who had had a serious myocardial infarction five years previously and was now retired. He was concerned about his physical health and feared dying. He felt a total failure as a father because his son, John, age 35, was an alcoholic, had failed in his marriage, and had never used his education nor been self-supporting. John maintained a marginal existence by doing small, menial jobs and was subsidized by the patient for rent, food, car insurance, and so forth. The patient felt angry and guilty about giving his son money, which he felt was being spent on alcohol. Ralph also worried about his own responsibility to society, since John had been involved in auto accidents while drinking. By the time Ralph came to the group, he felt John was about to hit skid row, and against the wishes of his wife and daughter, he wanted to have his son come and live with him. Ralph's wife and daughter pointed out that when he had had a heart attack five years before and was unable to help John, the latter had finally gotten a job and curtailed his drinking.

Ralph came for five sessions over a ten-week period, and during which he was able to express his feelings of frustration and failure in his relationship with his son. Although the group was empathic, they were also very confronting and challenged his behavior in infantilizing John. Over the ten-week period of time, Ralph was able to get some perspective, seeing that he had done his best and needed to set limits with John. He seemed to invest himself more in his retirement, his marital relationship, and his relationship with his daughter and grandchildren.

Rose, a 58-year-old, divorced woman, had been depressed, had recently been discovered to have high blood pressure, and was very concerned about her physical health. After ten years in a pressured administrative position, she decided to quit and find another job. She was determined not to continue in her present work, since her mother had also had high blood pressure, had had several strokes, and had died at the age of 62.

Divorced in her 30s from a professional man, who had been irresponsible and a heavy drinker, Rose had raised her three children, now adults, alone. She had never had the "real opportunity to remarry." Rose was pleasant, agreeable, and likeable but led a rather lonely life with no close friends. Her major investments were in her children, two older sisters, her job, apartment, and social acquaintances of a rather casual nature.

Her goals in the group were to put her present job into perspective and to examine her behavior in the group in an attempt to expand her contacts socially. The group immediately confronted her with the fact that she was much too compliant and self-effacing and encouraged her not to quit her job. Rather, they suggested she make appropriate and legitimate demands on her boss, who appeared to be tyrannical and overly controlling. She used their suggestions and found, for the first time, that her demands were met. She continued to be more assertive and, to her delight, found that her job was quite satisfying. She changed her mind about finding other work, recognizing that at her age it would be difficult to find a suitable job and to adjust to it. She learned to be more expressive in the group and found that this improved her interaction with her children, her sisters, and her casual social friends. In expressing her anxiety about her hypertension to the group, she was assured that her high blood pressure could be kept under control with proper medical care. She utilized 20 sessions over a 24-week period. Seen in a follow-up several months later, she was still doing very well.

Felice, a 50-year-old, unmarried woman, was acutely depressed and anxious when referred by her internist. On initial interview she wept, stating that her apartment had recently been burglarized. She was the youngest of four, with three older and favored brothers. She had been overprotected and was slated to care for her parents in their old age. Felice came from Europe to the United States in her 30s "to grow up finally" and separate from her family. She would visit her family abroad almost yearly and felt very guilty that her mother, now 83, wanted Felice to return and care for her, even though her three sons were nearby. It was clear that Felice related her apartment's being burglarized to some very traumatic memories and reactivated feelings stemming from World War II.

At about the same time as the burglary, she was devastated when a platonic male friend married another woman. She also saw her menopause as a final and irrevocable reality indicating the end of her feminine and productive life and her desirableness as a woman.

Felice attended the group weekly for several sessions, establishing immediate rapport with the members, the older ones providing positive parental surrogates. She expressed her anger and grief at the apartment break-in, the loss of her male friend, and the hopelessness of finding another. The group gave her much positive reinforcement and sympathy. They encouraged her to do what she wanted regarding her mother; they reality-tested that her mother had three sons near her, and was quite old, and would not live forever. She was encouraged not to return to Europe permanently. As her depression and anxiety lifted, she returned briefly, visited her family, and was surprised by her brothers' support of her decision to stay in the United States. They assured her that they would care for their mother's needs. This patient utilized seven sessions over an 18-week period and did not return for treatment. At her last visit, she was continuing her career as a teacher and was hoping to extend her current social relationships and to be more open with others.

The structure of the late midlife group is ideally suited for people dealing with the practical realities of later life. For these individuals, many of whom have lost or are in danger of losing things and/or people who are

or once were important parts of their social support system, the group provides a constant meeting, even when the therapist is away. Furthermore, it
is a place where one's sessions (time) can always be allocated so as to have
some time remaining.

The format of this group never addresses the time-limited nature of
the process as directly as does that of the young adult or midlife groups.
For the later midlife group members, who are presumably at one level,
dealing with issues of personal mortality, this issue may be far too intense
to confront directly, particularly in a time-limited format with a variable
membership.

CONCLUSIONS

This chapter has described three types of short-term (i.e., time-limited)
groups based on an adult developmental model. Our approach is in sharp
contrast to most other psychodynamic group treatment modes, which are
predicated on the assumption that patients do not make significant
changes without prolonged group therapy. Short-term group psychotherapy, as it is described here, capitalizes on the fact that people are constantly changing over the course of their lives, and that there is, within each of
us, a thrust toward maturation and development.

By bringing together, within the context of a time-limited group experience, patients who are dealing with similar life issues, by maintaining a
focus on these age-related concerns, and by assuming that a natural process of change which is instituted within the group can be carried forth and
more fully refined outside of the group, we have been able to develop a
coherent, planned, psychodynamically oriented, brief group treatment
approach.

As economic realities become increasingly important in the delivery
of mental health care, group therapy and, in particular, short-term group
therapy approaches may gain wider acceptance and importance. We hope
that others can use our efforts in this area as a starting place, and that further
refinements will follow widespread experimentation with such techniques.

ACKNOWLEDGMENTS

We wish to express our deep gratitude to Mary Clifford, Alan Gurman,
Rita Perlman Wilson, and Don Wertlieb, who read and commented upon

earlier drafts of this chapter, and to Deena Bridger, who typed what must have seemed like endless revisions.

REFERENCES

Barten, H. H. *Brief therapies.* New York: Behavioral Publications, 1971.

Bond, G., & Lieberman, M. A., Selection criteria for group therapy. In J. P. Brady & H. K. H. Brodie (Eds.), *Controversy in psychiatry.* Philadelphia: Saunders, 1978.

Budman, S. H. Avoiding dropouts in couples group therapy. In A. S. Gurman (Ed.), *Practical problems in family therapy.* New York: Brunner/Mazel, in press.

Budman, S. H., Bennett, M. J., & Wisneski, M. J. Short-term group psychotherapy: An adult developmental model. *International Journal of Group Psychotherapy, 1980, 30,* 63–76.

Budman, S. H., & Clifford, M. Short-term group therapy for couples in a health maintenance organization. *Professional Psychology, 1979, 10,* 419–429.

Budman, S. H., Clifford, M., Bader, L., & Bader, B. Experiential pre-group preparation and screening. *Group,* in press.

Budman, S. H., Demby, A., & Randall, M. Short-term group psychotherapy: Who succeeds and who fails? *Group, 1980, 4,* 3–16.

Budman, S. H., Feldman, J., & Bennett, M. J. Adult mental health services in a health maintenance organization. *American Journal of Psychiatry, 1979, 34,* 392–395.

Budman, S. H., Randall, M., & Demby, A. *Outcome in short-term group psychotherapy.* Manuscript submitted for publication.

Butcher, J. N., & Koss, M. P. Research on brief and crisis-oriented therapies. In S. L. Garfield & A. E. Bergin (Eds.), *Handbook of psychotherapy and behavior change* (Rev. ed.). New York: Wiley, 1978.

Erikson, E. H. Growth and crises of the healthy personality. In *Identity and life cycle.* New York: International Universities Press, 1959. (Monograph 1)

Grunebaum, H., & Solomon, L. *Toward a peer theory of group psychotherapy: II. Developmental stages of peer relationships.* Manuscript in preparation.

Gutmann, D. G. Parenthood: A key to the comparative study of the life cycle. In N. Datan & L. Ginsberg (Eds.), *Developmental psychology.* New York: Academic Press, 1975.

Hartley, D. *Therapeutic alliance and the success of brief individual psychotherapy.* Paper presented at 87th annual convention of the American Psychological Association, New York, September 1979.

Hoeper, E. W., Nyez, G. R., Regier, D. A., Goldberg, I. D., Jacobson, A., & Hankin, J. Diagnosis of mental disorder in adults and increased use of health services in four outpatient settings. *American Journal of Psychiatry, 1980, 137,* 207–210.

Jaques, E. Death and the mid-life crisis. *International Journal of Psychoanalysis, 1965, 46,* 502–514.

Jung, C. J. The stages of life. In J. Campbell (Ed.), *The portable Jung.* New York: V. King, 1971.

Klein, M. A contribution to the psychogenesis of manic–depressive states. In M. Klein, *Contributions to psychoanalysis.* London: Hogarth Press, 1948. (Originally published, 1935.)

Levinson, D. J., Darrow, C. N., Klein, E. B., Levinson, M. H., & McKee, B. *The seasons of a man's life.* New York: Knopf, 1978.

Malan, D. H. *A study of brief psychotherapy.* London: Tavistock Publications, 1963.

Mann, J. *Time-limited psychotherapy.* Cambridge: Harvard University Press, 1973.

Muslin, H., & Epstein, L. J. Preliminary remarks on the rationale for psychotherapy of the aged. *Comprehensive Psychiatry,* 1980, *21,* 1–12.

Myers, E. D. Age, persistence and improvement in an open out-patient group. *British Journal of Psychiatry,* 1975, *127,* 157–159.

Neugarten, B. L. Time, age and the life cycle. *American Journal of psychiatry,* 1979, *136,* 887–894.

Piper, W. E., Debbane, E. G., Garant, J., & Bienvenu, J. Pretraining for group psychotherapy: A cognitive–experiential approach. *Archives of General Psychiatry,* 1979, *36,* 1250–1256.

Sethna, E. R., & Harrington, J. A. A study of patients who lapse from group psychotherapy. *British Journal of Psychiatry,* 1971, *119,* 59–69.

Sloane, R. B., Staples, F. R., Cristol, A. H., Yorkston, N. J., & Whipple, K. *Psychotherapy versus behavior therapy.* Cambridge: Harvard University Press, 1975.

Small, L. *The briefer psychotherapies* (Rev. ed.). New York: Brunner/Mazel, 1979.

Strupp, H. H. Success and failure in time-limited psychotherapy. A systematic comparison of two cases: Comparison 2. *Archives of General Psychiatry,* 1980, *37,* 708–716.

Tuckman, B. W. Developmental sequence in small groups. *Psychological Bulletin,* 1965, *63,* 384–399.

Ursano, R. J., & Dressler, D. M. Brief vs. long term psychotherapy: A treatment decision. *Journal of Nervous and Mental Disease,* 1974, *159,* 164–171.

Vaillant, G. E. *Adaptation to life.* Boston: Little, Brown, 1977.

Winnicott, D. W. *Playing and reality.* New York: Basic Books, 1971.

Wolberg, L. R. (Ed.). *Short-term psychotherapy.* New York: Grune & Stratton, 1965.

Yalom, I. D., *The theory and practice of group psychotherapy* (2nd ed.). New York: Basic Books, 1975.

CHAPTER 13
THE TREATMENT OF WOMEN IN SHORT-TERM WOMEN'S GROUPS

Barbara Sabin Daley
Geraldine Suzanne Koppenaal

Pioneering clinical work has been done in a number of areas in group psychotherapy during the last decade. We believe that a focus of particular value has been the recent growth of interest in short-term groups. Describing a short-term group model, authors have emphasized the value of careful screening, a present focus, limited goals, patient responsibility, and an active supportive therapist (Bernard & Klein, 1977; Waxer, 1977). In the Harvard Community Health Plan (HCHP) model described by Budman and his colleagues (Budman, Bennett, & Wisneski, 1980, Chapter 12, this volume; Budman & Clifford, 1979), homogeneity in regard to patients' issues and developmental stages has been stressed.

Concurrent with the growing literature on short-term groups has been an increased interest in same-sex groups. Although brevity of treatment per se has rarely been discussed in the literature regarding women's groups, commonality of issues and an increased sense of support found in such groups are believed to hasten the development of cohesiveness (Aries, 1973; Nassi & Abramowitz, 1978). Such characteristics may make women's groups quite ideal as a brief treatment modality.

The popularity of women's groups has grown concomitantly with the development of the women's movement. Women's groups now operate within a variety of contexts. In particular, there has been the growth of women's consciousness-raising groups and psychotherapy groups. Theoreticians have further investigated an adult developmental model for women. New perspectives have been introduced, with a fresh view on traditional (primarily psychoanalytic) developmental models. Authors have

BARBARA SABIN DALEY and GERALDINE SUZANNE KOPPENAAL. Harvard Community Health Plan, Cambridge, Massachusetts. (Both authors contributed equally to this chapter; names are listed in alphabetical order.)

emphasized the sociocultural role changes women are facing and how those changes have affected age-specific tasks.

At HCHP, we have been treating adult women in short-term (15-session) group psychotherapy based on an adult developmental model for the past seven years. It is the purpose of our chapter to describe this treatment modality. To achieve this purpose, we first discuss women's issues that are appropriate for short-term group treatment. The authors hypothesize that such groups may be more appropriate for women at particular stages of female development. We describe how short-term women's groups are conducted, the role of the female group leader, and the process at various stages of group development. Case material is presented to illustrate how clients utilize the groups at respective stages.

REVIEW OF THE LITERATURE

There are a number of benefits in treating women in same-sex groups. A few of these, which we view as particularly significant to the psychotherapeutic treatment of women in short-term groups, have been selected for discussion. Authors in this area have indicated that, in comparison to cogender groups, women's groups facilitate more self-disclosure regarding personal feelings and significant relationships (Aries, 1973; Lynch, 1974; Nassi & Abramowitz, 1978); decrease the likelihood of women accepting stereotypical roles (Aries, 1973; Carlock & Martin, 1977; Lynch, 1974), and provide greater opportunity for role modeling and empathy for sex-specific conflicts (Aries, 1973; Brodsky, 1977; Halas, 1973; Lynch, 1974).

It has been reported that women disclose more material about personal feelings and significant relationships in women's groups (Aries, 1973; Lynch, 1974; Nassi & Abramowitz, 1978) and are more likely to bring up taboo subjects that would take longer to emerge in a cogender group (Brodsky, 1977). They may address such problems as wishing they had never married, not liking to care for young children, feeling more intelligent than their boss or husband, and being tired of boosting the self-esteem of others at their own expense (Brodsky, 1977).

Authors have proposed that in women's groups, there is less likelihood that the stereotypes of dependence, submissiveness, and acquiescence will be accepted (Aries, 1973; Lynch, 1974; Nassi & Abramowitz, 1978). In cogender groups, women are more likely to play a nurturing or seductive role in reaction to male initiative, whereas in same-sex groups, they tend to look more to themselves and other women for self-definition. In a similar vein, women in women's groups are seen as being more accepting of their aggression (Carlock & Martin, 1977).

Finally, and particularly noteworthy, women's groups are seen as providing a greater opportunity for role modeling and empathy for sex-specific conflicts (Aries, 1973; Brodsky, 1977; Halas, 1973; Lynch, 1974). For example, Gilligan (1977) and Mogul (1979) believe that some women share a common difficulty in their attempts to integrate their need to nurture others versus their need to nurture themselves. In part (according to Gilligan), this comes from the fact that the moral development of a woman starts from a position of caring. Women are self-defined as being concerned with, and committed to, the care of others. They see self-commitment as a rejection of femininity and feel that others could be hurt if they put themselves first. As a result, many women deny their own needs and have difficulty with autonomy and competition. They cannot resolve this conflict unless they realize that self-assertion does not necessitate destruction of themselves and others.

Gilligan supported this premise by drawing upon several authors' analyses of female early development. Chodorow (1978) went further, stating that a little girl is less likely to be pushed out of a pre-Oedipal relationship with the nurturing mother, for they are more alike, and thus the girl remains continuous with her mother. Girls remain a part of the dyadic, primary, mother–child relationship longer than boys and, therefore, continue to experience issues of merging, separation, and attachment. Consequently, women are less individuated than are men, and they have more flexible ego boundaries. Because girls, unlike boys, incorporate empathy as part of a primary definition of self, they have less need to deny pre-Oedipal relational modes. As a result, masculinity appears to be defined through separation from mother and further individuation from others more so than does femininity (Chodorow, 1974).

Other authors have also lent support to the notion that women define themselves as being part of a dyad and as being nurturers. Lever (1976) noted that girls in middle childhood play in smaller, more intimate groups, usually with a best friend, and are less likely to bring up disputes that might involve hurting one another. Girls' play demonstrates an atmosphere of cooperativeness, which facilitates the development of empathy and sensitivity necessary for understanding another person's needs.

It appears that the sex-specific "nurture-others-versus-nurture-self" conflict becomes paramount for women in their 30s. We view the treatment of women in short-term groups as being most appropriate at this time. It is in their 30s that women must come to terms with the integration or exclusion of childbearing and child rearing with some meaningful work (Mogul, 1979; Nadelson, Notman, & Bennett, 1978). Some women in their 30s appear to be struggling with the issue of being "deferred nurturers" or "deferred achievers" (O'Leary, 1977). For both groups, time is running out for making peace with the integration of these roles. The woman who delays childbearing until she is 30 or older, and who chooses to establish a career before having a family, is a deferred nurturer. Limited biologically, she faces interrupting her career and risking the loss of her former professional stature once childbearing is over. She is concerned that her identity might be absorbed by her husband and children. A deferred achiever is a woman in her early 30s who has had children and has postponed a career. She must deal with how the integration of a career will affect family life. A married woman with children often fears that by starting a career, she might provoke a husband's anger by becoming his competitor or by becoming less available as a homemaker or nurturer (Mogul, 1979). Furthermore, she may be confronted by what feels to be a hostile and competitive job market, from which she has most likely been away for ten or more years.

Women appear to experience a great deal of anxiety in the attempt to integrate the deferred-nurturing and deferred-achieving roles. Those who seek a professional career exclusive of childbearing feel the anxiety of such a choice, in that it deviates from their mothers' expectations or exceeds their mothers' achievements (Nadelson *et al.,* 1978). They may also view the necessary qualities for success (i.e., the ability to take risks, set goals, and compete) as being inconsistent with femininity. If the deferred-nurturing-versus-deferred-achieving conflict is resolved, a woman may be less likely to act out this dilemma unconsciously. A deferred nurturer might act out this conflict by not aggressively pursuing opportunities for career advancement because of guilt over the decision to delay having children. Conversely, a deferred achiever might subconsciously invite her family to discourage career pursuits. For women who have built their identities around feminine ideals of marriage and parenthood, but who never marry, the 30s may be a time of great depair, regardless of overt professional achievement.

WOMEN'S PSYCHOTHERAPY GROUPS VERSUS
CONSCIOUSNESS-RAISING GROUPS

There is often confusion in mental health circles as to the differences between women's psychotherapy groups and women's consciousness-raising (CR) groups. Similarities include the establishment of a supportive and confidential relationship, a specific setting, and a sharing of similar experiences (Nassi & Abramowitz, 1978). In both groups, there are empathy, available role models, and an awareness of sociocultural norms and their effect on women's conflicts and distresses.

The differences are related to the contrasting philosophy, focus, structure, process, and results. The philosophy of CR groups is that women's distress is primarily a social problem, and society is held responsible for distortions and prejudices (Brodsky, 1977; Kirsch, 1974; Nassi & Abramowitz, 1978). In psychotherapy, the problems of the individual are seen as being due, at least in part, to individual psychodynamics. While the focus of CR groups is to change society through expansion of one's awareness of what it means to be a woman in a prejudiced society, the focus of women's therapy groups is to change the individual through corrective emotional experiences (Brodsky, 1977).

The structure of the groups is different, in that CR groups have total peer equality, while in psychotherapy, there is an unequal hierarchy between therapist and patients (Kirsch, 1974). CR groups and therapy groups have a similar process early in the group's development, but this changes later. Both groups emphasize the creation of a culture fostering intimacy and trust and the recognition of commonalities. CR groups go on to analyze how women have been devalued in society, and how this position is maintained or altered. They then develop and discuss an ideology by which women can recognize the oppressive role of institutions (Nassi & Abramowitz, 1978).

In both CR groups and therapy groups, it is hoped that women will experience increased self-esteem as a result of the process. In CR groups, this may occur because members gain a political consciousness, become aware that their difficulty is rooted in the society, and learn what they can do to change it. In therapy groups, women may achieve greater self-esteem through examining and changing their unique characterological approaches to intrapersonal and interpersonal dilemmas. One study contrasting CR and therapy groups found that women entering CR groups had lower stress scores than a clinic population but higher scores than a normative sample of women (Kravetz, 1978).

HOW WOMEN ARE REFERRED TO GROUPS

In 1979, 700 women were referred to the mental health department at HCHP, Cambridge. Of these, 95 were referred to women's groups. The remaining women were either referred to other groups (such as those for young adults described in Chapter 12, this volume), seen in couples treatment, or treated in individual brief therapy. There are also specialized groups available, such as those for preorgasmic women.

A woman referred to a group must demonstrate that she has an ability to relate to other people. If a woman is to derive benefit from a short-term group, she must be able to interact with others (Budman *et al.,* Chapter 12, this volume). The clinician may evaluate this ability by exploring the person's history of relationships and ability to particpate in social or business groups.

If a therapist believes that a patient is appropriate for a group referral, time in the evaluation is spent preparing the patient for what she may expect in short-term group psychotherapy. An individual should be excluded from short-term women's groups if she is psychotic, borderline, or suicidal, or if she is a severe abuser of drugs or alcohol.

In preparing the patient for referral to a short-term group, the therapist often needs to discuss the benefits of group treatment. The therapist must deal with the patient's experience of rejection and rage at not having an individual therapist. Patients often view group therapy as sharing a nurturing parent with seven or eight others. Once the initial injury to the patient's self-esteem is addressed, she is usually able to recognize some of the more positive components of a group, such as (1) the support of peers and the sharing of common problems, (2) an opportunity to learn alternative ways of dealing with similar conflicts, and (3) a way of sharing interpersonal experiences which allows her to examine and validate her perceptions and behavior with others. The evaluating therapist then works with the patient to delineate specific issues upon which the patient can focus. (Development of a clear treatment focus is a necessary first step in any brief therapy.) The therapist may then describe what the patient can expect from a group.

After the patient has been informed of the technicalities of the group and has established a personal focus for group treatment, she is put on a waiting list for approximately three to eight weeks. When the group is about to begin, the patient meets with the group leader for one individual session. The patient's presenting problems are briefly reviewed again, with the aim being the establishment of a specific focus for group treatment. The leader discusses with the patient the length, size, place, and times of the group meetings. Candidates are asked to commit themselves to attend 15 weekly sessions. They are also requested to agree to confidentiality. It is emphasized that patients are responsible for sharing their problems in the group and for acting as participatory members in assisting others with problems. Further highlighted is the fact that patient improvement is the member's responsibility, and that the leader, as a facilitator, attempts to assist group members in achieving their goals.

SHORT-TERM WOMEN'S THERAPY GROUPS

Two observations initially led to our exploration of short-term therapy groups for women. First, as is true at most clinical settings, many more women than men were referred to the mental health department at HCHP. Therefore, waiting time for entry into a cogender group was much longer for a woman. Second, therapists observed that women shared developmental issues and questions that were very different than those of the male population. They regularly confronted such issues as choosing between career and childbearing, taking responsibility for one's own destiny rather than relying on a spouse or a parent to make life decisions, and not being able to be assertive without feeling guilty.

It appeared to us that women sought out the support of other female group members in dealing with these life events and the accompanying conflicts. They often tended to form a subgroup within the cogender group and addressed remarks and support largely to members of their own sex.

Given these observations, we began to run groups exclusively for women. We hypothesized that, in a limited time, female patients with common lifestyles and conflicts peculiar to their sex could more quickly address central difficulties in their lives. Furthermore, we believed removing the heterosexual component from the groups would allow for more intensive scrutiny of those issues common to women.

WHO IS REFERRED TO A WOMEN'S GROUP?

The patient referred to a women's group is generally in her early 30s. She has demonstrated the ability to form significant relationships. Her conflicts are intrapersonal as opposed to other directed, that is, emphasis has shifted from what others expect of her to what she expects of herself. The conflict evolves as "limiting one's responsibilities to others without abandoning moral concern" (Gilligan, 1977). The urgency of this dilemma is enhanced by the fact that the patient may feel that the remaining time for her to make major life decisions is limited.

> Karen was a 36-year-old, white, married woman who came to the mental health department complaining of "feeling anxious." She was having difficulty falling asleep at night and had lost weight in the preceding two months. Karen had been married at the age of 22. She had never worked and had depended on her husband for financial support as well as social status within the community. She identified herself totally with the role of wife and mother. After attending her fifteenth college reunion, Karen began to think about alternatives to her current lifestyle. She became fearful and anxious and felt guilty that she could consider "abandoning" her husband by establishing personal interests not related to the family. After she had attempted to avoid the conflict for several months, the anxiety generated by her denial became too oppressive, and she sought help. She was referred to a women's group, so that she might work on this developmental dilemma of nurture-versus-autonomy.

For other women who have established careers early in life, the issue of whether or not to have a family may be addressed. They must make choices about the role that their professions will play in their lives in the future.

> Mary was a 32-year-old, white, single, female associate at a law firm. She was living with her boyfriend of three years. She came to the mental health department to seek assistance with "anxiety attacks," which she had been experiencing for the past three months. These attacks had begun when she had started to seriously discuss possible marriage and family with her lover. She stated that she loved him and could not imagine marrying anyone else. She was doing very well at her job, however, and was afraid that if she worked part time for the years she was having children, hope for a future in the firm would be destroyed. She felt guilt about "wasting her education" if she did not work full time and try to get ahead. Yet, at the same time, she experienced a sense of obligation to her mother and her partner to start a family. Mary was referred to a women's group so that she could examine her own needs, independent of her family and her lover. She also wished to address the guilt that she experienced in relation to those needs.

Often, women referred to the groups have just had their last child enter school. They are faced with the conflict of whether they should pursue a more traditional role, involving staying home with the children, as their mothers had often done, or establish an independent career outside the home.

> Leslie was a 35-year-old, white, married, mother of three children, ages eight, six, and four. She had been married for 11 years to a physician in the area. She sought treatment because she had been feeling weepy and depressed for the previous month and a half. Her usual methods of cheering herself up had become ineffective. She was unable to name a precipitant for the sadness, stating that she got along well with her husband and children and considered herself fortunate in having a good family life.
>
> Her youngest child had started school several months prior to Leslie's first mental health appointment. At about the same time, the patient's younger sister, age 30, had come for a visit. The sister was progressing rapidly in her career as a businesswoman. It was at about the time of the sister's visit that Leslie began to question her own future. She started to feel helpless, trapped, and enslaved by her husband and family. The guilt that she experienced because of these feelings only led her to attempt to nurture her family more, often at the expense of her own needs. She was accelerating her nurturing behavior at a time when her children were beginning to want to separate from her.

Another major reason that women are referred to short-term women's groups is that they have sustained some major crisis peculiar to women (e.g., rape, abortion, or divorce and single parenting). Women's groups can be very important sources of support when a woman faces, for example, the pain of separation. The woman must define herself as a single person, not as part of a couple, and must overcome preconceived myths about divorced women, such as that they are sexually promiscuous and embittered. She worries about her attractiveness and wonders if she will be able to form another relationship. Women's groups are useful in helping such a woman to separate emotionally from her former spouse and to experience herself as a powerful person in her own right, not only through another person.

THE PROCESS OF A WOMEN'S GROUP

A women's group achieves a superficial cohesion very quickly. In the first session, women become excited and relieved to find that others share their difficulties. Each member eagerly shares the surface details of her life and is gratified by the support that she receives from other members. The therapist, at this point, is quite active, encouraging each member to participate in the group process and to try to keep her original focus for the group in mind.

At this point in the life of the group, members look predominantly to the therapist for support and approval, and they address most remarks to her. It is essential that the therapist keep returning responsibility for remarks and support back to the group. Many women have had difficulty because they have evaluated themselves through their mother's or their husband's eyes, and this pattern is rapidly displayed as authority-centered dependency. In the first four sessions, the therapist becomes the powerful person, who is able to judge the value of their contribution to the group. Her approval or lack of it becomes the barometer by which the patient judges her own contribution.

> Martha was a 32-year-old, white, married woman who was very interactive in her first three group sessions. Most often, she supported other group members. Her interventions, however, were all punctuated by a glance toward the therapist. She constantly sought approval for her contributions to the group. The therapist called her attention to this process, suggesting that Martha also looked to her husband and mother to define her role within the family. Martha then spoke about her fears of disapproval. She was also able to see that she abdicated most of the control over her life to her husband, and before him, to her mother, and that she viewed the therapist as a similar authority figure.

In the first three sessions, the therapist establishes the format for the remaining period. By returning the responsibility for actions within the group to the members, she is implying that each member is responsible for her life in the group. In addition, by carefully processing a member's response to her, the therapist can help the patient examine behavioral patterns early in the course of the group.

In approximately the fourth or fifth group session, members are beginning to know, and can thus feel supportive, of each other. Often in their lives, being supportive has meant totally subverting their own needs in the service of others. There is much talk about members not wanting to take time for themselves because someone else in the group is in such pain and needs support. Part of the willingness to nurture the "more needy" member entails relief that one's own life is not quite so problematic. A member may also be silently furious, however, that someone else is receiving so much attention. At this stage in the group, most patients are unable to verbalize that anger. Instead, they may attack the therapist for not running a more structured group, in which everyone can participate. We view this attack as "asking permission" of the powerful figure to take time in the group. At this point, it is important for the therapist to actively process what is happening. She may point out to the patient that perhaps the latter has difficulties asserting her needs and feelings outside the group as well as inside. She may then help the patient explore feelings of anger that are a result of her needs not being addressed. How the patient seeks permission from others outside the group in an effort to fulfill her needs may also be examined.

> Florence was a 31-year-old, white, married woman who quickly volunteered information about her life, while encouraging others to talk about themselves. At the beginning of the fifth session, she became very angry with the therapist, stating that she wanted more structure in the group meeting and suggesting that the leader provide topics for discussion. Florence went on to describe her feelings of being disapproved of by the leader. "I never feel like I'm saying the right thing." When the therapist suggested that perhaps she had experienced these feelings of insecurity and inadequacy with other people in her life, Florence became very tearful and described her relationship with her mother. She had fashioned her behavior to please mother most of her life, yet she never felt that she was "good enough" to make her happy. Florence wanted to help her mother recover from the grief experienced after the loss of her father; however, she felt helpless in this pursuit. Her rage at the therapist reflected much of the anger she had experienced toward mother yet was unable to express. Florence was able to share her feelings of sadness and helplessness with the group, and she began addressing her remarks much more to other members. Having expressed her anger toward the group leader and her mother, she was now able to begin to separate from both of them.

> Adrien was a 35-year-old, white, divorced woman who had remained quiet in the first three group sessions. During the fourth session, she became very angry with the therapist for allowing another woman to dominate that meeting. She suggested that everyone in the group be allotted a certain amount of time each week. The leader suggested to Adrien that perhaps she had difficulties making her needs known not only in the group but in her life outside the group, and, furthermore, that Adrien could learn to assert her needs within the group without such sanction.

Between the eighth and twelfth sessions, women in a short-term group begin to discuss topics from earlier sessions in much more depth. As they trust each other more, the emphasis in the group shifts from an interpersonal seeking of consensus, support, and similarities to intrapersonal probing and exploration. Women discuss their feelings of being inadequate, isolated, and fearful of censure. They may also explore how these feelings dictate their actions in the group. Florence, for example, was able to talk about the pain and rage involved in separating from her mother. She discussed how this fear of disapproval and subsequent censure and abandonment interfered with her ability to commit herself to a major career decision, and how these feelings impeded her work in the group. She also began to experience the fact that she could contribute to relationships within the group in roles other than that of the nurturer.

The interaction in the group at this stage has shifted from patient–therapist to patient–patient. The exchanges in the group often mimic sibling interactions. Women express fear of hurting another member of the group or of depriving her of adequate time. The therapist encourages members to address their feelings of competitiveness within the group and their fears of their aggressive instincts.

> Phyllis was a 32-year-old, white, married woman who was the eldest of three children. She had always felt very protective of her younger siblings and often sacrificed time she would have like to spend with friends in order to care for them. Her pattern of behavior in the group was very similar to that in her family of origin: she protected members who she thought were being attacked, and she tried to rescue others from their pain, always offering a tissue if a member started to cry. If a patient became angry, she attempted to diffuse the rage by suggesting that "everything would work out in time."
>
> In the tenth session, another group member, Mary, became very angry with Phyllis, telling her that she, Mary, had a right to her own feelings and that they would not be resolved with a tissue. Phyllis became tearful. She began to get in touch with the anger that she felt toward her siblings for not appreciating her efforts to nurture them. Phyllis was invited to consider alternative roles that she could have in relationships. She then discussed her fear of her own anger and rejection if she were to aggressively seek to meet her own needs. The group was very supportive of her and pointed out that if they were able to tolerate her pain and anger, other people outside the group could do the same.

The therapist takes a less active role in these later sessions and restricts herself largely to processing comments.

In the 12th through the 15th session, the group must work through termination. Often, the members attempt to collectively deny the fact that the group must end, discussing continuation of the group outside the auspices of HCHP. This period of termination allows each member to address other losses that she has experienced.

> Barbara was a 36-year-old, white, married woman who persistently changed the subject when the issue of termination was brought up. When the therapist brought this to her attention, she talked about what the group had meant to her. She expressed trust in the group members. She spoke of having come to "depend" upon the weekly meetings and then went on to talk about losses of

other people she had trusted. She addressed her fear of driving people away and was subsequently able to express her anger at the therapist for ending the group. In addition, she was able to address the anger that she felt toward her mother, who had died two years previously of cancer.

In the final sessions, group members take stock of what they have learned in the group. They often fear what will happen to them when the support of the group is withdrawn. Members sometimes revert to their early dependency on the therapist for reassurance. The therapist must address this regression and the fears about the group ending.

Some members are unable to benefit from a short-term women's group. They are unable to tolerate the intensity of the brief treatment model. When other group members confront them about behavioral styles and possible change, they usually become angry and subsequently withdrawn and sometimes drop out of the group in the first eight sessions. The therapist must actively address this loss with the group. She should encourage the other members to discuss their feelings of anger, guilt, and possibly relief about the person's choice to leave.

At the last session of a group, members are usually ready to say goodbye to each other. The therapist is active in helping each person formulate what she has learned from the treatment.

CONCLUSION

In the past six years, women between the ages of 25 and 40 have been treated in short-term, 15-session, women's psychotherapy groups at HCHP. Upon closer examination of these groups, it appears that they effectively address the needs of women in a particular developmental stage of life.

People referred to women's groups are predominantly in their 30s, although a few are in their late 20s. Most of these women have formed significant relationships in their lives and are currently married, divorced, or living with a primary partner. The emphasis of their difficulty has shifted from interpersonal exploration to an intrapersonal need for self-definition of nurture-versus-autonomy. The urgency around these intrapersonal conflicts is great, since the women perceive that time to make a major life change is running out. They no longer have limitless time to have children or to choose a career. Although interpersonal relationships are a concern to women in this stage of development, they are more concerned with establishing their own sense of identity, importance, and power, apart from their families of origin and immediate families. Much time in a women's group is spent empathizing with, and working through, fears and conflicts associated with change and independence. Most women in these groups find it very comforting to know that other women have experienced similar doubts, feelings of isolation, and conflicts between dependence and independence.

Further explorations as to how short-term women's groups compare with cogender groups could be useful. It appears that various short-term groups may be able to serve patients at different developmental stages, each reflective of particular issues.

We believe that an adult developmental emphasis allows for rapid cohesiveness and a pursuit of the focal work within the context of time-limited group treatment. The application of such a model to a variety of life-stage issues for both men and women is limited only by the interest, knowledge, and imagination of the reader.

ACKNOWLEDGMENT

We wish to express our thanks to Simon Budman for his suggestions and support during the completion of this chapter.

REFERENCES

Aries, E. J. *Interactional patterns and themes of men's, women's and mixed groups.* Unpublished doctoral dissertation, Harvard University, 1973.

Bernard, H., & Klein, R. H. Some perspectives on time-limited group psychotherapy. *Comprehensive Psychiatry,* 1977, *18,* 579–584.

Brodsky, A. Therapeutic aspects of consciousness raising groups. In E. Rawlings & D. Carter (Eds.), *Psychotherapy of women.* Springfield, Ill.: Charles C Thomas, 1977.

Budman, S. H., Bennett, M. J., & Wisneski, M. J. Short-term group psychotherapy: An adult developmental model. *International Journal of Group Psychotherapy,* 1980, *30,* 63–76.

Budman, S. H., & Clifford, M. Short-term group therapy for couples in a health maintenance organization. *Professional Psychology,* 1979, *10,* 419–429.

Carlock, C., & Martin, P. Sex composition and the intensive group experience. *Social Work,* 1977, *22,* 27–32.

Chodorow, N. Family structure and feminine personality. In M. Rosaldo & L. Lanpliere (Eds.), *Women, culture and society.* Stanford: Stanford University Press, 1974.

Chodorow, N. *The reproduction of mothering.* Berkeley: University of California Press, 1978.

Gilligan, C. In a different voice: Women's conception of self-found morality. *Harvard Educational Review,* 1977, *47,* 481–518.

Halas, C. All women's groups: A view from inside. *Personnel and Guidance Journal,* 1973, *52,* 91–95.

Kirsch, B. Consciousness raising groups as therapy for women. In V. Franks & V. Burtle (Eds.), *Women in therapy: New psychotherapies for a changing society.* New York: Brunner/Mazel, 1974.

Kravetz, D. Consciousness raising groups in the 70's. *Psychology of Women Quarterly,* 1978, *3,* 168–186.

Lever, J. Sex differences in the games children play. *Social Problems,* 1976, *23,* 478–487.

Lynch, C. Women's groups. *Family Therapy,* 1974, *1,* 223–228.

Mogul, K. Women in midlife: Decisions, rewards and conflicts related to work and careers. *American Journal of Psychiatry,* 1979, *136,* 1139–1143.

Nadelson, C., Notman, M., & Bennett, M. Success or failure: Psychotherapeutic considerations for women in conflict. *American Journal of Psychiatry,* 1978, *135,* 1092–1096.

Nassi, A., & Abramowitz, S. Raising consciousness about women's groups: Process and outcome. *Psychology of Women Quarterly,* 1978, *3,* 139–156.

O'Leary, V. *Toward understanding women.* Monterey, Calif.: Brooks Cole, 1977.

Waxer, P. H. Short-term group psychotherapy: Some principles and techniques. *International Journal of Group Psychotherapy,* 1977, *27,* 33–42.

SECTION V
MARITAL AND FAMILY THERAPY
AS BRIEF TREATMENT

CHAPTER 14
CREATING A FOCUS FOR BRIEF MARITAL OR FAMILY THERAPY

Warren Kinston
Arnon Bentovim

INTRODUCTION

The trend and ability drastically to shorten psychotherapeutic work with children and adolescents became evident only with the development of theories and techniques which recognized the parents, the extended family, and the social network as both targets for change and agents of change. In contrast to the United States, where family therapy originated from research into young adult schizophrenia, child guidance clinic workers in the United Kingdom branched into this field as part of their efforts to increase the efficiency of their interventions. The value of marital and family therapy has been broadly established by a large variety of methodologically adequate studies which were done mainly in the mid-'70s (Gurman & Kniskern, 1979). The field is still in its infancy, however, with theoretical and technical issues wide open, and so, in this chapter, we invite the reader to explore with us rather than learn from us.

Within the broad rubric of "family therapy," many treatment approaches have been used. Most of the shorter methods require an active technique, with the therapist engaging directly with the family members, setting family tasks, openly acting as a model of healthy functioning, providing video-tape feedback of interactions, interfering with dysfunctional behavior patterns, advising or consciously double binding. Even those techniques more directly emerging from psychoanalytic theory, as described by Ackerman (1958), Dicks (1967), Zinner and Shapiro (1974),

WARREN KINSTON. Brunel Institute of Organization and Social Studies, Brunel University, Uxbridge, Middlesex, England.
ARNON BENTOVIM. Department of Psychological Medicine, The Hospital for Sick Children, and the Tavistock Clinic, London, England.

and Boszormenyi-Nagy and Spark (1973), involve considerably more therapist activity and direction than is customary in individual psychoanalytic therapy. Some techniques highly specific to family life have also been developed (e.g., constructing and analyzing family genograms and sculpting the family). In this chapter, we are unable to describe in detail the technical armamentarium of the experienced family therapist and shall assume the reader has or can obtain some familiarity with work in this field (Guerin, 1976; Haley, 1971; Madanes & Haley, 1979; Selvini-Palazzoli, Boscolo, Cecchin, & Prata, 1978; Papp, 1978). We will be focusing on a conceptual approach to the application of the various techniques.

In our work with families conjointly over the past 15 years at the Department of Psychological Medicine at The Hospital for Sick Children (London, UK), we have become convinced of the value of family intervention in general and of the need for the therapist to be able to apply a range of techniques, irrespective of his orientation as an "individual" therapist. Diagnostic work in the department is multidisciplinary and usually takes place in a family setting. Whenever possible, treatment aims are rapidly clarified so as to harness the potential for change associated with the first meeting between a disturbed family and the professional. Without a clear purpose and overall strategy, it is easy to dissipate this charge; work becomes diffuse, and family members opt out of attendance. A particular problem is the emergence during family work of hidden problems and demands, most commonly in relation to long-standing but carefully avoided severe marital disturbance. Although we are a child-based facility, we now regard marital therapy as an essential part of our service.

The success in shortening individual psychoanalytic therapy by using a focal approach, as developed theoretically and practically by Balint and Malan at the Tavistock Clinic in London (Balint, Ornstein, & Balint, 1973; Malan, 1963, 1976), suggested the application of a similar model to family therapy. In association with his model, Malan (1959) developed a methodology for the assessment of improvement on an "individualized" basis. We regarded monitoring of outcome as essential in the young and enthusiastic phase through which family work was passing, and we attempted to apply Malan's methodology. Clearly, there were practical and conceptual hurdles to be surmounted in making the transition from a psychodynamic individual focus to a "family focus."

In 1973 we set up a workshop to monitor and supervise the treatment of families through the use of a brief focal approach. An experienced staff member of the Tavistock Clinic's brief psychotherapy workshop agreed to act as consultant and group leader during the first year. The workshop survived his departure and continued operating for a further 18 months. In all, 29 families were considered. At that time (1975), we paused and reviewed the outcome in all the families, our methodology, and the operation of the workshop. Full details were published, including brief details on every family and lengthy discussion of one family and one marital case (Bentovim & Kinston, 1978; Kinston & Bentovim, 1978). A new workshop was convened in 1978.

In this chapter, we shall briefly review the methodology, as originally developed, and outline the difficulties we encountered. We shall then turn to recent developments in our conceptualization, together with illustrative case material.

THE INITIAL ATTEMPT: METHOD, RESULTS, AFTERMATH

Table 1 compares the assessment procedure which Malan developed for brief individual psychodynamic therapy with that which we devised for families.

The workshop accepted any outpatient case, excluding psychotic children; this meant that "problem" cases were often brought. Without experience, it seemed unwise to reject families as unsuitable, and this indiscriminate acceptance may have played a part in the quarter of the families who did not engage.

In a general discussion in the workshop, hypotheses were developed—using a minimum of psychodynamic theory—which could encompass the reason for referral and presenting symptoms, salient facts about the history of the family, its members, and the families of origin, and observations of family interaction. These focal hypotheses then became the reference point for therapeutic progress and the source of criteria by which the success or failure of outcome could be judged. These criteria were objective, that is, socially sharable facts. The workshop then determined a focal plan,[1] which aimed at providing the therapist with guidance as to how changes were to be brought about. Techniques were not specified, but at that time, action methods, such as sculpting, were excluded. The duration and frequency of treatment sessions for the successful completion of the

[1] In our early work, we confused the two meanings of *focus* by referring to "focal hypothesis" and "focal plan." The latter term has now been dropped and has been replaced by "therapeutic plan."

TABLE 1. *Comparison of Individual and Family Methods*

Brief individual psychotherapy[a]	Brief focal family therapy[b]
A. Basic details: • Name, age, occupation • Complaints	A. Basic details: • Names, ages, occupations, school • Presenting problems
B. All known disturbances: • Symptoms • Relationships	B. All known disturbances: • Symptoms in any member • Observations of interaction
C. Personal history: • Childhood experiences • Recent events	C. Family history: • Family life cycle • Recent events • Families of origin
D. Focal hypothesis to explain B in the light of C	D. Focal hypothesis to explain B in the light of C
E. Criteria for the results of therapy	E. Criteria for the results of therapy
F. Therapeutic plan developed and implemented; patient subsequently followed up	F. Therapeutic plan developed and implemented; family subsequently followed up
G. Disturbances under B reexamined at follow-up	G. Disturbances under B reexamined at termination and follow-up
H. Assessment of results: compare E with G	H. Assessment of results: compare E with G

[a]After Malan (1976).
[b]After Kinston and Bentovim (1978).

focal plan were also estimated and formed the basis of the contract offered to the family. The family was not necessarily informed of the details of the focal hypothesis or plan.

This approach resulted in an unspectacular 66% remission of symptoms in the index child, which edged up to a very respectable 87% success if those families who failed to engage are excluded. These results are typical of psychotherapy research. When the family as a whole was considered in the light of the desired criteria, however, only 50% of those who engaged showed improvement. About one-third of our cases received marital therapy (with or without family therapy), but this was not related to outcome. Two findings were noted: first, psychiatric illness in a parent was a poor prognostic sign, and second, the greater the improvement in the family as a whole, the greater the improvement in the index child.

The research workshop and its findings deeply influenced routine clinical work. Our current policy is to consider every referral for brief family therapy when an intact family exists in the clinical picture. If admission of a family member is necessary (e.g., anorexia nervosa, schizophrenia, child abuse), long-term work is expected. If such external holding is not required, families are assessed with the intention of providing between six and ten sessions over four to six months. The usual interval between sessions has been reduced from three weeks to two weeks.

An individual approach is the treatment of choice when one member has some special difficulty or problem with which the family is managing acceptably. More often, the individual approach is a treatment by default when various family members refuse to attend, when the notion of a family problem is unacceptable to the members, when one member is grossly rejected, or when a partial approach to a multiproblem family is desirable.

Implementation of a clinical approach such as ours had immediate teaching implications, and in order to meet these obligations, we commenced a clarification of both method and theory.

FOCAL HYPOTHESIS

There are two crucial tasks for the construction of a focal hypothesis:

1. the collection of the base of relevant data which the hypothesis is to explain
2. the use of this data to construct a hypothesis

The problem of collection of the relevant data was noted in our early papers. Facts become "salient" only in the light of a sophisticated understanding of the problems to be overcome. A major difficulty in our workshop was the lack of a generally accepted, conceptual framework of families useful for family therapy. Neither the developments from psychoanalytic theory nor the precepts of the various systems-type theories were integrated effectively, and resistance to conceptualizing at the family level was marked. Even more difficult was the collection of accurate, relevant, clinical descriptions of family interaction. Our therapists lacked a vocabulary and any systematic mode of observation. Discussions about families *qua* families were seriously limited and appeared crude and simplistic in comparison with the richness and complexity of descriptions of the individual.

In order to tackle this problem, we embarked on a conventional research effort which operated independently of our ongoing clinical work. We have commenced the reporting of this work, which is still in progress (Kinston, Loader, & Stratford, 1979; Loader, Kinston, Burck, & Bentovim, 1980). We now have confidence, however, that a clinically adequate, systematic account of family interaction can be provided and can serve as the empirical base for our theoretical, therapeutic, and research efforts (Bentovim, 1979b).

The ability to "see" family interaction, combined with insufficient integration of family theory, had led us to be relatively conservative in the application of therapeutic techniques. As our knowledge and skill developed, therapists felt freer and operated more flexibly with a variety of techniques that were less bounded by their own needs and anxieties and more suited to the needs of the family. This evaluation is characteristic of the practice of psychoanalytic marital–family therapy; that is, it has become "largely 'analytic' in the way it organizes the complex material at hand and conceptualizes the nature of [disturbance], but is, of necessity, quite pragmatic, if not eclectic, in its selection of actual therapeutic interactions" (Gurman, 1978).

This chapter is predominantly concerned with the second issue stated above: Can therapists determine "salience" amidst the welter of facts at hand? Given accurate and sufficient historical and current interactional-state data, can therapists develop focal hypotheses? Will these hypotheses serve to guide treatment, and will they allow the development of empirical criteria of improvement?

We remarked that in our early review, the focal hypotheses appeared to be somewhat haphazard, ranging from minutely detailed, such as:

> The parents' unresolved maturational problems are being projected onto the children. The parents, being unable to find their own identity, have obtained security by self-idealization. They are frightened of the rage they have inside themselves and so are unable to be caring to the children.

to highly generalized:

> The family has conflicts over dependency and assertiveness.

and from grandly theoretical:

> Failure of integration of sexuality and aggression is resulting in isolation of family members.

to simply descriptive:

> Here we have an overprotective mother, a passive father, and a son with early
> separation experiences.

This chapter reflects our tentative preliminary steps toward bringing order
into this chaos.

WHAT IS A FOCUS?

It is crucial to differentiate between *focus* as a term generally used in brief
therapy and as it relates to the "focal hypothesis."[2] All brief methods use
a focus or a focused approach; that is, they make a delineated issue the
centre of therapist activity (Ursano & Dressler, 1974). It would be difficult, indeed, to imagine any alternative. A typical example in the family
therapy field is the highly focused, brief work of Weakland, Fisch, Watzlawick, and Bodin (1974). *Focus,* in the sense we use it, is a figurative adaptation of its optical meaning, namely, "that point at which an object must
be situated in order that the image produced by the lens will be clear and
well-defined" *(Shorter Oxford English Dictionary).*

A focal hypothesis refers to an "ad hoc clinical theory" developed to
clarify or bring into focus a large number of disparate and apparently
unrelated phenomena. It integrates and provides continuity to the manifestations of the person or family. It also serves as a beacon to guide the
therapist as he or she becomes involved in the detailed specifics of work
with the individual or family. For this reason, it must be brief and highly
pertinent and, despite the high level of abstraction, must evoke in the therapist the full complexity that gave birth to it.

In the individual, the historical background gave meaning to present
symptoms and disturbed relationships in a manner consistent with psychoanalytic theories. This meaning is not just an extra frill or pretentious addition, but something which has profound implications for the patient.
Armstrong, Yasuna, and Hartley (1979) showed that focal hypotheses
could be developed on patients assigned to behavior therapy as well as psychodynamic therapy. Behavior therapists choose to ignore the disturbances which are not directly related to the symptom or specifically com-
plained of, so they naturally do not consider changes in these.

The criteria for improvement, as developed from the focal hypothe-

[2]See Footnote 1.

sis, inevitably encompasses not just the symptom, but the whole range of disturbances identified by a professional. The aim is to produce not a "perfect" person, but one who, despite the effort, pain, conflict, and depression, will choose constructive solutions to difficulties which previously were avoided, projected, or destructively enacted. The appreciation of these new solutions (e.g., whether they are genuine or false) is best considered in the light of the focal hypothesis. Improvement according to focal hypothesis criteria is not nonspecific. It is, rather, the reverse: it is highly specific and represents improvement in aspects of the person which are judged central to an ongoing problem that has persisted subclinically for years. These considerations are applicable to family disturbance.

There is a crucial difference between the individual and the family in therapy. At an interview, it is impossible to observe directly and unambiguously the person's mental processes, but it is possible to observe the family interaction. The individual therapist has to lay much weight on the person's self-report and, of course, takes advantage of any behavior or relating evident in the session. The person's compulsively repeated self-defeating patterns of behavior manifest over the weeks, months, or years of the therapy and follow-up period. Part of the difficulty in assessing the results of individual analytic psychotherapy is that outcome may not be certain for many years, due to factors beyond the person's control.

The family, on the other hand, immediately presents its dysfunction. Its way of being is expressed synchronically rather than diachronically. Because of this, an improvement in interaction at the termination of therapy is a reasonable expectation if success is to be claimed. Long-term maintenance of improvement is important but can often be considered as a separate issue. In our view, family therapy aimed only at a symptom or a particular dysfunctional interaction (e.g., poor communication) is like behavior therapy. It might produce amelioration in a limited and important way, but it will do so without altering fundamental and long-standing problems in the family which are capable of change or resolution. Although it *might* result in alteration of underlying difficulties and widespread improvement, our contention is that this is neither aimed for nor inevitable nor considered in outcome evaluation. To examine this claim further, we must embark on a conceptual excursion into the nature of meaning within a family. If the clinician is to construct a helpful focal hypothesis, it is crucial that he or she be aware of the systems of meaning which arise out of and are constitutive of the family's interaction and life together (Harris, 1980).

FORMS OF MEANING

SURFACE ACTION

The most overt form of meaning refers to what the therapist observes when viewing a family, and what he or she hears from them in reports of themselves, each other, and events and episodes of family life. *Symptom* is the usual medical term for a presenting complaint. In the families we see, these are often descriptions of behavioral disturbance in a child. One example is the C. family, in which Janie, 10½ years old, the oldest of three children, was referred with severe abdominal pains. These were psychological in origin: physical investigation had shown no abnormality, and they recurred with each discharge from hospital.

There are a large number of other terms, however, which can be subsumed by the concept of "surface action." The overt behavioral patterns of interaction and events of family life have commonly been referred to as the "family system." We refer to a current cross-sectional view of the family as the "family state" (Kinston *et al.,* 1979). The repetitious quality of actions and reactions has led to ideas like defense, rule, and role. It is clearer to speak of surface rules or regulative rules to distinguish them from another use of the term described below. Similarly, in our work with disturbed families, the term "label" or "labeled role" is often more applicable.

Janie was the symptom carrier and was labeled "the patient" in the C. family system. Observation of the whole family immediately revealed repetitious patterns of behavior:

- Whenever the father spoke to his daughter or approached her, he was seductive. He asserted that "you can be firm with boys but not with girls" and demonstrated this by his differential handling of Janie and her younger brothers (Paul, 8 years old; Billy, 1½).
- His wife never forcefully contradicted her husband's belief or opposed his treatment of the children.
- Janie tracked her mother and was demanding, clinging, and babyish. This difficult and immature behavior developed after the birth of her youngest brother.
- Mother did nothing to make a more satisfactory boundary between herself and Janie and made no demand for age-appropriate behavior.

A circular reinforcement of the principle that one must be seductive rather than firm with girls is evident as the meaning of the interaction.

When a family comes to treatment, it is essential that the therapist rapidly home in on the crucially pathological interactions, such as described in the C. family. These surface actions have a number of well-defined characteristics:

1. Extreme repetitiousness, often to the point of defining the family.
2. Independence from external events. The patterns of surface action appear to be set off at random or haphazardly.
3. Circular causality. The patterns are self-maintaining, as each segment leads to the next and finally back on itself.
4. Compulsiveness. Simple requests to the family to stop behaving this way cannot be complied with for any significant length of time, and often not at all.
5. The surface pattern appears to run the family. It has a dominating and urgent quality which overrides apparently destructive consequences.

Surface patterns of action with such qualities, although readily regarded as "meaningful behavior" by family and outside observers, inevitably result in the family losing flexibility and adaptability. The family loses the capacity to respond creatively to significant external stresses and internal demands of family development, and it loses a sense of meaning, which keeps futility at bay. All therapists will have had the experience of seeing how an apparently meaningful behavior produces, on its nth pointless repetition, a sense of meaninglessness.

A typical attempt to get the C. parents to discuss seriously how to get Janie back to school went as follows:

MOTHER: I can't see her going back to school willingly.
FATHER: We have to keep trying to persuade her.
MOTHER: How long do you keep trying?
FATHER: You have to keep on trying?
MOTHER: For six months?
FATHER: Yes, try for six months—and if you do not succeed, try something else.
MOTHER: And if it doesn't work?
FATHER: You just have to keep on trying.

During this discussion, Janie butted in haphazardly and interfered with the communicative flow. The parents could not adhere to therapist requests that they prevent Janie's interference and decide on a time limit. This pointless, self-maintaining, endless interaction occurred within a most serious context: local school authorities were being advised to go to court and take the matter out of the family's hands.

Only rarely is a family referred for system dysfunction, although increased popular awareness of the family nature of problems is starting to alter this pattern. It is usually referred because of a symptomatic individual (index patient) or following a gross inability to deal with some particular stress (the precipitant). The recognition of system dysfunction at the surface action level is correctly regarded as a task for the expert clinician, who uses his or her clinical judgment of pathology, which is based on training and experience with many families. The clinician particularly relies on some notion of what form of family interaction would be requisite, in light of the total context within which the family interaction manifests. This context includes physical, personal, social, and cultural realities.

DEPTH STRUCTURE

The clinician need go no further than recognizing surface action. He or she will have pinpointed pathology and can claim to have a focus for work—focus, that is, in the simple descriptive sense. There are a number of puzzles still left if the clinician wishes to notice them. Even if the system is self-maintaining, why does the family not switch to another self-maintaining but more productive system? Why is the dysfunction so noticeable to the clinician and not to the family? How does the family come to act in this particular way and not some other (also pathological) way? Sometimes these are academic questions, but sometimes they are crucial to therapeutic efforts.

A human being, when given a puzzle, can either turn away and decry it as unimportant or attempt to give it meaning. This constructive act is performed using two methods. The puzzle can be *investigated,* that is, repeatedly probed using methodologically sound, deductively based research strategies. This method, almost by definition, is completely unsuited to the clinical setting. Alternatively, the puzzle may be *interpreted;* that is, an account may be provided to make sense of the object of study. This hermeneutic approach is central to the psychoanalytic tradition (Ricoeur, 1970) and, some would say, to all the social sciences (Steele, 1979). Such accounts are "depth" activities: they form part of the theory construction phase of conventional scientific method and can themselves be used as a basis for deductions and nonclinical investigative efforts. They structure the confusion or obscurity.

To say that the family system required interpretation is to claim not only that the interaction is in some way puzzling or confusing, as argued above, but also that it occurs within a coherent-meaning field, within which this puzzle might be resolved or said "to make sense." This "sense" or meaning must be for both the family members and the clinician. Any interpretation, no matter how "good," which is incomprehensible to the clinician (perhaps because of emotional or intellectual blocks or cultural differences) is therapeutically useless. Similarly, the family members must, at least to some degree, accept the interpretation, if it is to be useful.

The reading of meaning is a routine part of family life from the moment of birth (Bentovim, 1979a). To be a human being is to experience one's situation in terms of meanings, and family interaction which occurs in a background of desire, feeling, and expectation is inevitably charged with meaning. The family typically states its problem in the form of an interpretation; for example, the symptom may be stealing, but for the family, stealing means he is "sick," and then with further clarification, he is "bad," and with still further clarification, he is "like grandfather." Unlike in individual psychoanalytic therapy, the family does not have interpretations formally administered. Nevertheless, every statement and action of the therapist will carry the unspoken, even unformulated account. The only alternative would be a haphazard or chaotic series of unconnected interventions.

The technique of reframing is an attempt to replace one reading or interpretation of events by another. Like clarification, this is possible because there is not a one-to-one correspondence between meaningful behavior or surface action and depth meaning. A number of interpretations may underlie a surface pattern, and a number of surface actions may emerge from a particular meaning. Depth meanings are constitutive of family reality. Table 2 lists frequently used terms and the commonly attributed correspondences between surface and depth levels of understanding.

The C. family seemed to share a meaning like "confronting or frustrating females is dangerous or painful." Such a meaning made sense of the quality of the marital relationship, in which there was a lack of directness and in which conflict was routinely diffused. Depth meanings are powerful, and so in the C. family, the therapist used the above meaning to avert the short-term crisis. In the long-term, it would have been necessary

TABLE 2. *Correspondences between Surface and Depth Levels of Family Interaction*

Action	Structure
Symptom	
Behavior	
Overt	Covert
Events	Meaning
Interaction	Dynamic
Game	Authenticity
Theme	Myth
Surface rule	Depth rule
Regulation	Constitution
Labeled role	Identity
System	Shared interpersonal reality
Generated experience	"True" experience
Mechanical relatedness	"True" relatedness
Mission	Individuation
Defense	Affect–idea complex

to modify it. The therapist first helped mother reframe her daughter's state and regard it as "rebellious" rather than "ill." Then she was brought to confront the father, who had to either come into conflict with his wife or agree with her and be firm with Janie. Either alternative was believed by him to be dangerous. In the event, he sided with his wife, and Janie immediately returned to school without any protest. The existence of long-term problems was manifested by the simultaneous recurrence of an old somatic complaint of Paul's.

We hope it is not necessary to argue or, indeed, belabor the point that family interaction is fundamentally interlinked with deep meanings, and that this meaning is not equivalent to surface action. The family is both a collection of individuals linked through time and a social unit, and meaning has to be considered from each of these vantage points. We have labeled these two sorts of meaning, respectively, "common meanings" and "intersubjective meanings."

COMMON MEANINGS

Common meanings are rooted in the psychic lives of the individual family members. Each member has his or her own unique experience, much of which remains unconscious or private and not directly relevant to the concerns of other family members or the family therapist. There are certain core meanings, however, which are shared at the time of marriage and develop in common afterward; when children appear, they assimilate and contribute to these. These common meanings are exchanged and shared, unconsciously and by example and instruction, and include beliefs, views, guiding principles, fears, expectations. They are the roots of belonging, loyalty, and cohesion within the family. Common meanings are essential for comfortable communication, pleasurable participation in interests, and tolerance of each other's pain. They are the basis for consensus and easy conflict resolution and for a coherent response to the environment. When a member leaves the family, he or she can take these meanings without disrupting the family and can use them in the creation of a new family.

Common meanings predominate explicitly and sometimes disastrously in enmeshed families. In the K. family, 13-year-old Sheila presented medically with life-threatening obesity and was admitted for rapid weight loss and psychological treatment. The parents, an older brother of 26, and an older, spastic sister of 24 were seen together with Sheila. Both the parents and the brother were extremely obese.

The surface action was characterized by total agreement among family members, particularly on the importance of mothering. Mother was the core of the family's way of life, and all members expected her complete availability. If mother were not present, father acted as mother. The mothering figure did not allow any frustration. Family members spoke whenever they wanted, irrespective of interruption of discourse. Similarly, they ate whenever they wanted.

The depth meaning was common to all members; that is, it had the quality of an individual psychological statement rather than a system-based statement. We phrased it as follows: Separation, or any threat of separation, is equivalent to total abandonment and death. All members avoided knowing that obesity (which stemmed from action expressing this meaning) was life threatening.

The following excerpt came after an attempt to confront the family with the consequences of their actions:

MOTHER: My heart is as sound as a bell. There is not the slightest chance of having a heart attack. They put things on my arms and legs [ECG] and she, the doctor, said that surprisingly enough my heart is sound as a bell—considering I smoke 40 cigarettes a day.

FATHER: They went through her and me with a toothcomb. She has got some high blood pressure, but her heart is as strong as a horse and so is mine.

This interchange took place after father had mentioned in passing that his wife had been recently diagnosed as having syringomyelia.

When the family changed, they did so in concert:

FATHER: We realize that we were killing her with our love—and that we can help keep her weight down.

MOTHER: Sheila now knows what she can and can't eat.

FATHER: We've been regimenting ourselves. We can't eat as we used to. We don't want to eat like that.

MOTHER: She didn't go to bed until we did; she is going to go to bed at nine o'clock now.

SHEILA: I want to go to bed at ten o'clock.

MOTHER: You've got to do what you're told. By giving you this leeway, we're killing you. She knows it's for her own good.

The enmeshed family moves like a mass from one set of common meanings to another. Short-term work cannot undo gross enmeshment, but what it can do is provide the family with a carefully predetermined opportunity to abandon some particularly destructive common meanings for others of their own choice.

We may contrast the snowballing of pathological common meanings which occur in enmeshed families with those that occur in other families which lack shared common meanings.

The L. family presented with Tom, 9 years old, showing a variety of oppositional and bullying behaviors. He also stole food and money, concentrated poorly at school, and was emotionally cold. This behavior had been present to some extent since his adoption at the age of 9 months. His younger brother, Bill, was born two years later following administration of fertility drugs to the mother. Bill was born with a minor penile abnormality and clicking hips, which led to several hospitalizations. He clung to his mother during the interview, and the parents reported he had sleeping problems.

Surface action was dominated by the parents' intellectual, self-centered communications, which left little room for the children to express themselves. Instead of positive emotional bonds between the parents, there was a sense of conflict underlying a glib exterior. Mother and Bill were overly close, and father and Tom overtly antagonistic. Father spent much time attempting to "help" Tom talk or do things, but he always failed.

There was a vein of disagreement running through the parental discussion. Mother wanted to have more children, while father did not.

Either course of action could have been easily defended and pursued by the family as a whole. No decision was reached, however, and the therapist's investigation of the problem revealed extremely divergent meanings underlying the idea of "having a child."

Father's early family life had been dominated by the presence of his mentally retarded sibling, who had required a great deal of care. Father felt that his whole childhood had been destroyed by this. He could perceive the current problems in the family only as a repetition of his own childhood, and he expected the next child to be as severely handicapped as his sibling.

Mother, as an only and asthmatic child, had received excessive attention to the point of being overprotected. She saw the mother–child relationship as a state of blissful perfection. She could not imagine a repetition of the events that father expected or even further difficulties of the type that were currently existing. She simply expected a re-creation of warmth and closeness.

Lack of common meanings led to interpersonal distance. Therapy involved bringing such divergent meanings out into the open and moving away from the superficial disagreements.

INTERSUBJECTIVE MEANINGS

Intersubjective meanings, by contrast, are not the property of any single member but instead are rooted in the family life and are part of the self-definition of the family as a whole. Powerful common meanings lead to the development of a web of intersubjective meaning. This notion is not a new one in family theory and has been referred to with a number of concepts. The shared interpersonal reality has sometimes been called the "family matrix" or the "family identity." Contrast terms to surface concepts include "underlying dynamics" or "constitutive rules." Whereas surface action may be manipulated or artificially generated, underlying meaning refers to "true" experience or "true" relatedness. The idea of a "family myth" clearly expresses the notion that the family has its own reality. It has been noted that members of healthy families appear weaker when seen separately at interview, while in poorly functioning families, a separate interview reveals strengths (Lewis, Beavers, Gossett, & Phillips, 1976). This is because the family reality has an obscuring effect on members' psychic reality.

Understanding the intersubjective meaning was central to therapy with the N. family. Jason was an 18-year-old, only child who presented with a variety of self-destructive behaviors, including excessive drinking, drug abuse, accidents, and educational failure.

The surface action had some clear pathological characteristics. Father was constantly critical and yet anxious about his son's efforts, which he compulsively undermined. This was not only observed but also reported:

> I came back from holiday and, although I heard that Jason had really done well when we were away—he was working regularly, earning and saving his money and had no problems at all—I went into the restaurant where he was working and when I saw his excessively short haircut I was almost sick and I said without thinking: "God—that's terrible!!" I felt awful for having said that but I just couldn't help it.

Inevitably, father and son constantly rowed. They were always competing with each other. Often the son worked father up until he got out of control and then walked out on him. Mother stood by without intervening. She consciously thought to herself that she was not going to be like her own mother, who had continuously squabbled with her stepfather. She would support first the father and then the son. This undermined the parental coalition as well as both the men. Here is a typical sequence:

SON: It was much easier to make money when you were young, Dad, than it is for me nowadays.
FATHER: What do you mean? There are so many ways of raising money now than when I was young. It's much easier for you than it ever was for me.
SON: You just can't get a mortgage these days. Now you could quite easily before.
FATHER: You always get money from a bank for a good scheme—it's a question of working hard.
MOTHER *(to father)*: Oh, Jim, you know that is just not true. You really can't give Jason a break.

The repetitive pattern of interaction acquired meaning in the context of patterns revealed in the family histories. Both parents had fathers in special roles. Father's father died early and was greatly idealized by father's mother. Mother's father left the family at an early age and was as greatly denigrated. The parents never mourned their fathers; instead, they preserved them and the relationships involving them in the intersubjective reality of the current family. Father, for example, found himself having impossible ideal expectations for Jason, similar to those he had felt from his father, but then found himself a denigrated figure when mother's support went to her son.

There was also a pathological and powerful common meaning in this family, namely, that to fail in what you really want to do is absolutely catastrophic. This resulted in none of them really daring to attempt to achieve or be effective in ways they would really have liked and in all of them suffering with low self-esteem.

AVOIDANCE OF MEANING

We drew attention to the qualities of pathological surface actions, emphasizing that they appear to be "required" by the family. This requirement results in a loss of meaning and a loss of the appropriately interpretive and flexibly responsive mode of functioning that characterizes and is essential for health social functioning. We must ask why family members should be so foolish as to allow this. The only reasonable explanation or interpretation is that the family sustains this loss as a by-product. In order to avoid some particular aspect of human experience, the family finds itself caught in a pattern in which the essence of all human experience is lost.

This struggle between "the required" and "the avoided" has been noted in group therapy interactions (Ezriel, 1956). Before a family accepts treatment, it must judge the extra cost of the avoidance maneuver as outweighing the benefits. Sometimes, when this cost–benefit issue becomes clearer during therapy, the family may opt for their original choice; for example, it may become apparent that a son's delinquency is relieved only by facing mother's depression, but father may not be prepared to tolerate this. Making such unconscious choices explicit introduces the notion of responsibility, humanizes interaction, and, by appealing to a sense of dignity, may benefit family members.

The issues which family members may have difficulty facing run the gamut of human experience: commitment, intimacy, loss, separation, individuation, painful affects, disappointment, change, historical reality. When the avoided issue is confronted, possibilities open up, and the family regains control and a sense of order and progress.

Let us return to our earlier examples. The C. family, but not being firm with girls, avoided direct expressions of conflict. Making boundaries, being firm, and using angry feelings in a constructive way was, for them, painful and anxiety provoking. The L. parents did not face what it meant to adopt a 9-month-old infant with previous poor-care experiences. To avoid being overwhelmed, these parents ignored the emotional implications of almost everything they talked about. This led to a general meaninglessness and loss of reality in tackling the human issues. The N. family, as well as fearing attempts to achieve, avoided an awareness of the achievements the members actually had made. They could not face disappointment.

REQUISITE ACTION

To ascertain whether an avoided issue has been faced and resolved requires a return to the level of surface action. The aim of therapy is not insight or hypothetical juggling with insubstantial entities, but actual changes in family life. By consideration of the underlying meaning structure of the family, it is possible to specify, within broad limits, changes in family interaction which are suitable and desirable for the particular family. The resultant surface action we call "requisite." This approach avoids the danger of specifying some normative, "ideal" interaction to which families would be expected to conform. Because of the open-system nature of the family, a variety of forms of surface action may contain and express the therapeutically achieved resolution of underlying meaning.

The criteria for improvement do not make explicit what surface action is requisite. Judgment is therefore necessary to assess whether the particular actions chosen as a result of therapy do actually meet the criteria. Inevitably, family reports of how they feel and what they think are important evidence.

The reader can obtain a feel of the issues from consideration of the S. family. Mother had been a vivacious and unusually capable woman. Two years before the consultation she suffered brain damage in a road accident that occurred while her husband was driving. Despite much loss of intelligence, she retained some painful insight into her state. The family scene altered dramatically. Father, already busy as a physician, successfully took over domestic responsibilities. John, 17, strong and grown-up, also appeared to cope well. Anne, 15½, showed rebelliousness and commenced an unsuitable sexual relationship. She felt prematurely pushed into adulthood and felt her right to happiness had been taken away. Joseph, 13, was displaying bravado and failing academically. Sharon, 4, had regressed.

The family system involved Sharon being allocated the role of something for mother to look after and for which she could feel responsible. Father talked about his wife as if she were not there, and mother fitted in with this. All members avoided expressions or thoughts of anger, and there was general support for father. It appeared to the therapist that the family had been unable to assimilate the appalling alteration in mother's state into the operating meaning system. This, in essence, was the focal hypothesis. The members did not mourn the loss of the mother they knew, and they showed an inappropriate form of concern for this brain-damaged person. These observations were the basis for criteria of improvement.

To judge change against criteria, the therapist must decide whether observed alterations do indicate assimilation of the event. Requisite change involves the family members showing acceptance and integration of the situation as it is. In the case described above, the youngest daughter needs to be given proper mothering, and Anne provided with appropriate controls. Mother should be treated as still real, although different in some ways. Her rehabilitation should be considered and implemented either at home or in an outside setting. Father needs to provide himself with periods of quiet and calm to reflect on the best methods of handling the difficult emotional problems as well as the practical ones. He also needs to reflect on and integrate his personal loss. While all this goes on, it is expected that the children will be unhappy and angry but not guilty and self-destructive.

FAILURE TO CREATE A FOCAL HYPOTHESIS

The focal hypothesis is created, rather than found, in an act of ad hoc theory construction; hence, the opposition of raw empiricists. We must now briefly consider the inability of a therapist to find the structure which links and integrates the family manifestations: complaints, surface action, depth meanings, historical events.

There are a number of possibilities requiring scrutiny. First, the therapist may not have collected the relevant evidence; for example, he or she may have poorly documented the events in the recent or distant family history or may have prevented the family from interacting freely. Second, the therapist may have an insufficient understanding of the various theories of individual and family functioning. Third, the therapist may find him- or herself, for personal or cultural reasons, unable to operate within the meaning field of the family. Finally, and most difficult to admit, the therapist may be unable to conceptualize and theorize. This ability is not a requirement and might even be a handicap for many trained workers.

The insight required to integrate observation and theory and to know when theoretical knowledge is insufficient is itself not formalizable. This means that there can never be a manual with step-by-step, foolproof instructions, and that not just anyone can engage in this work. This is not elitism but an inevitable extension of the conception of theory formation as the central activity of the therapist working within our model. Theoretical development will progress through clinicians, with sufficient capacity for abstraction and conceptual modeling, resolving their own states of ignorance.

Our view encompasses that of the empiricists, such as pure systems theorists and behavioral theorists, and in no way minimizes therapeutic efforts stemming from their work. Their contribution is incorporated within our concept of surface action. Crucially, our criteria for the assessment of change are specific and objective, that is, defined social events. The criteria can be used with *any* modality of treament or in association with *any* theoretical stance (Armstrong *et al.,* 1979). These criteria may be unknown, unnoticed, or unimportant to the family, unlike the symptom or the focused-upon surface action, and therefore can sometimes provide stringent and convincing evidence of therapeutic effect.

Construction of a focal hypothesis does not imply treatability or suitability for brief family therapy. It represents the first step in a comprehension of the family and its disturbance. In the next section, we introduce a formal classification of focal hypotheses.

STRESS AND MEANING

The recognition of an event as stressful depends on existing meaning systems based on urges for survival, well-being, and attachment. Other meaning systems are required for the psychological handling of stress and the activation of any appropriate action. Both recognition and resolution of stress are frequent and possibly continuous experiences, which are mainly unconscious. Systems of meaning develop during childhood and subsequently undergo relatively minor modifications. Alteration in adulthood has been noted following massive trauma (Kinston & Rosser, 1974). Psychoanalysis also aims at a major revision of meaning.

In family therapy, we refer to the parents and children who present for help as the "family of procreation" and the previous generation (i.e., grandparents, parents, and siblings of parents) as the two "families of origin." In the families of origin, the parents obtained personal experiences and family life experiences which resulted in unique systems of meaning. Marital choice depends on both similarity (common meanings) and complementarity (intersubjective meanings). Children are born into this marital reality and immediately alter it. Events which occur in the family of procreation have minimal adverse effect on the children if the parents can sustain the mental impact and connote them positively. Children cannot be totally shielded from traumatic events, and the healthy processes of acceptance, integration, resolution, and working through of meaning are usually incomplete in childhood, at least to some degree, and are the basis of vulnerability to stress in adulthood.

Healthy families adequately nurture and socialize the children and provide psychosocial protection and support for all members. Surface action is often not optimal but is adequate in terms of communication, decision making, and so on. Underlying this action is a functional web of common and intersubjective meanings. Such families could be treated, but they rarely request it.

Our research has led us to propose a formulation, still tentative and under scrutiny, of the nature of meaning and surface action in families who attend our clinic. It appears possible to distinguish families where the primary stress has occurred in the families of origin from those where attendance is due to an event in the family of procreation. In other cases, the presentation implicates both the families of origin and procreation, either because events in the previous generation have so affected matters that events in the family of procreation are precipitated, or because family-of-procreation events have activated buried, but not dead, family-of-origin issues. Table 3 shows how this classification is applied to the five families reported in this chapter.

Three mechanisms for the handling of meaningfulness can be distinguished in order to explain the formal characteristics of the operative meaning systems in the family. These mechanisms can apply to events in either the family of origin or the family of procreation, although with greatly differing final results. They are:

1. denial, nonassimilation, or ignoring (e.g., the S. family's response to the traffic accident)
2. repetition without resolution or working through (e.g., the N. family's re-creation of attitudes toward fathers)
3. depositing or reversal (e.g., the G. family's attempt to overcome deprivation)

Although these mechanisms are not independent of each other, and the trichotomy, like the dichotomy of a precipitant mainly in the family of ori-

TABLE 3. *Relevant Stress and Its Site*

Family	Family of origin[a]	Family of procreation[a]
S.	No relevant stress	Traffic accident and brain-damaged mother
C.	(Pathological pattern used in therapy and not treated)	Birth of sibling
K.	Obesity and separation problems	No relevant stress
N.	Idealization and denigration of father	No relevant stress
L.	Deprivation due to neglect and overprotection	Damaged adopted and biological children

[a]The boxed sections indicate the location of therapeutic work with the family.

gin or procreation, is a simplification, this approach does seem to make sense when applied clinically and is some improvement beyond our earlier research. Table 4 summarizes the classification.

We suspect that particular characteristics and forms of family interaction in the presenting family (i.e., the family of procreation) can be linked with each of the categories in Table 4. If the classification is confirmed in further work, we may have a key to assist therapists in their conceptualization of family disturbance and the construction of focal hypotheses.

CONCLUSION

In this chapter, we have clarified and elaborated on our method of formulating focal hypotheses for use in brief marital or family therapy. The focal hypothesis is an ad hoc clinical theory which captures the essence of the family and integrates its complaints and overt interaction, the source and site of its stressful events, and its deep common and intersubjective meanings. Such a focus serves as a beacon to guide intervention and facilitates relevant evaluation.

TABLE 4. *Classification of Family Pathology*

Site of stressful events[a]	Handling of meaning-fulness of events by family members involved	Characteristic of operative meaning system in presenting family[b]
Family or origin and family of procreation	Accepted, integrated, resolved, worked through	Functional web of common and intersubjective meanings
Family of origin: • Events which have affected both parents as children and hence their ways of being and systems of meaning	Denied, ignored, not assimilated	No meaning, loss of meaning, artificial meaning
	Repeated, accepted, not resolved, not worked through	Shared, pathological common meanings and repetition of intersubjective meanings
	Depositing, reversal	Reversal of past intersubjective meaning
Family of procreation: • Events which affect mother and father as adults and require integration within already operating systems of meaning • Events and the parental response which affect the next generation • Events that may be past or current (e.g., handicap, accident, stage in family life cycle)	Denied, ignored, not assimilated	Displacement of meaning, falsity of meaning
	Repeated, re-created	Lack of shared common meaning
	Depositing, reversal	Shared common meaning that x is bad or contains all bad things
Family of origin and family of procreation: • Events in the former and the resulting systems of meaning that precipitate events in the latter • Events in the latter that activate undealt-with issues in the former	(Combinations from the above)	

[a]Source of details of the focal hypothesis, that is, depth meaning system or depth structure.
[b]Psychic reality/inner experience; "family reality."

REFERENCES

Ackerman, N. W. *The psychodynamics of family life: Diagnosis and treatment of family relationships.* New York: Basic Books, 1958.

Armstrong, S., Yasuna, A., & Hartley, D. *Brief psychodynamic psychotherapy: Interrater agreement and reliability of individually specified outcomes.* Paper presented at the European Conference of the Society for Psychotherapy Research, Oxford, 1979.

Balint, M., Ornstein, P. H., & Balint, E. *Focal psychotherapy: An example of applied psychoanalysis.* London: Tavistock Publications, 1973.

Bentovim, A. Child development research findings and psychoanalytic theory—An integrative critique. In D. Shaffer & J. Dunn (Eds.), *The first year of life.* New York: Wiley, 1979.(a)

Bentovim, A. Towards creating a focal hypothesis for brief focal family therapy. *Journal of Family Therapy,* 1979, *1,* 125–136.(b)

Bentovim, A., & Kinston, W. Brief focal family therapy where the child is the referred patient. I: Clinical. *Journal of Child Psychology and Psychiatry and Allied Disciplines,* 1978, *19,* 1–12.

Boszormenyi-Nagy, I., & Spark, G. M. *Invisible loyalties.* New York: Harper & Row, 1973.

Dicks, H. V. *Marital tensions.* New York: Basic Books, 1967.

Ezriel, H. Experimentation with the psychoanalytic session. *British Journal of Philosophy of Science,* 1956, *7,* 25–41.

Guerin, P. H. (Ed.). *Family therapy.* New York: Gardner, 1976.

Gurman, A. S. Contemporary marital therapies: A critique and comparative analysis of psychoanalytic, behavioural and systems theory approaches. In T. J. Paolino, Jr., & B. S. McCrady (Eds.), *Marriage and marital therapy: Psychoanalytic, behavioral and systems theory perspectives.* New York: Brunner/Mazel, 1978.

Gurman, A. S., & Kniskern, D. P. Research on marital and family therapy, progress, perspective and prospect. In S. L. Garfield & A. S. Bergin (Eds.), *Handbook of psychotherapy and behavior change: An empirical analysis* (2nd ed.). New York: Wiley, 1979.

Haley, J. *Changing families.* New York: Grune & Stratton, 1971.

Harris, L. Analysis of paradoxical logic: A case study. *Family Process,* 1980, *19,* 19–34.

Kinston, W., & Bentovim, A. Brief focal family therapy where the child is the referred patient. II: Methodology and results. *Journal of Child Psychology and Psychiatry and Allied Disciplines,* 1978, *19,* 119–143.

Kinston, W., Loader, P., & Stratford, J. Clinical assessment of family interaction: A reliability study. *Journal of Family Therapy,* 1979, *1,* 291–312.

Kinston, W., & Rosser, R. Disaster: Effects on mental and physical state. *Journal of Psychosomatic Research,* 1974, *18,* 437–456.

Lewis, J. M., Beavers, W. R., Gossett, J. T., & Phillips, V. A. *No single thread: Psychological health in family systems.* New York: Brunner/Mazel, 1976.

Loader, P., Kinston, W., Burck, C., & Bentovim, A. *Systematic description of family interaction.* Manuscript submitted for publication, 1980.

Madanes, C., & Haley, J. Dimensions of family therapy. *Journal of Nervous and Mental Disease,* 1979, *165,* 88–98.

Malan, D. H. On assessing the results of psychotherapy. *British Journal of Medical Psychology,* 1959, *32,* 86–105.

Malan, D. H. *A study of brief psychotherapy.* New York: Plenum Press, 1963.

Malan, D. H. *Toward the validation of dynamic psychotherapy: A replication.* New York: Plenum Press, 1976.

Papp, P. *Family therapy: Full length case studies.* New York: Gardner, 1978.

Ricoeur, P. *Freud and philosophy: An essay on interpretation.* New Haven: Yale University Press, 1970.

Selvini-Palazzoli, M., Boscolo, L., Cecchin, G. F., & Prata, G. *Paradox and counterparadox.* New York: Jason Aronson, 1978.

Steele, R. S. Psychoanalysis and hermeneutics. *International Review of Psycho-Analysis,* 1979, *6,* 389–412.

Ursano, R. J., & Dressler, D. M. Brief vs. long-term psychotherapy: A treatment decision. *Journal of Nervous and Mental Disease,* 1974, *160,* 164–171.

Weakland, J. H., Fisch, R., Watzlawick, P., & Bodin, A. M. Brief therapy: Focused problem resolution. *Family Process,* 1974, *13,* 141–168.

Zinner, J., & Shapiro, R. The family group as a single psychic entity: Implications for acting out in adolescence. *International Review of Psycho-Analysis,* 1974, *1,* 179–186.

CHAPTER 15
BEHAVIORAL MARITAL THERAPY AS BRIEF THERAPY

Robert L. Weiss
Neil S. Jacobson

A distinction between and among forms of therapy in terms of duration often implies that therapies can be miniaturized only at the risk of providing lesser benefit. It was somewhat startling in this context to be invited to consider behavioral marital therapy (BMT) as a form of *brief* therapy. The unstated assumption seemed to be that marital therapy normally might be viewed as long-term therapy. Yet, most forms of marital therapy are reported to last from six to ten sessions (Beck, 1976; Gurman & Kniskern, 1978). Determining whether BMT has any special claim to being short-term is of less practical consequence than carefully considering whether the conditions of theory and practice can lead one to conclude that marital therapy requires long-term involvement, say, ten months or more of weekly sessions.

Our emphasis will be on BMT. We accept the axiom that BMT is brief by design, not by default. Our presentation is directed to the practitioner and student of marital therapy who does not have substantial familiarity with developments in BMT. We have chosen to omit a review of specialized research data on this or that aspect of BMT, since these writings are available elsewhere (Jacobson, 1979a; Jacobson & Margolin, 1979; Weiss, 1978, 1980). Our applied focus is in keeping with the aim of this volume, which is to facilitate the application of health services, broadly defined, through explicitly designed, time-limited interventions. Our discussion will proceed along three lines: BMT in contrast to other therapies, current examples of BMT approaches, and BMT as brief therapy by design.

ROBERT L. WEISS. Department of Psychology, University of Oregon, Eugene, Oregon. NEIL S. JACOBSON. Department of Psychology, University of Washington, Seattle, Washington.

CONTRASTING BMT WITH OTHER THERAPIES

In this section, we examine some of the assumptions which guide BMT and then compare them with other forms of therapy.

SOME DIMENSIONS OF CHANGE

That which is selected for change depends, in part, upon one's theory of human misery, determinants of thought and action, and one's assessment of the relative plasticity of both. Certainly, one influential approach to therapy is based upon a deterministic, developmental view of individuals, meaningfully described in terms of relatively enduring structures of personality, which are variously defined as traits or other dispositional constructions. Other points of view emphasize intraindividual potentialities, which therapy is designed to release, actualize, or otherwise potentiate. These points of view represent human complexity in often highly integrated theoretical statements, which lead to the view that symptoms are conflict manifestations of organized, explainable structures and functions associated with unconscious conflict; they also make recommendations for including an expressive component of therapy. Affect and idea, feeling and behavior, must come together in order for one to be restored to a level approximating adequate adjustment or mental health.

Within these points of view, the role of cognition is quite central; some form of insight is crucial to effecting change. The explicit goal of changing cognitions (attitudes, beliefs, etc.) is regarded as difficult but not impossible to attain.

When these individualizing theories are brought to bear on committed, intimate relationships, such as marriage or other forms of adult intimacy, the locus of change still remains largely within the person, although of late, there is increased recognition of how individual psychodynamic functions play out, as it were, in the context of committed intimacy (Gurman, 1980; Meissner, 1978).

Alternatively, one can conceptualize the determinants of human behavior more in terms of coping with the demands of more immediate situations. Rather than viewing adequate change as requiring some reorganization of mental structures or functions—requirements of the personality point of view—it is possible to adopt the view that behaviors manifested currently are problematic in their own right and best described as manifestations of coping. Various situational views of behavior belong at this level. The determinants of behavior, from this situationist perspective, are described by transactional patterning, that is, the ways in which the members of a relationship mutually constrain their adaptive options. Most forms of therapy which make any attempt to construe transactions rely on mechanisms for describing relationship interdependencies which derive from the attempts of the partners to accommodate to one another.

This brief description of the bipolar extremes available as models of human behavior helps us focus the dimensions of change endorsed by therapists. If therapy seeks to effect changes on a structural or personality level, it is reasonable to assume that whatever the neurological basis of the original learning, a concerted effort of time will be required to effect change now. Recognizing this, some points of view "settle for next best"; that is they retain basic assumptions of the role of structure and dynamics but are content to effect changes at a more "superficial level." This is the popular notion of dealing with symptoms only, taking a calculated risk that treatment outcome is less than complete.

BMT makes no assumptions about the "depth" of symptoms, but rather views problematic behaviors (including obsessional thoughts) as current adjustments interfering with one's functioning. It is not a great complication of behavioral theory to suggest that one deals with removal of symptoms, thus defined, in a manner that protects the client or makes it beneficial for the client to change. Thus, if symptomatic behaviors appear to limit greatly what a person is now able to accomplish, removal of the symptomatic behavior must be preceded by consideration of whether skills exist for accomplishing new goals. A couple, for example, may develop rituals which seem to function to prevent their becoming sexually intimate. One must consider some of the more typical fears about intimacy (e.g., rejection, making a fool of oneself) as part of the planned intervention to increase intimacy.

One tenet of BMT is that behavior can be functional (i.e., it can accomplish ends) without also requiring an intrapersonal motivational basis for the action. Couples sometimes create exquisite mutual dependencies, which we observe as "symptomatic" or "neurotic" or simply unappealing to ourselves. The point at issue is whether one assumes that the partners sought each other out for the purpose of enacting their intraindividual symptomatology, or whether their observable, "symptomatic" (often ritualized) interactions are maintained by more immediate consequences. Thus, for BMT, marital distress is seen in terms of transactional patterns which actually prevent the relationship from being beneficial in nonritualized ways. So-called "stable–unsatisfactory" relationships are said to be beneficial to the partners, yet the observer is struck with the barrenness of these constricted, nonrewarding kinds of intimacy. The existing transaction may protect the partners from changing as persons and, in that sense, may be said to be protective of them.

The issue for BMT is whether it is possible for the partners to participate in adult intimacy without their evoking the feared inevitable outcomes or without their experiencing the devastation of being without coping skills. If their symptomatic interactions prevent them from changing, it is not helpful to posit theoretical justifications for this state of affiars. What is helpful is to assess whether we can make change worth their while. Intimacy may fail for many reasons, but it behooves us, as practitioners, to avoid enshrining justifications for the failures by means of theories of the inevitable. Indeed, as we point out below, BMT may be ideally suited for creating test conditions to assess a couple's ability to make necessary changes.

To be sure, both the trait and systems points of view are thought to be appealing, since they provide a means for describing patterning in relationships. There is an economy of thought in being able to explain events as lawful outcomes of antecedent events. BMT approaches can deal with patterning in exchanges either by techniques for describing the statistical structure of interactions (Gottman, 1979) or, more clinically, in terms of analysis of situational control (Jacobson, 1978c; Weiss, 1978).

BMT thus seeks change along the dimension of relationship transactions, and while cognizant of patterning in relationship transactions, it does not rely upon personality structures as the locus of such changes.

DEFINING CRITERIA FOR RELATIONSHIPS

As Weiss and Margolin (1977) have observed, one of the difficulties of any form of marital therapy is defining successful outcome. Traditionally, investigators have relied on measures of marital satisfaction as the criterion for outcome. It is unfortunately still the case that many presumed necessities for a satisfying relationship, whether these be skills, personality attributes, cognitions, or whatever, have not been shown empirically to be either necessary or sufficient characteristics of "successful" marriages. For example, it is generally accepted in clinical circles that communication skills are vital to relationship success, yet until very recently, there has been no empirical support for that belief.

Rather, successful relationships are often defined by exclusion: whatever was known about distressed relationships should be absent from nondistressed relationships. Yet it has long been recognized that health is not just the absence of illness. One of the consequences of adopting a behavioral view of marriage is that the criteria of successful intimacy are *not* provided by one's theoretical model (Jacobson, in press; Weiss & Margolin, 1977); other models posit various forms of normalcy or maturity from within the theory itself. At the present time, we simply do not have a well-developed behavioral–analytic model of modern marriage at various life stages (cf. Goldfried & D'Zurilla, 1969, for such an approach to college student adjustment). What this would require is a careful sampling of the domain of critical adjustment in maintaining adult intimacy, and a taxonomy of how these were handled by people who are judged to be effective in their intimacy.

Nonetheless, it is easy to point to available criteria, which are quite limited. Longevity of a relationship may define sufficiency criteria but not the quality of a relationship. Satisfaction measures are highly tried to societal definitions of marriage roles, the more traditionally oriented person finding a better fit in marriage. There is some developing concern for using the quality of physical health as a means of judging marriage relationships. (There is a sizable literature on the effects of divorce on health status, cf. Bloom, Asher, & White 1978.) Depression has been shown to be a concomitant of distressed marriages (Weiss & Aved, 1978). A measure of health status which is sensitive to perturbations of marriage has yet to be reported.

A promising lead is to define marital relationship competencies in a form which is testable (Weiss, 1978; Weiss & Birchler, 1978). By positing relationship accomplishments thought to be necessary to a well-functioning marriage, we can assess how well couples meet these objectives pre- and postintervention. We shall consider these in a later section on examples of BMT interventions.

TARGETS OF BMT

To complete this analysis of assumption underlying BMT as brief treatment by design, we turn to a consideration of the likely targets of BMT. We propose a four-item hierarchy for use in defining targets of marital therapy.

Responses

Brief therapy is often seen as crisis intervention. The aim is to make a rapid change in behavior in order to alleviate an immediate crisis. According to this definition, the focus is on responses made by partners, in the hope of reducing some conflict. Such a focus on responses is useful to stop some situation which is likely to escalate and be detrimental to the partners.

This is only one aspect of BMT, however, not its primary objective. For example, a couple may benefit temporarily from a therapist injunction about their continuing, open-ended discussions of their problems. "I am going to ask you to agree not to discuss your plans for moving this entire week!" "This week the whole issue about whether you should separate or not is to be put on the back burner; no discussions of this sort until we meet again."

Skills

BMT typically is carried out at the level of training skills. If the focus is communication skillfulness, for example, a host of specific communication techniques will be grouped under the rubric of communication skills training. These may involve teaching partners to make new responses in a wide variety of their situations together (e.g., helping identify the mechanics of good listening, such as eye contact and utterances), the aim here being to establish a repertoire of responses which can serve a variety of situations.

Unlike response targets, skills training assumes that the training will continue outside of the therapy, that it will persist beyond it or generalize to a nontherapy environment. For example, we might focus on some aspect of communication requiring specific speaker–listener skills: "I want you to make an opening statement to Jim about something you found interesting about your day, Joan, and Jim, I want you to make a response that would effectively encourage her going further into her feelings about the event. Jim, you don't have to agree that the event was a winner, just that you are going to be a helpful listener."

Whenever skills training is the targeted level of intervention, the assumption is made that one has a reader learner, an assumption most often violated by conflict-related behaviors of the couple. Preventing a couple from falling back on their use of aversive control techniques (criticisms, baiting comments, trait names) can also be accomplished at either a response or skills training level and may have to precede the teaching of other skills.

Competencies

Unlike either responses or skills, competencies refer to higher organizations of skills directed toward accomplishing a generic end. In the model of BMT proposed by Weiss (1978), four classes of competency were identified as discrete relationship accomplishments: objectification, support-understanding, problem solving, and behavior change. A couple may be said to have greater or lesser skillfulness in each of these areas of accomplishment.

Competencies are like skill traits, in that they can be thought of as transcending specific content, as defined by contexts (see below: Contexts). A couple may have difficulty objectifying all sorts of transactional events (e.g., whether one was *really* interested in sexual experimentation, whether they subscribe to particular marital myths). Similarly, support-understanding competencies can transcend specific contents, although here, too, it is more advisable to work with behaviors in situations. A person in our system is not "a considerate partner," for example, but rather a partner who shows appreciation, listens and offers support, is nonverbally affectionate, and recognizes the intellectual (e.g., artistic) contributions made by the other at parties, and at home. (We refer to this specificity below in the competency by content matrix). Let us define each class of competency in turn.

Objectification refers to the ability to make reliable discriminations in one's behavioral environment. Early behavioral approaches refer to this as discrimination training. Given the propensity of couples to fall back upon inferences about one another, we posit such discrimination skills as a major part of what is required for successful interaction. Similarly, being able to label the degree of situational control over behavior is further evidence of objectification skills.

Support-understanding refers to the affiliative, consideration, and supportive functions of adult intimacy. A relationship requires these competencies to accomplish closeness and to communicate supportive understanding for the partners. We include affection, sexuality, and the gratifications attendant upon being understood by one's partner as ideal examples under this heading.

Problem solving refers to accomplishment of objectives. It is product oriented and concerned with distributing resources and generating relationship rules, all in the service of accomplishing goals. Supportive functions may be important to the quality of intimacy, but they are not outcome oriented in the sense reserved for problem solving.

Finally, *behavior change* is meant to describe these accomplishments, which focus on how change within a relationship comes about. To the extent that a couple learns to rely on formal behavior change tactics, such as negotiation, contracting, and bilateral exchanges, they are bringing about change within the relationship by orderly, positive-based procedures. These outcomes are to be contrasted with the more typical reliance on aversive control procedures, which themselves become patterned as relationship dysfunctioning.

An important theoretical difference between BMT and other approaches to marital therapy is related to the issue of whether behavior change competencies can be taught within a relationship. Both dynamic and systems models suggest that relationships resist change (although for different conceptual reasons). To explicitly teach relationship change tactics assumes, as we noted above, a willing learner. Gurman and Kniskern (1978) argued that a limitation of BMT is the assumption that relationship changes can be brought about by tactics directed at responses, when, in fact (following Watzlawick, Weakland, & Fisch, 1974), change requires restructuring the rules which govern a relationship. Furthermore, the argument goes, rules can be changed only by forces outside the relationship (system) itself.

In working with couples, one is quickly educated in what might be referred to as resistances (cf. Jacobson & Margolin, 1979; Weiss, 1979, 1980). Because of its technological explicitness, BMT readily attracts the criticism that it is antihumanistic, that there is too much emphasis on manipulation, direction, preoccupation with structure, homework assignments, and not enough emphasis on choice. Beginning BMT practitioners often complain of problems of noncompliance, notably, that couples fail to complete assignments. At a somewhat more abstract level, noncompliance appears to be less technique based and more a matter of illicitly holding to the status quo—illicit in the sense that there appears to be a collusion not to change, even though a couple appears for marriage therapy.

The issues of noncompliance or "resistance" appear, at first glance, to support the Gurman and Kniskern (1978) argument that behavior change competencies cannot be taught within marital relationships. Weiss (1980), however, addressed these issues as problems of cognitive restructuring. It is possible to identify "efficacy expectations" or belief barriers, which prevent change within a relationship. Given certain cognitive sets about relationship transactions, each partner may deem his or her behavior appropriate to survival. An active part of BMT is reframing cognitions which the therapist identifies as maladaptive to achieving relationship benefits. To be sure, given a current status of extreme reward devaluation, prolonged experience with stereotyped interaction patterns, and noncontingent aversiveness (failures to recognize positive helping behaviors), one does not retain credibility by suggesting the couple seek new ways to be exciting to one another! But there are identifiable ways for decentering, as it were, by the use of therapist-created problems, active reframing, and the prescribing of tasks which produce "behavioral insights." For example, a couple may be asked to detail all the ways they can make fail some activity suggested by the therapist. By bringing "involuntary acts" under voluntary control (i.e., one knows what to do to make something fail!), it becomes necessary to change the cognition about involuntariness.

We mention these issues at this point to help dispel some beliefs held about BMT, which make it sound far more mechanistic than is necessary, and to alert therapists of other persuasions that the differences between BMT and other models may be more a matter of the systematic emphasis within BMT than the way in which the therapist encourages compliance.

Contexts

The discussion of competencies purposely ignored content: objectification about what, or problem solving related to which content? We can choose to use either a fine or coarse screen in how we define contexts. In any event, contexts refer to the specific areas of marital interaction. In previous discussions, some 12 content areas were used to define the context of interaction (Weiss, 1978); one could also work with fewer categories, including affectional, communication, and instrumental areas of interaction (Jacobson, Waldron, & Moore, 1980). Conceptually, the goal is to discriminate contexts for transactions which reflect the content of competencies. Thus, we might be concerned with how a relationship problem-solves (competency) when issues of child care (context) are at stake; or we could isolate objectification skills (competency) as applied to the communication process (context).

It is important to note that contexts and competencies can be arranged as a matrix of rows and columns, so that if we take 12 contexts (indicative of areas of marital interaction) and 4 categories of competencies (relationship accomplishments), a 48-cell matrix results. Like a map, the 48 cells define specific targets for intervention and help determine whether one is operating at a response, skills, competency, or contextual level. As we indicate below, the matrix is also useful for assessment of relationships.

CURRENT EXAMPLES OF BMT APPROACHES

In this section, we describe the rationale and technological applications of BMT within the broader context of brief therapies. This section is not intended as a procedural manual for therapists, but rather as a vehicle for demonstrating both the breadth and flexibility of this approach to couples and relationship disharmony.

THE EMPIRICAL BASIS OF BMT

It should be recognized that BMT does not derive from a single theory of human behavior. It has evolved from a set of behavioral principles, the social psychology of exchange, and considerable clinical research experience with couples in conflict. In its current forms, BMT is considerably more cognitive than its first beginnings (cf. Jacobson & Margolin, 1979; Weiss, 1978, 1980). It was in the late 1960s and early 1970s that the first systematic statements about what was to become BMT were published (cf. Patterson & Hops, 1972; Stuart, 1969; Weiss, Hops, & Patterson, 1973). These early formulations combined the following ingredients:

1. an emphasis on beneficial exchanges, using concepts from social exchange theory (Thibaut & Kelley, 1959)
2. a model of coercion (Patterson & Reid, 1970), which described reciprocity in conflict relationships, based on the use of aversive control procedures
3. concepts of reinforcement and punishment applied to dyadic interactions, which showed that partners actually reinforce one another for use of aversive control procedures, and that this could be used to explain escalations of conflict
4. beneficial exchanges operating in a relationship according to rules of *quid pro quo,* which led Stuart (1969) to employ specific "contracting" procedures to couples in conflict
5. behavioral principles of shaping, discrimination training, and reinforcement of the control of behavior, which were expanded to couples, as were techniques designed to provide specific behavioral training

Thus, numerous techniques were developed to increase both the stimulus and the reinforcing control of exchanges of benefits within a relationship, such as tracking discrete pleasing and displeasing behaviors (cf. Azrin,

Naster, & Jones, 1973; Weiss *et al.,* 1973). Early attempts to change relationship behaviors made the desired behavior of one partner contingent upon the occurrence of a similarly desired behavior from the other (Azrin *et al.,* 1973; Stuart, 1969). Other forms of behavior change contracting relied on specific rewards for change rather than on those provided by changing a targeted (distressing) behavior (e.g., Jacobson, 1977; Weiss, Birchler, & Vincent, 1974.

Given this melange of separate techniques, to what extent did they all grow out of careful experimental documentation? Within BMT, assessment and intervention go hand in hand; behavioral technology is outcome oriented, in the sense that techniques are designed to produce immediate changes on the response target level. If changes are not produced, the intervention (technique) itself is changed. Many of the elements of the technical armamentarium did, indeed, show a desired relationship with marital distress (cf. Birchler, Weiss, & Vincent, 1975; Jacobson, 1978a, 1979b; Vincent, Weiss, & Birchler, 1975; Wills, Weiss, & Patterson, 1974). The point of an early paper (Weiss *et al.,* 1973) was to demonstrate that the modular arrangement of techniques could be effective with couples. Since so many techniques were employed, however, it was not possible to isolate, at any one time, which were the most active ingredients. Jacobson's research (1978a, 1979b) was designed to isolate specifics about behavior change contracting and problem solving. Margolin and Weiss (1978) made a similar attempt to manipulate attributions about the tasks themselves (i.e., by defining the tracking of pleasing and displeasing events, individually or bilaterally, to heighten either a monadic or dyadic focus).

The earlier studies (Weiss *et al.,* 1973) also introduced other techniques that had much in common with non-BMT communication approaches to marital therapy, such as the techniques that Guerney (1977) described as conjugal therapy. What were considered to be the therapeutic ingredients differed: techniques for training paraphrasing or reflecting were *not* seen as ends in themselves, but only as adjuncts to accomplishing the behavioral training, which, in the earlier publications, reduced to behavior change contracting.

A number of behaviorally oriented assessment techniques (cf. Jacobson & Margolin, 1979; Weiss & Margolin, 1977) grew out of this activity. Some of these are more appropriate for laboratory use, since they require technical equipment and trained coders. Others require daily tracking of events outside the laboratory, while still others have a format more like that of traditional self-report questionnaires.

Here, then, is a partial listing of what various BMT techniques are thought to accomplish:

Stimulus Control

All instances of objectification, as defined above, are examples of stimulus control. Here the intent is to increase discrimination between and among environmental and behavioral events. For example, couples often benefit from situational control of their behavior, such as restricting certain acts to certain places or increasing capability to label events. Thus, discrimination training, whether focused on communication or on the benefits of the relationship, promotes use of cue control in behavioral transactions (e.g., "Remember, we said we were *not* going to discuss problems before going to sleep?"). Whenever a couple makes use of ways to bring their own behavior under rule control, such as creating an agenda prior to a problem-solving session, it is an instance of stimulus control.

Reinforcing Control

Behaviors are often under the control of their consequences. Consequences can alter the rates at which we are likely to repeat some action on future occasions. The scheduling of consequences is equally important, however, with behaviors that are reinforced on an intermittent schedule being more resistant to change. Many spouse conflicts are under the control of stimulus–response chains, which involve a patterned unfolding of successive responses. These are often automatic or overlearned, so that finding ways to break these chains is beneficial to couples. Shifting behavior to stimulus control (rule control) is one technique. (It is also important to note that some behaviors, such as affection, lose their reward value if overly programmed.)

Partners can be taught ways to increase their rewardingness for one another. BMT makes very explicit attempts to increase beneficial exchanges.

Behavioral Rehearsal

When interactions become highly stereotyped, they unfold automatically. Couples often respond with the first thought that comes to mind, or so it seems; they are highly practiced in what they predict their partner will do next. Thus, merely suggesting that they engage in weekend activity can be the cue for an argument. Behavioral rehearsal is one way of helping couples generate menus of alternatives. By overtly examining alternatives, the chances of reacting reflexively diminish enormously. Many techniques are designed to put a delay between what appears to be an eliciting stimulus from the partner and one's response.

Problem Solving

BMT is characteristically problem-solving therapy. The emphasis is on negotiating, on learning communication techniques which have a high payoff for the individual; in a sense, couples learn assertive techniques. They are taught, for example, to make pinpointed "I" statements instead of abstract, trait-like accusations; so "you're damn lazy" becomes "I would like you to help me in the yard for one hour next Saturday." Couples frequently resent having to ask for some behavior from the other. "If he or she *really* loved me, I wouldn't have to ask." Or a partner may complain bitterly that the other does not spend enough time with him or her. These kinds of demands for change, of either attitude or overt behavior, can be cast into a dyadic, problem-oriented frame, as part of teaching appropriate problem-solving skills. Spending enough time translates to the quality, not quantity, of time together; by increasing the quality of what happens together, we satisfy both partners and avoid the trap of siding with the demand for one thing at the expense of the other.

Behavior Tracking

Couples are often asked to track a set of their relationship behaviors. Tracking is seldom therapeutic in its own right, but it does provide the therapist and the couple with a basis for increasing self-control over troublesome issues. For example, in dealing with anger and fighting within BMT, one creates a demand for the partners to identify the situational and behavioral cues that precede an overt outburst of hostilities. Tracking these cues makes it easier to elicit couple compliance for ways of dealing with anger prior to the point of blowup.

Tracking is also utilized to establish the empirical connection between daily relationship events and daily marital satisfaction. Couples are often surprised to see a demonstration of the empirical relationship between what they do (and do not do) together and their satisfaction on any given day.

More than any other approach to marital therapy, BMT has relied on experimental investigations to develop and test its theoretical principles (cf. Gottman, 1979; Jacobson, 1979a; Weiss, 1978), validate its assessment procedures (Jacobson, Elwood, & Dallas, 1981; Weiss & Margolin,

1977), and evaluate the efficacy of its treatment procedures (Azrin, Besalel, Bechtel, Michalicek, Mancera, Carroll, Shuford, & Cox, 1980; Gottman, 1979; Harrell & Guerney, 1976; Jacobson, 1977, 1978a, 1979b; Jacobson & Anderson, 1980; Liberman, Levine, Wheeler, Sanders, & Wallace, 1976; Margolin & Weiss, 1978). This emphasis on empirical validation probably is the greatest strength of BMT.

Jacobson and his associates have investigated the efficacy of BMT in a series of controlled experiments. In studies evaluating a treatment program which combined a specific form of communication training (problem-solving training) with contingency contracting procedures, the efficacy of BMT was consistently demonstrated with mild, moderate, and severely distressed couples. These changes were maintained in follow-ups ranging from six months to one year and were replicated across a variety of assessment procedures, including self-report questionnaires, frequency counts made by spouses of "pleasing" and "displeasing" behaviors in the natural environment, and observations of communication skills taken in the laboratory. Jacobson and Anderson (1980) determined that the model of communication skill training practiced in BMT investigations (including behavior rehearsal, modeling, and verbal or video-tape feedback) was necessary for the acquisition of problem-solving skills.

These results have been replicated and extended in a variety of independent, published investigations (Azrin et al., 1980; Gottman, 1979; Liberman et al., 1976; Margolin & Weiss, 1978) and in a number of unpublished doctoral dissertations and yet to be published studies (see Jacobson, 1978b, and Jacobson & Weiss, 1978, for a summary of these studies). The vast majority of these studies have demonstrated the effectiveness of BMT. As we have mentioned elsewhere, not all these studies provide such support, and, as yet, there is very little direct evidence that BMT is *more* effective than alternative approaches to marital therapy (cf. Jacobson, 1978b; Jacobson & Weiss, 1978). BMT is the *only* approach to treating relationship problems which has rigorously evaluated its treatment procedures, however, and the primary techniques described in this section, when delivered as a modular treatment package, seem to be very effective.

PLANNING BMT INTERVENTIONS

Intervention into a couple's relationship requires considerable planning, usually in the form of pretreatment assessment. The required commitment of time and effort, on both the therapist's and the clients' parts, is sometimes discouraging. Given the complexity of most adult intimate relationships, however, it is equally surprising to note that therapists are willing to start intervention before knowing in detail how a particular relationship functions, that is, knowing its strengths and weaknesses. In our view, all marital therapy is strategic, in the sense that it requires a master plan for intervention, which then marshals specific tactics for accomplishing explicit outcome goals. An excessive preoccupation with this or that technique (e.g., contracting) is less likely to facilitate change than are a thorough understanding of one's options and a commitment to ongoing evaluation of clients' willingness to carry out instructions (Jacobson & Margolin, 1979).

As already noted, there are differences among the proponents of the various packages now available for BMT. In this section, we attempt to highlight major similarities across approaches, which may do violence to any particular package.

The purpose of the initial contact with a couple is to establish the basis for continued sessions. The therapist seeks evidence that the clients are interested in continuing their own relationship, on the expectation that things could be more beneficial. One behavioral indication of this might be their willingness to devote time to therapy, since it requires them to engage in many out-of-session activities. Is there evidence of an illicit contract? Does one person seek to use therapy as a "respectable" exit from the relationship? It is not unusual for the partners to see the other person's behavior as the cause of the difficulty, but are there indications that the partners could adopt a slightly different set, a dyadic focus?

Initial sessions often provide relief to couples who badly need the structure that BMT can provide. Couples frequently express relief that they will not be expected to drag out old unresolved, painful, historical events. The therapist's optimism and inclination to view difficulties as skills deficits, rather than as personality anomalies, is often particularly helpful.

Thus, the initial session with a couple should provide considerable stimulus control for (a) how their "problem" is defined, (b) the likely course of continued association with the therapist, and (c) considerable reassurance that they will be the first to know whether therapy is helping. The initial session also establishes the rationale for more formal assessment procedures, such as self- and spouse-reporting forms.

These interviews differ from other initial interviews, in that here the content of the session is the *process* of dealing with therapist-posed issues. The content is not contained in answers to specific, historically oriented questions, history being of interest only in defining strengths for a continued relationship or in allowing the therapist to reframe a problem. Thus, if the mates are unable to speak positively about one another, it might be well to move them to a time in the past (perhaps their initial days together) when they enjoyed one another. Do they nonverbally recreate those happy feelings, or are they totally perplexed by the task? Their reaction provides important information.

Establishing a therapeutic contract is the goal of initial sessions. Marital therapy can become wide ranging, and couples can relapse into nonproductive rehashings of past hurts, injustices, and cruelties. If allowed to continue, the therapist can only be a spectator to these descriptions (and often enactments) of past events. BMT is managed by the therapist, which means that issues which are judged as being able to lead to change become session topics. The therapist and clients may appear to be at opposite ends of the argument as to what therapy is to accomplish, however, with clients seeing marital therapy as a last ditch attempt to change a recalcitrant other and not as an opportunity to renegotiate aspects of a relationship which has heretofore been unsatisfactory. The beneficial focus of BMT suggests that partners can see the possibility of gaining value from the other. The therapist may find it necessary to take a position that says, in effect, "How amazing that you let things deteriorate to the point where you get little satisfaction. My interest in working with you would be to promote the benefits you get from such a relationship, even at the expense of encouraging you to be selfish!" It then becomes a matter of technique as to how one structures benefits so that they are reciprocal, that is, so that one person does not draw down the account at the expense of the other.

Therapeutic contracts are tacit agreements between parties about the purpose of sessions and the roles each person is to play. A basic ground rule states that therapy will be forward moving, focusing on solutions rather than problems. (This often identifies couples who would rather discuss problems than solutions.) Such contracts provide structure and help keep all parties on target. They are constant reminders that regardless of how intensely negative a partner may feel about some event, the therapy agreement is to find a solution which maintains benefits within the relationship. It is not so much an injunction against feelings as it is a dedication to being productive and active in the search for more beneficial outcomes.

Therapeutic contracts set a time frame for marital therapy—typically eight to ten sessions. It is much easier to stay focused on problem x or y, as defined, than to attempt to unravel problem a or b. If the therapist does, indeed, provide gains for the couple, the likelihood increases that they will stay on target.

In planning initial sessions, it is important to identify the ways in which a couple has turned the positive aspects of being supportive and protective of one another into rigidly patterned, aversive transactions. For example, couples will spend considerable amounts of time justifying their actions to whomever will listen. Each person believes that he or she is well intentioned but not understood. It is far better strategy to focus on the development of objectification skills (being able to state what one wants now) than on a better understanding of past complaints. In so doing, it becomes immediately clear that a statement of what one wants now is very difficult to formulate: "Well, after all these years, she *should* know what I want! I shouldn't have to say it." Preoccupation with the past can functionally block ability to make discriminations in the present.

Most BMT programs stress some form of objectification training. The focus may be on communication itself (e.g., developing pinpointing skills, active paraphrasing, assertive "I" statements) or on the objectification of behavioral environments and how these control relationship outcomes. The aim is to make the couple experts on themselves. It is important in such training to separate "description" from "agreement." Couples in distress often cannot adopt an as-if stance: merely mentioning that one would like something is perceived as a challenge to the other to provide it! A justification ensues as to why he or she will not provide it, with countercomplaints about not caring and so forth. Before encouraging further negotiation of positions, the therapist needs to ensure that alternative positions have been developed.

Building menus of alternatives often relieves the pressure and curtails this pattern of cross-justification. For example, a couple may be engaged in an accelerating discussion of recreation—why mutually enjoyable recreation "always" fails, how one or the other is a genetically inferior athlete, and the like. This discussion usually is based on past experience with fixed activities (e.g., he wants to go fishing, she wants to look at antique stores). Creating a menu of alternatives requires the couple to generate other possible enjoyable activities, from the most farfetched to the most mundane. Knowing what possibilities are contained in the deck makes it easier to find an agreeable activity. One spouse, hearing that the other would consider it fun to do *x* or *y*, might well lead to the surprised inquiry, "*You* would be willing to go there?" The therapist quickly follows up with how little they actually know about each other's "secret" desires, and that maybe the more important task is to get more of these unknowns out in the open rather than to justify past refusals.

Caring is, of course, what intimacy is all about. Helping couples develop caring (support–understanding competencies) requires active reframing of intentions. It is most likely that couples will read their absence of affectional behavior as an intentional omission, and seldom do they label it as a skill deficit. The problem may be, in part, situational, in that couples may fail to arrange their time together in ways which promote closeness. Too often, affection is made a demand for performance in an otherwise nonsupportive environment. Teaching affectional exchange skills is difficult because of such performance anxiety being combined with fears of rejection. Since everyone shares such feelings, it is easier to make this training dyadic. Lack of affectional behavior may be part of a larger problem of limited behavioral repertoires. An important part of therapy planning requires that we find ways to change the routine context of transactions in order to allow for new behaviors.

It is important to help couples discriminate between a caring response and a problem-solving response. It is no less caring to acknowledge that one's partner is feeling badly, even without knowing specifically what to do about it. It is almost like a formula, which states, "If I acknowledge how you feel, then I will be obligated to change myself in some way." This automatic substitution of caring for problem-solving behaviors often produces distancing between partners. I *can* acknowledge your concern without also knowing *how* to solve it. But offering problem solving to a person who is seeking caring (e.g., understanding, sympathy) is a greater breech. Not only does one person feel badly about *x* or *y,* but now he or she has to feel worse at having failed to utilize the correct (as suggested by the other) solution! No wonder such attempts to "be helpful" backfire so badly.

Problem solving runs through all forms of BMT. In some cases, it is made quite explicit with structured exercises. Problem solving cannot take place if the agenda is not clear, if there is not a sense that the issue can be resolved and that the people involved are operating in good faith. This suggests that it is not a good tactic to introduce problem solving per se when resentments and frustrations of not being heard are still prepotent. Problem solving involves a considerable degree of stimulus control (e.g., agenda sessions devoted to agreements about which issues will be addressed later). The actual negotiation required during problem solving has to be based on a track record of successes at the other levels of competencies, such as objectification and support–understanding. Strategically, this means holding off some of the identified "big problems" until such time as problem solving can succeed. It is also true that the magnitude of problems may change as one accomplishes skills at the earlier, less complex levels.

Behavior change encompasses formalized methods for bringing about agreed upon changes and, therefore, is best left to the later stages of intervention. The same logic applies here as with problem solving. One wishes to build on strengths, and earlier accomplishments make behavior change agreements somewhat easier. The general rule is to ensure that such agreements are first carried out with the active involvement of the therapist. It is as if the couple were contracting with the therapist as the mediator. With practice, the couple takes over more responsibility for themselves and uses the therapist as a consultant to their own agreements.

It is not possible, of course, to lay out all the techniques that one uses in accomplishing these objectives of BMT intervention. (The reader is referred to Jacobson & Margolin, 1979, for a more technique-oriented presentation.) We have attempted to show the sectors about which the therapist plans intervention. The approach is modular, conceptualizing a hierarchy of specific tactics, all of which are orchestrated by our conception of relationship competencies. BMT is directive, it is focused, and it is highly reciprocal. As clients move along, the therapist includes more skills content. Many of the specific techniques of BMT may be familiar from other points of view. This is not at all disconcerting, since the strategic elements of BMT focus on how the techniques are sequenced. Proper ordering of modules, for example, reduces the need to deal with every issue that a couple will be able to mention.

BMT: APPROPRIATE FOR WHOM?

As we have stressed, BMT is change oriented: it is designed to enhance coupling benefits within a behavior exchange mode. It requires active participation of partners, which itself is taken as an indication of relationship commitment. The skills training, which most see as characterizing BMT, requires identification of deficits in relationship transactions. Thus, if one partner is removed from the exchange process (e.g., by being severely depressed), heaping skills training onto the relationship is unlikely to be useful. The same criterion would apply to the decision to undertake any form of relationship therapy. On the other hand, some problems, such as overuse of alcohol, may exist within the very context of the relationship, so that relationship therapy would be the treatment of choice. There are really two issues to consider when answering the question, for whom is BMT appropriate?

The first issue concerns whether relationship therapy is appropriate at all. As a working assumption, we encourage practitioners to err on the side of an affirmative answer, since most problems are germane to one's intimate relationship, if such a relationship exists. Many problems show a reciprocity or homeostatic balance within the marriage relationship. For example, as one partner becomes less severely depressed (e.g., alcoholic, anxious), the other may either adopt some of those very behaviors or be seen as driving the system back toward those symptoms. Having a functioning partner may, indeed, threaten a person who has organized his or her adult intimate life around "taking care of the other."

If it is decided that relationship therapy is a reasonable intervention, the question relevant to BMT is whether the relationship could exist on a more obviously beneficial level of exchange. Could active change lead to divorce? For some couples, marital therapy does offer that risk, especially whenever one member is seeking permission to divorce. But the longevity of relationships should be respected in the light of the alternatives either partner may have. Our own values enter into such decisions, and we need to be constantly alert to prejudices about "adequate" relationships.

On the other side of the coin is the view that one can "save" all marriages. This is clearly not the case, and BMT can lead to this conclusion faster than less planned approaches. Thus, knowing who will not benefit from BMT is equally important.

In our experiences, BMT is generally applicable for clients who are still sufficiently involved to put in the effort required by an active program. The danger here is that therapists often can be far more active and involved than the partners themselves. BMT is a good bet, however, whenever issues related to self-esteem are present, whenever the partners still control one another's destiny (e.g., can produce affective ups and downs), and whenever there is any sign that pleasure is something both seem to want but are unable to attain. We often hear that couples in BMT must be highly intelligent or highly organized or particularly articulate. This is more apparent than real. We have worked with a wide range of couples at diverse intellectual levels, and the therapeutic issue remains the finding of a common ground of relevance to which change can be related.

Thus, in the absence of clear-cut evidence to the contrary, our recommendation is to err in the direction of assuming BMT is applicable to any couple for whom relationship therapy is a viable alternative. Indeed, we go somewhat further by suggesting that most problems can be actively construed as relationship oriented.

The directiveness, planning, and technological emphasis required by BMT are germane to certain training issues. Two problems seem to confront the beginning BMT therapist learning an active form of intervention. They are (1) dyadic focus and (2) assessment.

Dyadic Focus

Most therapists have a solid background in individual therapies. Their tendency is to rely on content or immediate affective expressions of *individuals*. Conjoint therapy, which is the recommended format for BMT, provides an opportunity to see people engage in their problems. The addition of another person in the room makes it a social situation, in which coalitions with the therapist are actively sought. Not only will a couple explain their difficulties, they will act them out for the therapist and seek therapist agreement, even though this would put the other person down. People in such settings make very extreme statements ("There is *nothing* you can do that would ever please me!"). Dealing with this kind of communication is different from hearing about it secondhand. Dyadic focus refers to adopting a minisystems point of view, whereby the therapist actively encodes transaction outcomes. Unfortunately, the usual tendency is for therapists to ask each person questions and then to somehow add these answers together to form a dyadic conclusion.

Learning to view interactions as dyadic transactions is difficult and not intuitively obvious. If one wanted to know about affection in a relationship, one could ask each person how he or she felt about that aspect of their togetherness. Alternatively, one could raise a new issue for the dyad, for example, by suggesting that all relationships have to provide support and understanding to the partners, the therapist wonders how "you people have solved that problem." The couple's response to this higher level issue is what the therapist wants to observe. Do they define their relationship outside of this support "requirement"? Is support not necessary to them? Indeed, that would be a strange situation for marriage therapy.

Causality is nonlinear, and therapists working with couples would do well to grasp alternative ways of constructing problem presentations.

Becoming familiar with cognitive restructuring procedures is also helpful in this work. As individuals, each person is convinced that his or her interpretation of marital failures is the correct (i.e., most functional) one. More often, it is the transactional stereotype that is the "problem," and one needs to identify ways of making inroads on a competency level.

BMT is quite compatible with many systems notions. It simply makes very explicit how one would intervene on a technique level. Communication skills training can be used to bolster the reward value of the partners, while it also accomplishes the mechanics of how to talk and listen in a reinforcing manner.

Assessment

As noted above, most practitioners are reluctant to systematically assess a relationship. Assessment is important for a number of reasons, not the least of which is to communicate therapist interest in structure. Assessment provides a way of modeling a work set for the couple. To be sure, there are numerous opportunities when emotional upheaval detracts from that work set, so it is wise to have that as a clearly defined objective.

The interview is not a particularly good vehicle for obtaining factual information about a couple. It is far better as a means for observing interaction and assessing commitment.

It is perhaps easiest to introduce assessment in the form of self-report inventories, as a pre- to posttreatment change index. These devices have been described in the literature, and the reader will find them discussed in Jacobson and Margolin (1979).

BMT: BRIEF THERAPY BY DESIGN

Thus far, we have presented an overview of BMT, in the process of which we have examined theoretical assumptions, empirical foundations, and basic treatment goals and strategies. In this concluding section, we make explicit what has been an implicit perspective taken throughout the chapter—that BMT is a brief therapy by design, not by default. The implications of this view are that BMT is inherently brief, not as an acceptable but less than optimal substitute for a more "in depth," long-term approach, but as the most desirable of alternative frameworks for conducting marital therapy. Our justification of a brief therapy framework is subdivided into a feasibility inquiry, followed by a consideration of why brief therapy is optimal.

FEASIBILITY OF BMT AS BRIEF THERAPY

In the psychotherapy literature, the more intractable the clinical problem, the longer the treatment length assumed to be necessary to ameliorate the problem. This equation of dysfunctional complexity with treatment length is an equation based on faith, not on hard data. From the social casework literature, there is evidence that marital and family problems can be dealt with just as effectively—and perhaps even more effectively—in a brief, as opposed to an extended, casework framework (Reid & Shyne, 1967). Although there have been no direct comparisons between brief and extended treatment in regard to BMT, the outcome investigations reviewed earlier attest to the feasibility of successfully treating a substantial majority of moderately distressed couples in 6 to 12 treatment sessions (Azrin *et al.,* 1980; Jacobson, 1977, 1978a; Margolin & Weiss, 1978; Stuart, 1969; Weiss *et al.,* 1973). Although it is also clear that some couples require more than 12 sessions for treatment to be successful, particularly when one or both spouses suffer from severe behavioral dysfunction in addition to the relationship problems (cf. Jacobson, 1979b), there is an abundance of evidence that most couples can be helped significantly within a brief therapy format.

That this is the case is not particularly surprising. The skills that are required in order to improve the functioning of a marital relationship are not overwhelmingly difficult to acquire, provided spouses are willing to accept them. The art of marital therapy consists largely in creating a therapeutic environment which supports desirable changes in the relationship. The skills required of the therapist in preparing the couple to work toward these changes do not depend on "time" per se; rather, the requisite therapist behaviors can be enacted expeditiously and over a surprisingly brief period of time. As we argue in the paragraphs below, it is not only feasible but desirable and perhaps even necessary that the therapist exercise the option of moving the couple directly and quickly toward change within a brief therapy format.

DESIRABILITY OF BRIEF THERAPY

When BMT is conducted within a brief therapy format, both therapist and clients must discipline themselves. Within the constraints of a time limit, therapy is automatically structured, and the unfolding of therapy must be directively orchestrated by the therapist. To respond adequately to the demands of this format, clients must treat marital therapy almost as a full-time job. Whatever tendencies they have to resist the therapist's influence, whatever ambivalence they might experience in regard to change, will surface more quickly. Most clinicians would agree that behavioral resistance which has surfaced is less pernicious than resistance which remains covert. Having surfaced, this resistance is then more easily subject to therapist influence (Jacobson, in press; Weiss, 1979, 1980).

Let us examine these points separately. The importance of therapist self-discipline cannot be overemphasized. When the duration of therapy is brief and time limited, a fairly explicit agenda is required. The therapist must prepare and structure the sessions, and subgoals for each week can be discriminated within the overall treatment goals. Not only is time utilized more efficiently this way, but therapy is rendered more accountable. At any point in time, progress can be assessed by both therapist and clients; progress can be measured in terms of both immediate and ultimate treatment goals.

Clients' energies are also mobilized immediately within a brief therapy format. Clients are more likely to direct their efforts toward change, because they perceive both the therapist and the therapy technology as credible, a by-product of the therapist's structuring skills. They are also more likely to work hard because they must—their treatment contract requires it.

Jacobson and Margolin (1979) argued that an imprinting phenomenon occurs during the early stages of therapy. Consider brief therapy's antithesis—open-ended and extended therapy. Almost by definition, time does not emerge as an issue. The structure of the extended format allows inertia to intrude on the process of change, with little apparent cost to the ultimate treatment goals. No matter how forcefully the therapist may direct his or her interventions, the structure provides a powerful message, namely, that there is no hurry. This provides an opening for reticence and conflict about change to intrude, but in such subtle ways that it may not be noticed for weeks or months.

The therapist is also placed in a bind when what is therapeutic conflicts with the structure of the treatment format. Sessions can be impotent without much apparent cost. The therapist can be slothful, either in the preparation or in the conduct of a therapy session, without much difficulty in rationalizing, because, after all, there is plenty of time.

Unfortunately, more is at stake than simply wasted time. What is implied in the notion of imprinting is that precedents are established during the early stages of therapy which are not easily discarded later. Once the structure of therapy permits lethargy on the part of either therapist or clients, it is most difficult to convert that lethargy into an effective working alliance directed toward behavior change.

In marital therapy, spouses are almost always ambivalent about change (Gurman, 1978; Haley, 1963; Jacobson & Margolin, 1979; Weiss, 1979). This ambivalence is complicated and has been subjected to numerous interpretations in the literature (Barton & Alexander, 1981; Birchler & Spinks, 1980; Gurman & Knudson, 1978; Haley, 1963). In our view, however, this ambivalence is usually best understood in terms of the greater salience of the short-term costs of behavior change relative to the potential long-term benefits of such change. Each spouse enters therapy with transactional patterns designed to maximize the ratio of positive to negative outcomes. In order to raise the ratio to the point where it exceeds the threshold necessary for a subjective report of marital satisfaction, each spouse must engage in new behaviors which temporarily reduce their satisfaction. The long-term payoffs are not guaranteed, and what is more important, they are delayed.

Consider the directive that each spouse increase the frequency of pleasing behaviors during the ensuing week. The assignment requires effort: each spouse must concentrate on pinpointing behaviors in his or her repertoire that the other spouse finds pleasing and then generate these behaviors at a higher frequency. Neither spouse can be sure that the other will reciprocate; in other words, the overall consequences of compliance with the assignment are uncertain. Therefore, one would expect spouses to be ambivalent and behavioral resistance to be a rather common occurrence.

The brief therapy format almost guarantees that resistance will surface quickly; the very structure of the agenda and the therapist's directiveness concretizes and specifies those behaviors that are expected of spouses. The time constraints actually demand that these behaviors occur within a narrowly specified time period. Compliance with the therapist's directives is usually unambiguous.

The faster resistance surfaces, the more quickly it is subject to the therapist's influence. Hidden agendas cannot be attacked until evidence for their existence surfaces. Resistance is destructive either if the therapist is unaware of it or if its existence must be inferred. The brief therapy format operationalizes resistance, so that its occurrence is usually clear both to clients and to the therapist.

It should also be pointed out that the very structure of a brief therapy format can often eradicate resistance by allowing for such a precise, unambiguous determination of its existence. Extended therapy formats allow for a subterfuge of cooperation, so that spouses can both resist and simultaneously deny that they are resisting. BMT conducted within a brief therapy format, however, *demands* that clients engage in change-promoting behaviors at specified times, and noncompliance is a clear and blatant violation of the treatment contract. Clients who would otherwise resist change must now subject themselves to being labeled "bad clients" as a cost of following through on antitherapeutic maneuvers.

The essence of our position is that brief therapy either counteracts spouses' likelihood to resist or guarantees that resistant behavior will emerge early in therapy, where it can be subjected to the therapist's influence. When combined with the other advantages of brief therapy, outlined above, it should be apparent why we choose by design, not by default, to engage in BMT within a brief therapy form at. We feel it necessary to add that brevity is insufficient in and of itself; brevity has its effect only when combined with a directive, highly structured, technologized approach to marital therapy which is oriented toward behavior change. BMT is all these things. That is why, in our view, BMT and brief therapy constitute both a stable and a satisfactory marriage.

REFERENCES

Azrin, N. H., Besalel, V. A., Bechtel, R., Michalicek, A., Mancera, M., Carroll, D., Shuford, D., & Cox, J. Comparison of reciprocity and discussion-type counseling for marital problems. *American Journal of Family Therapy,* 1980, *8,* 21–28.

Azrin, N., Naster, B., & Jones, R. Reciprocity counseling: A rapid learning-based procedure for marital counseling. *Behaviour Research and Therapy,* 1973, *11,* 365–382.

Barton, C., & Alexander, J. A. Functional family therapy. In A. S. Gurman & D. P. Kniskern (Eds.), *Handbook of family therapy.* New York: Brunner/Mazel, 1981.

Beck, D. B. Research findings on the outcomes of marital counseling. In D. H. L. Olson (Ed.), *Treating relationships.* Lake Mills, Ia.: Graphic Publishing, 1976.

Birchler, G. R., & Spinks, S. H. Behavioral-systems marital and family therapy: Integration and clinical application. *American Journal of Family Therapy,* 1980, *8,* 6–28.

Birchler, G. R., Weiss, R. L., & Vincent, J. P. A multimethod analysis of social reinforcement exchange between maritally distressed and nondistressed spouse and stranger dyads. *Journal of Personality and Social Psychology,* 1975, *31*(2), 349–360.

Bloom, B. L., Asher, S. J., & White, S. W. Marital disruption as a stressor: A review and analysis. *Psychological Bulletin,* 1978, *83,* 867–894.

Goldfried, M. R., & D'Zurilla, T. J. A behavioral analytic model for assessing competence. In C. D. Spielberger (Ed.), *Current topics in clinical and community psychology* (Vol. I). New York: Academic Press, 1969.

Gottman, J. M. *Marital interaction: Experimental investigations.* New York: Academic Press, 1979.

Guerney, B. *Relationship enhancement.* San Francisco: Jossey-Bass, 1977.

Gurman, A. S. Contemporary marital therapies: A critique and comparative analysis of psychodynamic, systems, and behavioral approaches. In T. J. Paolino, Jr., & B. S. McCrady (Eds.), *Marriage and marital therapy: Psychoanalytic, behavioral, and systems theory perspectives.* New York: Brunner/Mazel, 1978.

Gurman, A. S. Behavioral marriage therapy in the 1980's: The challenge of integration. *American Journal of Family Therapy,* 1980, *8,* 86–96.

Gurman, A. S., & Kniskern, D. P. Research on marital and family therapy: Progress, perspective, and prospect. In S. L. Garfield & A. E. Bergin (Eds.), *Handbook of psychotherapy and behavior change: An empirical analysis* (2nd ed.). New York: Wiley, 1978.

Gurman, A. S., & Knudson, R. M. Behavioral marriage therapy: I. A psychodynamic-systems analysis and critique. *Family Process,* 1978, *17,* 121–138.

Haley, J. Marriage therapy. *Archives of General Psychiatry,* 1963, *8,* 213–234.

Harrell, J., & Guerney, B. Training married couples in conflict negotiation skills. In D. H. L. Olson (Ed.), *Treating relationships.* Lake MIlls, Ia.: Graphic Publishing, 1976.

Jacobson, N. S. Problem solving and contingency contracting in the treatment of marital discord. *Journal of Consulting and Clinical Psychology,* 1977, *45,* 92–100.

Jacobson, N. S. A review of the research on the effectiveness of marital therapy. In T. J. Paolino, Jr., & B. S. McCrady (Eds.), *Marriage and marital therapy: Psychoanalytic, behavioral, and systems theory perspectives.* New York: Brunner/Mazel, 1978. (a)

Jacobson, N. S. A stimulus control model of change in behavioral marital therapy: Implications for contingency contracting. *Journal of Marriage and Family Counseling,* 1978, *4,* 29–35. (b)

Jacobson, N. S. Behavioral treatments for marital discord: A critical appraisal. In M. Hersen, R. M. Eisler, & P. M. Miller (Eds.), *Progress in behavior modification.* New York: Academic Press, 1979. (a)

Jacobson, N. S. Increasing positive behavior in severely distressed adult relationships. *Behavior Therapy,* 1979, *10,* 311–326. (b)

Jacobson, N. S. Marital problem: Direct strategies for inducing compliance. In J. Shelton & R. Levy (Eds.), *Systematic behavior assignments.* Champaign, Ill.: Research Press, in press.

Jacobson, N. S., & Anderson, E. A. The effects of behavior rehearsal and feedback on the acquisition of problem solving skills in distressed and nondistressed couples. *Behaviour Research and Therapy,* 1980, *18,* 25–36.

Jacobson, N. S., Elwood, R., & Dallas, M. The behavioral assessment of marital dysfunction. In D. H. Barlow (Ed.), *Behavioral assessment of adult disorders.* New York: Guilford Press, 1981.

Jacobson, N. S., & Margolin, G. *Marital therapy.* New York: Brunner/Mazel, 1979.

Jacobson, N. S., Waldron, H., & Moore, D. Toward a behavioral profile of marital distress. *Journal of Consulting and Clinical Psychology,* 1980, *48,* 696–703.

Jacobson, N. S., & Weiss, R. L. Behavioral marriage therapy: "The contents of Gurman *et. al.* may be hazardous to our health." *Family Process,* 1978, *17,* 149–164.

Liberman, R. P., Levine, J., Wheeler, E., Sanders, N., & Wallace, C. Experimental evaluation of marital group therapy: Behavioral vs. interaction–insight formats. *Acta Psychiatrica Scandinavia,* 1976, suppl. 266.

Margolin, G., & Weiss, R. L. A comparative evaluation of therapeutic components associated with behavioral marital treatment. *Journal of Consulting and Clinical Psychology*, 1978, *46*, 1476–1486.

Meissner, W. W. The conceptualization of marriage and family dynamics from a psychoanalytic perspective. In T. J. Paolino, Jr., & B. S. McCrady (Eds.), *Marriage and marital therapy: Psychoanalytic, behavioral, and systems theory perspectives*. New York: Brunner/Mazel, 1978.

Patterson, G. R., & Hops, H. Coercion, a game for two: Intervention techniques for marital conflict. In R. E. Ulrich & P. Mountjoy (Eds.), *The experimental analysis of social behavior*. New York: Appleton-Century-Crofts, 1972.

Patterson, G. R., & Reid, J. B. Reciprocity and coercion: Two facets of social systems. In C. Neuringer & J. Michael (Eds.), *Behavior modification in clinical psychology*. New York: Appleton-Century-Crofts, 1970.

Reid, W. J., & Shyne, A. W. *Brief and extended casework*. New York: Columbia University Press, 1967.

Stuart, R. B. Operant-interpersonal treatment for marital discord. *Journal of Consulting and Clinical Psychology*, 1969, *33*, 675–682.

Thibaut, J., & Kelley, H. H. *The social psychology of groups*. New York: Wiley, 1959.

Vincent, J. P., Weiss, R. L., & Birchler, G. R. A behavioral analysis of problem solving in distressed and nondistressed married and stranger dyads. *Behavior Therapy*, 1975, *6*, 475–487.

Watzlawick, P., Weakland, J., & Fisch, R. *Change: Principles of problem formation and problem resolution*. New York: Norton, 1974.

Weiss, R. L. The conceptualization of marriage and marriage disorders from a behavioral perspective. In T. J. Paolino, Jr., & B. S. McCrady (Eds.), *Marriage and marital therapy: Psychoanalytic, behavioral, and systems theory perspectives*. New York: Brunner/Mazel, 1978.

Weiss, R. L. Resistance in behavioral marriage therapy. *The American Journal of Family Therapy*, 1979, *7*, 3–6.

Weiss, R. L. Strategic behavioral marital therapy: Toward a model for assessment and intervention. In J. P. Vincent (Ed.), *Advances in family intervention, assessment, and theory*. Greenwich: JAI Press, 1980.

Weiss, R. L., & Aved, B. M. Marital satisfaction and depression as predictors of physical health status. *Journal of Consulting and Clinical Psychology*, 1978, *46*, 1379–1384.

Weiss, R. L., & Birchler, G. R. Adults with marital dysfunction. In M. Hersen & A. Bellack (Eds.), *Behavior therapy in the psychiatric setting*. Baltimore: Williams & Wilkins, 1978.

Weiss, R. L., Birchler, G. R., & Vincent, J. P. Contractual models for negotiation training in marital dyads. *Journal of Marriage and the Family*, 1974, pp. 321–330.

Weiss, R. L., Hops, H., & Patterson, G. R. A framework for conceptualizing marital conflict, technology for altering it, some data for evaluating it. In L. A. Hamerlynck, L. C. Handy, & E. J. Mash (Eds.), *Behavior change: Methodology, concepts, and practice*. Champaign, Ill.: Research Press, 1973.

Weiss, R. L., & Margolin, G. Assessment of marital conflict and accord. In A. R. Ciminero, K. D. Calhoun, & H. E. Adams (Eds.), *Handbook of behavioral assessment*. New York: Wiley, 1977.

Wills, T. A., Weiss, R. L., & Patterson, G. R. A behavioral analysis of the determinants of marital satisfaction. *Journal of Consulting and Clinical Psychology*, 1974, *42*, 802–811.

CHAPTER 16
INTEGRATIVE MARITAL THERAPY: TOWARD THE DEVELOPMENT OF AN INTERPERSONAL APPROACH

Alan S. Gurman

To the current generation of psychotherapists in training, there would appear to have been a rapid upsurge of interest in brief methods of psychotherapy in the last decade. Actually, a more accurate historical perspective makes it clear that there really has been a *re*surgence of interest in the area. In addition to the oft forgotten fact that many of the early treatments by Freud himself were of quite short duration, an impressive number of influential psychotherapists, such as Alexander (Alexander & French, 1946), Ferenczi (1920/1950), and Rank (1947), offered models of brief therapy long before the 1970s. It is not surprising, of course, that most of these models were steeped in psychoanalytic thought, since, until about 10 to 15 years ago, the modal psychotherapist identified his or her theoretical orientation as "psychodynamic." Only in the last decade have alternative theoretical orientations won the allegiances of large numbers of professional therapists. While behavior therapy, for example, certainly had its beginnings more than two decades ago (Kazdin, 1979), it was not until the 1970s that it emerged as a pervasive and dominant force in the delivery of mental health services. Moreover, it has been only in the last decade that the apparent winner in the theoretical orientation sweepstakes has become the doctrine of eclecticism (Garfield & Kurtz, 1977).

Indeed, most of the relatively newer influential therapies (e.g., behavior therapy, Gestalt therapy, cognitive therapy, transactional analysis) are thought to be "brief" psychotherapies. But such a characterization is

ALAN S. GURMAN. Department of Psychiatry, University of Wisconsin Medical School, Madison, Wisconsin.

often confusing, if not misleading. For example, while behavior therapists emphasize the application of highly specific treatment methods to specific, carefully operationalized treatment goals, it is not outside the range of behavioral practice to treat some patients for well over 100 sessions (cf. Klein, Dittman, Parloff, & Gill, 1969). The confusion that arises as to whether a given therapeutic method should be classified as brief is reminiscent of a classic one-liner by comedian Shelley Berman. When asked, "How are you?" Berman's reply was, "Compared to what?"

THE MYTH OF BRIEF INDIVIDUAL PSYCHOTHERAPY

The point here is that psychotherapy is brief only with reference to some temporal standard. In order to consider meaningfully what constitutes brief marital therapy, we must first consider what constitutes brief psychotherapy in general. As the term is usually used, psychotherapy is thought to be brief when it is of significantly shorter duration than the ideal practice of individual psychoanalytic psychotherapy, and of psychoanalysis in particular, that is, multiple sessions per week over three years or more. This arbitrary criterion of brevity exists, of course, in the collective minds of professional psychotherapists. In the minds of most consumers of psychotherapy, quite a different state of definitional affairs obtains.

It has been established reliably that most people seeking psychotherapy in outpatient clinic settings expect their treatments to last less than three months (Garfield, 1971). Moreover, in such settings, the fact is that a very high percentage of individual patients terminate treatment in less than 12 sessions (Butcher & Koss, 1978; Garfield, 1971). Recent data suggest that treatments of about this length are not limited to lower socioeconomic patients (Lorion, 1973, 1974) but also characterize the general practice of psychotherapy conducted in private practice settings (Koss, 1979). Nor is this merely a recent trend. Almost two decades ago, Matarazzo (1965) observed that the "fact is that the majority of patients seen in any given week are typically seen for a grand total of fewer than ten sessions. . . . The general practicing psychotherapist treats on a continuing basis only a few patients for as long as a year, two, three, or longer" (p. 218).

Thus, on an empirical basis, not only is the notion of brief psychotherapy not new; it is, more importantly, a myth, inasmuch as most individual psychotherapy lasts only about 10 to 12 sessions. Therapists' traditional and idealized standards regarding treatment length notwithstanding, unplanned "brief" treatments are factually the convention. What is new is the notion of brief therapy by design (time-limited treatment) rather than by default (e.g., Mann, 1973).

THE COUNTERMYTH OF BRIEF MARITAL THERAPY

In contrast to the situation for individual psychotherapy, marital therapy has never had to contend with the struggle of finding ways to shorten the treatment process. By traditional standards of individual psychotherapy, marital therapy, like family therapy, has been overwhelmingly brief (Gurman, 1971, 1975, 1978). For example, in the first published review of the outcomes of marital therapy, Gurman (1971) found an average treatment length of only 17.45 sessions, and Gurman and Kniskern (1978b), in their comprehensive review of research on marital and family therapy several years later, found that treatment length was less than 20 sessions in about 70% of the studies reviewed. (Note that this figure was not skewed by the inclusion of treatments that were arbitrarily time limited for research purposes, since of the 35 studies used to compute this figure, only 2 set limitations on treatment length.) Moreover, data consonant with these research findings have come from sources as divergent as Framo (1981), who conducts psychodynamically based marital therapy in private practice and reported his average treatment length to be 15 sessions, and Andolfi (1978), who practices symptom-focused structural–strategic family therapy (Andolfi, 1979) in Italy and reported his average treatment length to be about 12 sessions.

Thus, in contrast to individual psychotherapy, the dominant theme in marital and family therapy has been that treatment which is brief by traditional therapeutic standards is expected, commonplace, and the norm. Therefore, to speak of "brief" marital therapy is both redundant, since the overwhelming majority of marital therapies are brief, and naive, since "long-term" marital treatment has virtually never existed as a temporal standard against which particular methods can be compared. Thus, to think of marital therapy methods as brief requires the adoption of a reciprocal assumption, or countermyth, unsupported by clinical data, of the existence of lengthy treatment as the standard of comparison.

It is interesting to speculate about the reasons why most marital therapy is of relatively short duration. Some appealing explanations may be grouped usefully under the headings of the contributions of the therapist, on the one hand, and of the patients, on the other. The major therapist contribution to the brevity of treatment is probably his or her emphasis on what Aponte and VanDeusen (1981) refer to as the sustaining structures of the presenting problem, rather than on its generating structures. That is, however a problem began and whatever its original dynamics and motivations, what is most important for producing change is to address the current relational patterns that undergird the problem presented. Thus, the therapist may seek to understand something of the historical development and evolution of the current problem—but only in order to plan change-oriented interventions, not in order to elucidate the reasons for past failures at producing change. Another way of stating this view would be to argue that if past transactions are relevant to the maintenance of the current problem, the interactional processes of the past will also be found in the present.

The patient's contribution to treatment brevity seem to involve two factors. First, as a group, people entering marital therapy have already been self-screened, by virtue of the very existence of the marital relationship, on one of the most important variables used in selecting patients for brief individual therapy, that is, a history of at least one meaningful relationship. As Sifneos (1972) noted, a "meaningful relationship" is one characterized by "shared intimacy, emotional involvement, trust, and also an ability to give and take" (p. 78). While all marriages certainly do not match this description, the odds are that for most couples, this description will have been true at some time in the history of their relationship.

The second patient contribution to brevity derives from the fact that the interactional sources of anxiety are not merely talked about in marital therapy but are present in the treatment setting, so that defenses are more identifiable, accessible to the therapist, and less easily denied by both patients.

The final patient contribution to treatment brevity centers on the symbolic meaning of the termination of the experience. The loss of the therapist at the end of marital treatment simply does not have the experiential salience of the loss of the therapist in individual psychotherapy (cf. Mann, 1973). The ever present, implicit threat of the real loss of the marriage partner is far more powerful and attracts a great deal more of each spouse's conscious and unconscious energy and attention. Thus, what the setting of time limits in individual therapy may facilitate in terms of heightened emotional arousal (Butcher & Koss, 1978) is enormously outweighed by the arousal, often quite consciously, of course, of the dangers to the very survival of the marital relationship.

TIME-LIMITED MARITAL THERAPY:
WHEN MEANS HAVE LITTLE MEANING

Given the discrepancies that have existed between idealized and actual treatment durations in individual psychotherapy, it is not surprising that both terminological and statistical confusion abounds when one seeks to determine what constitutes brief treatment. For example, should the term "brief therapy" be used to refer to the number of treatment sessions or to the total elapsed duration of treatment? For example, we may speak (albeit rarely) of a "standard" brief therapy of 10 to 15 weekly sessions; of a "clustered" brief therapy of the same number of sessions in a shorter period of elapsed time; of an "extended" brief therapy of the same number of sessions over a longer period; of "intensive" brief therapy, which has a limited duration but no limit on session frequency; or of "brief contact" brief therapy, involving brief sessions (e.g., 20 minutes) over an extended period of time! By traditional standards, all qualify as brief treatment, so there is no rational basis for asserting just what is and what is not brief psychotherapy.

Similarly, even with the use of the more restrictive term "time-limited therapy," consensus is difficult to achieve. Influential time-limited individual psychotherapies currently range from 12 sessions (Mann, 1973) to 40 sessions (Malan, 1976) to as long as one year (Sifneos, 1972). While, as noted, most marital therapy is brief, few marital therapists have set forth explicit time limits for their treatments. Among those marital therapists who have set such time limits, treatment durations do not vary quite as much as they do among time-limited individual psychotherapies. Stuart (1979), Weiss (1975), and Jacobson and Margolin (1979), all of whom are behavioral marriage therapists, limit treatment to 8, 19, and 12 sessions, respectively, and the "strategic" therapists of the Mental Research Institute limit treatment to 10 sessions (Weakland, Fisch, Watzlawick, & Bodin, 1974). Still, leading proponents of other methods of marital therapy, such as Stanton (1981), who do not set explicit time limits, rarely exceed six months of treatment and generally end treatment much earlier.

Thus, in both time-limited individual psychotherapy and marital therapy, there exists no magic number of treatment sessions to demarcate

the limits of brief therapy. What constitutes the essence of brief psychotherapy of any sort is not the setting of a time limit, which is necessarily arbitrary, but the establishment of a clear focus for the treatment. Since the
natural courses of marital therapy are overwhelmingly brief, by traditional standards, regardless of theoretical orientation (Gurman, 1978), it
is usually redundant to fix time limits for the treatment of marital discord.
The conceptually most sophisticated contemporary models of brief individual psychotherapy (e.g., Malan, 1976; Mann, 1973; Sifneos, 1972)
have clearly carried the connotations of condensing the classical psychoanalytic approach (i.e., using traditional analytic methods in a shorter
than standard time period) and of compromising with the constraints of
limited treatment time (by addressing more limited treatment goals than in
psychoanalysis).

      In contrast, no major method or model of marital therapy has origi-
nated in long-term practice. Moreover, most marital therapists simply
have not had to struggle with concerns of compromising treatment goals.
On the contrary, marital therapy, with rare exceptions (e.g., Bowen, 1976;
Kerr, 1981), has always encouraged and fostered the selection of limited
goals, whether the outcome criteria have emphasized symptomatic (e.g.,
Haley, 1963; Stanton, 1981; Weakland et al., 1974), behavioral (e.g.,
Jacobson & Margolin, 1979; Stuart, 1980; Weiss, 1978), or psychodynamic (e.g., Bentovim & Kinston, 1978; Framo, 1981; Nadelson, 1978)
changes.

TOWARD THE DEVELOPMENT OF
AN INTEGRATIVE MARITAL THERAPY

The need for a framework to bridge the gap between the theory and practice of marital therapy and the research on the outcomes of marital
therapy is no less immediate for the continuing development of the field
than is the need for the development of an integrative model of marital relationships per se and of their clinical treatment. To date, marital therapists with declared theoretical allegiances, especially the most influential
leaders in the field, have generally remained quite ignorant of developments within alternative treatment approaches. This is not surprising,
given the very different and, indeed, almost independent origins of those
methods (Broderick & Schrader, 1981).

      Psychodynamically oriented views and methods, of course, have
evolved from the thought and practice of psychoanalysis and psychoana-

lytic psychotherapy, beginning with confrontation of the issues arising in concurrent individual psychoanalytic treatment of married partners by the same analyst. Predictably, psychodynamic marital therapies have been advocated primarily, though not exclusively, by psychiatric clinicians (e.g., Dicks, 1967; Nadelson, 1978; Sager, 1976, 1981; Skynner, 1976, 1981). Strategic approaches to marital therapy (Stanton, 1980, 1981), on the other hand, while originating, in part, in psychiatric settings (Broderick & Schrader, 1981; Guerin, 1976), have generally denied the treatment relevance of almost all concepts central to psychoanalytic practice (Bodin, 1981; Stanton, 1981). They place nearly exclusive emphasis on the current interactional forces maintaining dysfunctional relationship patterns. Moreover, these methods were initially developed by clinicians who were mavericks within established mental health professions (e.g., Paul Watzlawick, Don Jackson) or whose initial professional training was not even in these professions (e.g., Jay Haley, John Weakland). In contrast, behavioral marital therapy, the most recent significant arrival on the scene, has been influenced primarily by the contributions of academic psychologists (e.g., Birchler & Spinks, 1980; Jacobson & Margolin, 1979; Stuart, 1980; Weiss, 1978), whose efforts have been directed toward developing treatment methods that link up clinical practice with empirical knowledge derived from general, experimental, and social psychology.

Understandably, these apparently incompatible treatment methods have found both conceptual and professional obstacles which have precluded their integration. To date, then, there have been few significant integrative advances in marital therapy, and, indeed, there have been few such attempts. The most common type of existing effort at integration has involved the incorporation of strategic concepts and treatment techniques within behavioral approaches (e.g., Birchler & Spinks, 1980; Stuart, 1980; Weiss, 1979). While some influential, psychodynamically oriented marital therapists have allowed that certain behavioral techniques (e.g., contracting) are not incompatible with the general aims of psychodynamic methods (Framo, 1981; Sager, 1981), contributions integrating behavioral and psychodynamic views have been rare (e.g., Gurman, 1980a, 1980b). Rare, as well, are those geared toward integrating the methods of all three approaches (e.g., Berman, Lief, Williams, & Green, 1980; Feldman, 1979; Gurman, 1978, 1980a, 1980b).

The rationale for encouraging such an integrative approach has several interdependent bases. First, the clinical choice of addressing either intrapsychic or interpersonal forces in marital relationships, to the exclusion of the other, can be made only on totally arbitrary grounds (Gurman,

1978, 1980a, 1980b; Gurman & Knudson, 1978; Gurman, Knudson, & Kniskern, 1978; Knudson, Gurman, & Kniskern, 1980).

Second, it is likely that treatment approaches which systematically consider and attempt to produce change on multiple levels of psychological experience will facilitate the development of interventions that are more flexible and responsive to differences between patients and will thus lead to more positive and enduring clinical outcomes. Moreover, an integrative approach may permit a matching of types of treatment intervention and the sequencing of interventions for different types of marital dysfunctions. While the research to date does not provide a basis for a clinically useful taxonomy of marital dysfunction that simultaneously addresses the various levels and domains of psychological experience (Gurman & Kniskern, 1978b, 1981), it is self-evident that any method of marital therapy which arbitrarily excludes any of these levels or domains as irrelevant to effecting meaningful change will, at the same time, unwittingly be limiting both theoretical and experimental advances in the field.

Third, treatment models which address such multiple psychological domains will necessarily lead to the adoption of research strategies which include multidimensional assessment of therapeutic change. In addition to facilitating a richer understanding of therapeutic change processes in general (Bergin, 1971; Bergin & Lambert, 1978), such multidimensional approaches can help decrease what often seems to be an unchangeable mutual mistrust and denigration between clinicians and clinical researchers.

Given this background and rationale, the rest of this chapter has the following aims: first, to present a brief statement of the major assumptions and treatment methods of psychodynamic, strategic, and behavioral marital therapies; second, to propose the beginnings of a working model for integrating these views in a manner that is clinically meaningful; and third, to set forth a number of treatment principles derived from this model and to note how these principles are especially relevant to the conduct of a focused treatment of married couples that is sensitive to its usual brevity.

THREE APPROACHES TO MARITAL THERAPY

This section simply sets forth the major characteristics of psychodynamic, behavioral, and systems theory approaches to marital therapy. A more elaborated, comparative discussion of these models, and a detailed critique thereof, can be found in Gurman (1978).

PSYCHODYNAMIC APPROACHES

Among the numerous contributions from psychodynamically oriented marital therapists (cf. Gurman, 1978), those of Sager (1976, 1981), Dicks (1967), and Skynner (1976, 1981) seem to offer the most fertile conceptual ground for an appreciation of the dynamics of intimate relationships.

Psychodynamic theories applied to marital relationships have a strong developmental emphasis and, in this way, stand in marked contrast to behavioral and systems views, which are largely mute on developmental issues (Gurman, 1979). In these models, marital choice is thought to be influenced to a significant degree by unconscious factors. These factors emphasize the maintenance of an organized (if maladaptive) sense of self, intrapsychic and interpersonal boundaries, and tolerable levels of anxiety in an ongoing, intimate relationship. As Skynner (1976) expressed these themes, "couples are usually attracted by shared developmental failures" (p. 43). For example, Barnett (1971) detailed the nature of the unconscious interaction in the commonly encountered obsessive–hysteric marriage: while for the hysteric, narcissism is largely in the service of dependency, and for the obsessive, dependency is in the service of narcissism, both spouses are primarily conflicted around the issue of establishing and maintaining a manageable, that is, personally tolerable, level of intimacy. Thus, overt style differences and apparently different needs in the relationship often reflect conflict over the same, more basic dynamic issue.

The unspoken processes by which such arrangements are upheld in relationships are referred to variously as "family projection process" (Bowen, 1966) or "collusion" (Dicks, 1967). This collusive process requires both partners' collaboration, wherein each implicitly agrees to form "contracts" that are beyond awareness (the overriding purpose of which is to meet the historically unfulfilled needs of each partner) and to protect the partner from those aspects of intra- and interpersonal experience that are laden with conflict (e.g., anxiety). Thus, these contracts (Sager, 1976, 1981) are oriented toward the maintenance of each partner's consistent self-perception, and the unconscious agreement is to "see" the partner as the partner needs to see him- or herself (Gurman, 1978; Gurman & Knudson, 1978; Knudson et al., 1980). In this light, it can be seen that repetitive, nonproductive conflict is goal oriented: it serves to prevent the awareness of unconscious anxiety stimulated by increases in relationship intimacy (Feldman, 1979).

Thus, object relations theory, as applied to marriages, focuses on "how interpersonal relationships determine intrapsychic structure in the mind and how these structures come to reactivate such relationships at a later date'' (Bentovim, 1981). A more cognitive and less "economic" model, such as Kelley's (1955) personal construct theory, would similarly point to the ways in which interpersonal interactions are channeled by the psychological constructs laid down earlier in life. In an object relations framework, the core source of marital dysfunction is each spouse's failure to see him- or herself and the marriage partner as "whole persons" (Dicks, 1967; Stewart, Peters, Marsh, & Peters, 1975); that is, conflict-laden aspects of one's self are repudiated, split off, and projected onto the spouse (or onto other family members), who "accept" the projections by behaving, in large measure, on congruence with them. Moreover, many of the mutual expectations spouses have of one another are logically incompatible. Thus, the elements of such collusive contracts may be simultaneously out of each partner's awareness, mutually exclusive, and unfillable by anyone. While all this sounds rather pessimistic, it is vital to recall, as many marital therapists repeatedly fail to do, that this unconscious collaboration has, as its main emotional purposes, both the mutual protection of each spouse and the rediscovery of repressed aspects of one's self. Thus, collusion, while geared toward overt conflict avoidance, is a potentially growthful collaboration, an adaptive effort to resolve individual conflicts through specific, accommodating, intimate relationships.

General Treatment Philosophy and Goals

The overriding aim of psychodynamically based, conjoint marital therapy is to interrupt collusive processes and, in so doing, to make explicit the multileveled expectations both partners have of themselves and their mate, so that these may be understood and negotiated at a conscious level of experience. Therapy, then, focuses on the restructuring of each spouse's self-perceptions and perceptions of his or her mate. An understanding of each partner's own past is viewed not as an end in itself, but as a means for facilitating an appreciation of how past experience influences current interaction. Thus, therapy necessarily has a developmental sensitivity. Still, rather few interventions have been described by psychodynamically oriented marriage therapists. In truth, marital therapy based on object relations (e.g., Dicks, 1967) and/or contract theory (Sager, 1976, 1981) is largely "analytic" in the way it organizes the complex material at hand and conceptualizes marital discord, but it is quite pragmatic and even eclectic in its choice of actual therapist interventions (Gurman, 1978; Nadelson, 1978). As Ables and Brandsma (1977) state, "theory is employed as a means of understanding and appraising individual dynamics manifest in present and interactional behaviors" (p. 2).

BEHAVIORAL APPROACHES

Several related models of marital interaction and therapy have been proposed in the last few years, the most prominent being those of Jacobson and Margolin (1979), Stuart (1980), and Weiss (1978). While these models vary somewhat in terms of behavior change principles, they share a common heritage of influence from social psychological and social learning theories. All the major behavioral treatment approaches are characterized by modular, sequential application of intervention techniques, with quite explicit criteria for movement from one stage of treatment to the next (see below: Treatment Philosophy and Goals).

The core of the behavioral conceptualization of marital conflict involves Thibaut and Kelly's (1959) exchange theory model of social psychological interaction, in which individuals strive to maximize "rewards" while minimizing "costs." In this model, social behavior in a given relationship is maintained by a high ratio of rewards to costs and by the perception that alternative relationships offer fewer comparative rewards and most costs ("comparison level of alternatives"). The potential for marital conflict exists either when optimal behavior-maintaining contingencies do not exist or when faulty behavior change efforts are implemented.

In the latter and more common context, two social reinforcement mechanisms are operative—coercion and reciprocity (Jacobson, 1981). Coercion describes an interaction in which both persons provide aversive stimuli that control the behavior of the other person, with negative reinforcement resulting from the termination of this state of affairs, thus maintaining the behavior of both people. Reciprocity, on the other hand, describes an exchange in which two people reinforce each other at an equitable rate, with positive reinforcers maintaining the behavior of both. Thus, marital conflict results from the use of aversive control tactics rather than the use of positive control, with the eventual outcome being a low rate of positive reinforcers exchanged by the spouses, such that each is less attracted to the other.

The social learning position also asserts that, as Lederer and Jackson (1958) phrased it, "nastiness begets nastiness"; that is, the use of aversive stimulation in interpersonal relationships tends to produce reciprocal behavior in the second person. Research has confirmed (Jacobson, 1981) both that the spouse who "gives" the highest rate of aversive stimulation also "receives" the highest rate, and that distressed couples can be differentiated from nondistressed couples by the mean rates with which aversive stimuli are exchanged. Moreover, couples in distressed relationships are characterized by both poor communication skills and poor problem-solving and conflict resolution skills.

General Treatment Philosophy and Goals

All behavioral marriage therapies begin with broadly gauged, systematic evaluation of marital interaction, often, though not exclusively, through the use of standardized assessment devices (see, for example, Jacobson, 1981; Jacobson & Margolin, 1979; Stuart, 1980). As is true in behavior therapy generally, the rationale for all planned treatment interventions is explained to couples, along with an explicit description of the phases or stages through which treatment will progress. Early interventions focus on developing in the couple an attitude—and a behavior consistent with this attitude—of trying to achieve mutual relationship goals; for example, Jacobson and Margolin (1979) emphasize the development of a "collaborative set," and Stuart (1980) introduces "caring days" in the first session. These interventions are geared toward increasing commitment to the relationship. Overriding treatment goals are to increase the use of positive reinforcement methods and to decrease the use of aversive consequences to obtain desired spouse behavior change.

Throughout treatment, pinpointing (i.e., the behavioral specification of each partner's wishes and desires) is encouraged and modeled. Communication skill training is systematically taught via verbal instruction and feedback, therapist modeling, role playing, and behavior rehearsal. Listening and reflective skills as well as expressive skills (e.g., the use of "I" statements) are common. Following the achievement of a reasonable mastery of these social skills, skills for contracting and negotiating behavior change are taught, practiced, and utilized along with a variety of skill procedures for dealing with conflict and for problem solving and decision making. Because of the explicitness of all therapeutic interventions, each course of treatment aspires to have the couple learn a variety of specific, relationship-enhancing skills that can be self-applied long after therapy ends. To facilitate this process of increasing the generalization and durability of therapy-induced change, explicit homework activities are used throughout therapy.

STRUCTURAL-STRATEGIC APPROACHES

While structural family therapy (Aponte & VanDeusen, 1981; Minuchin, 1974) and strategic family therapy (Bodin, 1981; Stanton, 1980; Watzlawick, Weakland, & Fisch, 1974) are often considered to be rather separate schools of treatment, they share many assumptions about human behavior and behavior change, therapist role, and treatment goals and, therefore, are increasingly becoming thought of as a single school (e.g., Andolfi, 1979; Kniskern & Gurman, 1980; Stanton, 1981). Both approaches are concerned with the rules, patterns, and redundancies of family behavior. To date, very little has been written about structural therapy with couples (cf. Heard, 1978; Stanton, 1980), largely because of its triadic and two-generational clinical emphasis (Gurman, 1978), whereas discussions of strategic marital therapy have appeared in the literature somewhat more often, despite its clinical origins with the families of schizophrenics (Bodin, 1981).

In the structural–strategic view, the symptoms of individual family members are both system maintained and system maintaining, and all individual problems are seen as manifestations of marital–familial disturbance. Marital conflict is viewed as the result of interaction, largely unaffected by intrapsychic (especially unconscious) forces. The psychological symptoms of a husband or wife are assumed always to have interpersonal meaning and, in fact, to function as communicative acts, so that a symptomatic individual cannot be expected to change unless his or her family system changes.

Marital and family systems are conceived as analogous to cybernetic systems, in which causality is circular rather than linear, and in which complex, interlocking feedback mechanisms and behavior patterns repeat themselves in sequence. Thus, an individual's symptoms serve as homeostatic mechanisms which regulate family transactions.

General Treatment Philosophy and Goals

Structural–strategic therapy is quite pragmatic, and its advocates draw upon a rather wide variety of interventions, including many from outside the structural–strategic school (e.g., behavioral). Treatment is decidedly symptom focused, and the treatment contracts negotiated with patients usually revolve around presenting complaints, which, for the purposes of establishing treatment goals, are defined in very concrete, behavioral terms. Predictably, therapy is very present centered, and the therapist is especially concerned with behavioral sequences which create the interpersonal context for the presenting problems. Interpretation is not used to foster either genetic or interactional insight, but rather to reframe or relabel behavior in order to give it a new meaning in terms of the problematic homeostasis.

As in behavioral marriage therapy, the structural–strategic therapist is extremely active in terms of both setting the agenda for treatment sessions and initiating what occurs within sessions. Gaining covert control of treatment is essential, and this control is established within the problem framework defined by the couple. While very little skill training is provided, as in behavioral marriage therapy, the cornerstone of the approach rests on the therapist's issuance of tasks and directives for the couple. These tasks may be designed to be carried out either within sessions, between sessions, or both (Aponte & VanDeusen, 1981; Stanton, 1981). It is hypothesized that out-of-session tasks shorten the process of therapy.

Interventions based on the assignment of tasks and directives are of two general types. Structural interventions are designed to produce direct change in the major interactional parameters of the marital relationship (e.g., by modifying the boundaries between spouses). Paradoxical interventions, which take a wide variety of forms (Stanton, 1981; Weeks & L'Abate, 1979), appear absurd because of their contradictory nature, such as prescribing symptoms (e.g., requiring a couple to continue to perform the very behaviors of which they complain). The use of paradox, in its multiple forms, assumes an enormous amount of resistance to change on the part of patients. The purpose of prescribing symptoms, for example, is to put the couple in a therapeutic bind: resistance leads to improvement, whereas compliance gives control to the therpist.

SOME CONCEPTUAL AND TECHNICAL PRINCIPLES FOR AN INTEGRATIVE APPROACH TO MARITAL THERAPY

As I (Gurman, 1978, 1979, 1980a, 1980b) and others (Berman *et al.*, 1980; Berman & Lief, 1975; Feldman, 1979) have emphasized, effective marital therapy does not set up an artificial dichotomy between individual change and relationship change. Berman and Lief (1975) put it straightforwardly: "The interrelationships between intrapsychic and interpersonal factors are at the heart of marital therapy" (p. 584). More than any other approach to marital therapy, psychodynamic–interpersonal models (e.g., Dicks,

1967; Framo, 1981; Sager, 1976, Skynner, 1981; Stewart *et al.,* 1975) generally have attempted to transcend the false dichotomy between individual–intrapsychic change and interactional–structural change (Gurman, 1978).

Moreover, only psychodynamic views of marital interaction, conflict, and change can incorporate the multileveled nature of intimate relationships (Gurman, 1980b). Behavior therapists, with extremely rare exceptions (e.g., Mahoney, 1979), do not even admit of the possibility of unconscious forces in interpersonal behavior (e.g., Jacobson, 1981; Jacobson & Margolin, 1979; Stuart, 1980), and structural–strategic therapists, while not generally denying the existence of the unconscious, assert that systematic attention to unconscious motivation is not only unnecessary for effective treatment, but possibly even antithetical to it (e.g., Bodin, 1981; Stanton, 1980, 1981).

It is essential, at this juncture, to make clear what is meant in this chapter by the term "psychodynamic." Paolino's (1978) discussion of the frequent synonymous use of the terms "psychodynamic" and "psychoanalytic" is most helpful in clarifying this distinction. He suggested that the term "psychodynamic"

> can be broadly defined as referring to theories that expand on the fundamental hypotheses [that a person's thoughts, feeling and behavior are based on complex interactions between the mind, body and external environment] by applying various specific *mentalistic* concepts that include dynamically interacting components of the mind . . . [the psychodynamic view] includes specific identifiable factors that are often in conflict and are psychological, powerful, usually unconscious, motivating forces of human behavior. (pp. 91–92)

In contrast, the term "psychoanalytic" can be used in reference to Freudian principles of psychic functioning and human behavior, the psychoanalytic instrument of scholarly investigation, and a body of techniques as a method of treatment. Thus, all psychoanalytic theories are clearly psychodynamic, but not all psychodynamic theories are psychoanalytic. As Mahoney (1979) emphasized, belief in the existence and influence of unconscious processes does not require advocacy of a psychoanalytic (or of any other particular) formulation.

Rather than order a full-course meal of a psychodynamic view of any flavor (which may only lead to feeling bloated), the pragmatically wisest clinical option is to savor, à la carte, those specific psychodynamic mechanisms which can give coherence to, and guide the actual practice of, conjoint marital therapy. This selective use of psychodynamic concepts characterizes the integrative treatment approach discussed here.

PSYCHODYNAMICISM, SYSTEMS THEORY, AND
SOCIAL LEARNING THEORY

Human (family) systems are composed not only of triadic and dyadic subsystems but also, by definition, of individual subsystems. These individual subsystems themselves operate along multiple dimensions (e.g., biochemical, physiological, motoric, cognitive, affective). Individuals, unlike machines, are also characterized by a hierarchy of levels of psychological experience (e.g., conscious, preconscious, unconscious). Clinical attention to nonconscious aspects of psychological experience is not precluded by an adoption of a human systems view of families and marriages. In fact, it can be argued that it is a perversion of the notion of "thinking systems" to arbitrarily ignore intrapsychic factors, both conscious and unconscious, in intimate relationships. As Duhl and Duhl (1981) put it simply, "It is hard to kiss a system."

Thus, the implicit interactional rules of a marital dyad (which, it must be noted, are not observable, but must be inferred) begin somewhere, particularly with the expectations, both conscious and unconscious, of each partner. Such patterned regularities do not evolve randomly or *de novo* from repetitive interactional sequences. Dyadic relationship rules evolve from a complex and subtle interplay of the implicit rules of individuals (Gurman, 1978; Gurman & Knudson, 1978; Gurman *et al.,* 1978; Knudson *et al.,* 1980). As Sager (1976) argues, the overt and observable interactions of conflicted couples represent attempted solutions of individual intrapsychic difficulties on the part of each spouse.

Linking such observations to those of behavioral marriage therapists (e.g., Jacobson, 1981; Jacobson & Margolin, 1979; Jacobson & Weiss, 1978) regarding the reinforcement- and punishment-based mutual control that characterizes relationships, Gurman (1978) and Gurman and Knudson (1978) have emphasized that the most salient and fundamental exchanges in marriage involve the reciprocal exchange, over time, of behaviors that confirm each partner's projections and maintain a relatively consistent self-perception. Thus, each partner has reinforcement value (Weiss, 1978) for the other, but such reinforcement value is only secondarily and derivatively at the level of overt behavior; its behavior-maintaining power is drawn primarily from its recurrent confirmation of each spouse's self-perception and perception of his or her mate. As Jackson (1965) exemplified this view, "the marital quid pro quo . . . is a *metaphorical* statement of the marital relationship bargain; that is, how the couple had agreed to *define themselves* within this relationship" (p. 12, italics added). In such a view, the central aspect of mutual reinforcement contingencies is not the details of how specific behaviors are consequated; it is a bargain about definition of self. Parenthetically, it may be noted that a failure to differentiate between the surface structure and deep structure meanings of quid pro quo illustrates how clinically meaningful evaluation of therapeutic outcomes may be precluded by not addressing multiple levels of therapeutic goals (Gurman & Kniskern, 1981).

Observations such as these, which suggest how the intrapsychic, systemic, structural, and behavioral parameters of relationships are interrelated, carry the further implication that the intrapsychic dimensions and consequences of relationship interaction must form the psychological foundation of a comprehensive understanding of couples in conflict. Such as understanding, however, is, by itself, quite insufficient as a basis for generating clinically useful strategies, and, indeed, there are few techniques in the practice of marital therapy that have derived directly from an appreciation of the psychodynamics of intimate relationships. In fact, as I discuss below, many of the standard techniques of psychoanalytic psychotherapy are either unusable or relatively impotent in treating couples. As I have pointed out elsewhere (Gurman, 1978), "psychoanalytically oriented marriage therapy is largely 'analytic' in the way it organizes the complex material at hand and conceptualizes the nature of marital discord, but is, of necessity, quite pragmatic, if not eclectic, in its selection of actual therapeutic interventions" (p. 466).

It is within the framework thus far created that we now turn to the consideration of a number of principles for the conduct of marital therapy. These principles have two prominent characteristics: first, they may facilitate an integrative approach to treatment (i.e., one that acknowledges the interplay among different levels of psychological experience in relationships), and second, they are consonant with therapeutic efforts to establish a focus which is useful for treatment and one which may aid the marital therapist in achieving maximal clinical improvement on multiple psychological dimensions in the brief amount of time that is, so often, all that is available.

With these aims in mind, I will set forth, in the rest of this chapter, a number of treatment principles, which pertain to the following areas:

treatment goals and assessment, early intervention and the therapeutic alliance, midphase issues (including transference and countertransference, resistance, and the use of specific techniques), and termination.

TREATMENT GOALS AND ASSESSMENT

In an integrative, focused marital therapy, an overriding goal is to achieve change in each partner as well as in the marital interaction. While any relationship is "more than the sum of its parts," it is crucial to remember that it also *has* its parts. The behavior of each spouse is not always under interactional control, some influential family therapy views (e.g., Stanton, 1980, 1981) to the contrary not withstanding. A good deal of everyday behavior, including marital behavior, is under the control of self-administered consequences (e.g., Beck, Rush, Shaw, & Emery, 1979; Kanfer, 1975). Moreover, even behavior with obvious relationship consequences is probably never completely under relational control.

The marital agoraphobic pattern (Goldstein & Chambless, 1978) offers an illustration of this point par excellence. The phobic spouse's deficits in identifying the antecedents to anxiety arousal exist independently of the dyadic struggle over dependency and power. Conversely, while one spouse's symptoms certainly very often have communicational meaning for the relationship and often reflect a disturbance in the relationship, they need not have such functional value. Finally, to complete the picture, one partner's symptoms may reflect both that person's disturbance and that relationship's disturbance. A corollary of the position taken here is that, again contrary to many notions in the family therapy field regarding behavior maintenance and change, while change in one spouse necessarily changes the marital system, system change is not always required in order for change to occur in one member of the marital system. It is also consistent with this view to note that the psychiatrically diagnosable "pathology" of one partner can be either the direct result of interactional patterns or the necessary antecedent conditions for the production of pathological–dysfunctional interactions. The practical treatment implication of the view espoused here is that the marital therapist must be conceptually and technically skilled to bring about both intrapersonal and interpersonal change, the appropriate interventions for which are often not identical. The implications of this view for the assessment of identified patient change has been discussed by Gurman and Kniskern (1981).

In parallel fashion, an integrative marital therapy seeks to achieve two clinically interrelated, yet conceptually separable, goals: more accurate interpersonal perception, and more whole self-experiencing. From an object relations view of conjoint marital therapy, these goals are, in fact, inextricable. As Dicks (1967) noted, a marriage which is successful and is capable of managing inevitable conflict requires "a flexible readiness *in each partner* to change their role behavior in response to the other's needs of the moment" (p. 31, italics added). This individual flexibility of responsiveness is directly correlated with the rigidity–flexibility of each spouse's (interpersonal) perceptual capacities. Thus, each spouse's object relations schemata, that is, the structure for organizing experience and giving meaning to interpersonal events, constrain the way in which interpersonal messages are received (perceived). Hence, a poorly differentiated individual is necessarily restricted in the variety of available "decoding channels" for processing information. This restriction within an individual has important consequences for dyadic interaction, in that "the restriction in variety of any part of the system limits the system as a whole . . . a reduction in the variety [of the system or its subsystems] . . . will limit the ability of the system to adapt to new circumstances" (Raush, Barry, Hertel, & Swain, 1974, p. 25). Thus, rigid object relations schemata make it likely that such individuals will see their spouses in terms of past relationships or past marital experience instead of as Raush *et al.* (1974) put it, as "real contemporary people."

What must be achieved in therapy, in order for such perceptual capacities to be enhanced, is a loosening and broadening of each spouse's schemata, that is, the implicit matrix of assumptions, expectations and requirements of intimate interpersonal contact. This fundamental developmental task is accomplished by each spouse's exposure or reexposure to those aspects of him- or herself and his or her mate which are blocked from awareness, and which constitute the most salient impasse to knowing each other as whole persons. This aim is achieved only if each spouse is helped to acknowledge the aspects of him- or herself and his or her mate that are beyond overt observation as well as those that are immediately observable. Moreover, therapy usually must build behaviors in each partner that have been absent from their relationship repertoire because of the specific requirements of the couple's collusive agreement and because of skill deficits attributable to prior learning histories.

Thus, the most important and most challenging task of assessment is to identify the central issues that tap into both the conflictual and the developmental aspects of the marital relationship. As Sager (1981) notes, not all areas of the marriage relationship need to be dealt with clinically, since disharmony is usually determined and characterized by a few major issues. Nor is it necessary or even appropriate to deal with all the identifiable areas of each spouse's individual conflict. Indeed, aiming for such therapeutic perfectionism tolls the death knell for any focused method of brief psychotherapy (Malan, 1976; Wolberg, 1965). It is the interlocking individual conflicts and their reciprocal interlocking defenses that require focused evaluation. When a marital relationship is in crisis, it is usually the case that the collusion, which previously was bilaterally adaptive, is being challenged by a threat to the consistency of one or both partner's (implicit) self-definitions. Thus, more often than not, the couple's presenting problem(s) will contain the clues to the identification of these central interlocking conflicts, albeit often in disguised or derivative fashion. For most couples, these conflicts will be identified as involving issues of power and control, independence–dependence, or closeness–distance.

Since time is usually limited in marital therapy, the appropriate stance of the therapist during the assessment phase of treatment is not the "evenly hovering attention" of the psychoanalyst, but a confidently structured and focused investigation directed simultaneously toward both individuals and toward their joint "marital personality," as evidenced in their interaction.

The most effective assessment model for rapidly assaying those aspects of the marriage that are most closely linked to the couple's presenting complaints requires a balanced use of both interactional and psychodynamic assessment perspectives and methods. Thus, what is required is a simultaneous assessment of:

- the functional relationships (Karoly, 1975) between the antecedents and consequences, both overt and covert, of particular discrete behaviors and interaction sequences
- the recurrent patterns of interaction occurring in varying relationship content areas, including the implicit rules governing these redundancies
- each spouse's individual schemata for intimate relationships, and the joint, unspoken, interactional contracts (Sager, 1976, 1981) linking the two

While the functional analytic assessment approach of behavior therapists, which is limited to a concern with overt behaviors, may appear to be irreconcilable with more inferential psychodynamic approaches, their compatibility is, in fact, limited only by the constraints arbitrarily imposed by individual clinicians (i.e., therapists' own schemata for assessment). If (as I believe must be done in order to provide an integrative treatment) a marital therapist regards his or her own expertly trained inferences regarding the unobservable psychological events within and between marital partners as data useful for understanding human behavior, then the issue of incompatibility becomes moot.

THE THERAPEUTIC ALLIANCE AND EARLY INTERVENTION

The marital therapist routinely faces the problem of being caught between a technical Scylla and Charybdis early in treatment. On the one hand, the time available for therapeutic work is quite limited, so that the process of change induction cannot be delayed for very long, while on the other hand, a working alliance between the therapist and patient must be developed in order for the anxiety-evoking process of change to begin. From an integrative view of marital interactional change, the therapist's task is to balance the attention given to the most salient aspects of the couple's dynamic struggle with that given to their presenting problem(s) and to do this without compromising the therapeutic approach and while fostering a collaborative alliance with the couple.

Obviously, a therapist does not "stage" treatment in terms of first developing an alliance and then intervening to produce change. On the contrary, early intervention must be aimed at both establishing an alliance and producing meaningful change. Thus, all early interventions directed toward producing change within the marriage must also facilitate the patient–therapist alliance. Moreover, as Jacobson and Margolin (1979) emphasize so convincingly, the first phase of treatment must also be geared toward increasing collaboration between the spouses. Given the high level of resistance to change common to most couples in therapy (Gurman & Knudson, 1978; Gurman et al., 1978; Knudson et al., 1980; Stanton, 1980, 1981; Stuart, 1980), accomplishing the latter goal of husband–wife collaboration is itself a major undertaking, and the simultaneous achievement of a working patient–therapist alliance often seems to be an insurmountable task.

Elsewhere (Gurman, 1980b), I have detailed a number of approaches and techniques for establishing a working patient–therapist alliance. Here, I will briefly discuss the three major targets of early alliance building in conjoint couples therapy. While in most cases, the therapist must attend to all three dimensions simultaneously, the following order of priority identification of the first two targets is consonant with the view taken earlier—that both individual and dyadic change must occur in an integrative marital therapy.

Therapist-Marital Partner Alliance

This alliance between the therapist and each marital partner is the initial one that must be established, usually in the very first conjoint session. The best practical criterion of these alliances having been realized is phenomenological: each spouse must feel that something of personal value has been gained in the first contact. The method(s) by which such felt satisfaction is obtained varies from individual to individual. Some patients experience an alliance with the therapist as the result of no more dramatic an intervention than the therapist offering empathy and warmth (Gurman, 1977). Others require more structured responding, in terms of interactional insight (e.g., identification of repetitive interaction sequences) or genetic insight, and still others require at least minimal direction for behavior change outside the treatment context. Moreover, a husband and wife of the same couple may require different experiences in the first session with the therapist to feel a sense of a developing working alliance. While therapeutic attention must be given to each spouse, it need not routinely be given in equal amounts. For example, in the common situation in which conjoint therapy is begun in the context of one spouse's symptomatic presentation (e.g., depression, phobia), rather than in the context of the relationship being mutually presented as problematic, the nonsymptomatic spouse may need either a good deal more or a good deal less alliance-building attention than the symptomatic spouse, and the therapist must be able to discern this difference almost at once.

Therapist-Couple Alliance

The second alliance that needs to be fostered early in treatment is between the therapist and the couple *qua* couple. While the couple does not, of course, have a palpable, organismic existence as a psychological entity apart from the separate existence of each partner, it does have a behavioral and dynamic relatedness of the parts, which must be considered functionally in its own right. Thus, the therapist must identify early the paired, unspoken language which simultaneously bonds the partners together and creates the medium for the emergence of the current continuing conflict. The therapist must learn to speak to both spouses at the same time, even when overtly addressing only one of them. While this connectedness between therapist and couple must obtain throughout the longer middle phase of therapy as well, the groundwork for its therapeutic use must be laid early in the treatment process, usually within the first three sessions.

This alliance is most rapidly established by speaking to the mutually contingent manner in which the spouses collude to keep aspects of themselves and of the other spouse out of awareness. In contrast to the middle phase of therapy, when interpretation of the collusive process may be appropriately aimed at eliciting rather high levels of anxiety in each partner (see below), the interpretive aim here is to give tentative public acknowledgment of the main way in which the partners' overt struggles reflect the growth-oriented purposiveness of their initial attraction and commitment to one another.

Interpretation oriented toward this dyadic process simultaneously serves to strengthen the therapeutic marital alliance. This therapeutic marital alliance is meant to refer not to an increased feeling of commitment to the marriage per se (e.g., to its indefinite continuation by each partner) but simply to a felt sense of getting down to work in the treatment. In order to foster this alliance with the couple *qua* couple, the therapist must, of course, have obtained sufficient understanding of each spouse's individual relationship history and of the couple's joint history to be able to place the current marital struggle in developmental perspective.

Such interpretations, quite early in therapy, usually address issues about which the couple has rarely, if ever, overtly spoken. Therefore, they require an empathic therapeutic context. Nonetheless, despite the concerns of many marital therapists that to engage in such interpretive probing as discussed here would be premature, the offering of such an understanding is rejected only infrequently by one spouse and rarely by both. While the underlying dynamic struggles in the marriage may have been repressed for years, the mere emergence and current presence either of an overt relationship conflict or of relationally relevant individual symptomatology signifies that the hidden agendas and conflicts are, in the couple's phenomenology, closer to conscious expression.

Husband–Wife Alliance

Although it is strengthened by the therapist's focus on the therapist–couple alliance, the husband–wife alliance requires additional intervention aimed toward an acknowledgment of differences in personality style and equalization of fundamental relationship strivings. Couples in crisis, of course, can be predicted, with confidence, to detail and even exaggerate the differences in their overt styles of relating to one another, responding to conflict in life in general, and so forth. While many of these differences are often not only quite real, but also easily perceptible in early contacts with the couple, they must not obstruct the therapist's vision, thereby causing a failure to recognize the spouses' similarities, if not commonalities, regarding their most basic, unspoken relationship fears and needs. As Meissner (1978) notes somewhat pejoratively, couples "tend to choose partners who have achieved an equivalent level of immaturity, but who have adopted opposite patterns of defensive organization" (p. 43). Skynner (1976) stated this view more neutrally: "Couples are usually attracted by shared developmental failures" (p. 43). Illustrative of this thematic similarity is Barnett's (1971) discussion, referred to earlier, of the unifying dynamic similarity regarding intimacy, in obsessive–hysterical marriages, which may seem, on the surface, very much marriages of opposites.

The therapist's concrete goal here is to confront the couple with the fact that while they behave quite differently with each other in conflict situations, each of them is fundamentally struggling with the same categorical individual conflicts, and each is seeking the same relationship ends. While taking this position may seem, to some therapists, to be a mere tactic to foster marital collaboration in the therapy, its efficacy (and possibly its psychological accuracy) is attested to by the sense of relieved acceptance it so often receives when offered to couples.

In the early phase of therapy, as noted above, the therapist must be working simultaneously to establish the three sides of the theapeutic alliance and to produce some behavior change that is consistent with the couple's stated purposes for seeking treatment. In working toward the latter, of course, the therapist further strengthens his or her alliance with the couple and with each individual spouse. In the majority of cases, the most appropriate position to take is to work toward producing rapidly at least some perceptible improvement in each spouse's overt behavior or, as Stuart (1979) put it, to "build behaviors consistent with the couple's stated goals." Often, but certainly not always, this requires focusing on the most coercive, destructive, and distance-generating behavior patterns. In general, this is not the proper time for using paradoxical interventions. (The rationale for this position will be discussed later in this chapter.) What is called for here are more direct interventions, such as behavioral tasks (e.g., Stuart's, 1980, "caring days" procedure), boundary-regulating instructions, and conflict management and containment techniques.

MIDPHASE ISSUES

Transference, Resistance, and Countertransference
While transference issues are considered irrelevant for overt discussion by many marital therapists, especially those with strict behavioral (e.g., Jacobson & Margolin, 1979; Stuart, 1980) or systems theory (e.g., Stanton, 1980, 1981; Watzlawick *et al.,* 1974) leanings, they obviously require careful thought in a treatment method concerned with individual differences and intrapsychic experience as well as with interpersonal transactions. Unlike the individual psychotherapy setting, in which only one physically real transference pairing (patient–therapist) exists (of course, ghost transferences also exist, that is, transferences to persons not physically in the room yet psychologically present nonetheless), in conjoint marital therapy there exist four transference pairs: husband–wife, wife–husband, husband–therapist, and wife–therapist (and more, of course, if a cotherapist is involved). To deal conceptually with this array of transference potentials, three major issues need to be considered: (1) the extent to which the transference between each spouse and the therapist can be fostered in conjoint therapy, (2) the presumed necessity of therapeutic regression for positive and lasting change, and (3) the use and role of transference analysis in the context of an active and generally brief therapeutic encounter.

Three characteristics are generally required of a psychotherapeutic treatment in order for a transference neurosis to develop. They limit tremendously the possibility of safeguarding the transference in couples therapy, however, and by traditional psychoanalytic standards, they virtually guarantee its contamination. They are (1) a long course of treatment, (2) limited participation of the therapist as a real object, and (3) relative constancy of the therapist's behavior. The limitations upon the development of transference neuroses imposed by the brevity of couples therapy are obvious. Moreover, the therapist's relative constancy and anonymity are difficult, if not impossible, to achieve in couples work. While the patient–therapist transference is thus diluted in marital therapy, this need not be destructive of the therapeutic encounter in general or, in particular, of the use of the patient–therapist relationship to further the therapeutic aims. This latter point is elaborated below. In addition to the fact that significant clinical changes have been documented in marital therapy in the absence of major therapeutic regression (Gurman & Kniskern, 1981; Jacobson, 1978), the issue is essentially moot, since, as already noted, transference neuroses have little likelihood of developing, given the structured aspects of most couples therapy. This is especially due to the requirement for a clear focus (or series of foci) which is developed in an active collaboration between patients and therapist, thereby largely demystifying the role and person of the therapist.

Transference reactions, as distinct from transference neuroses, do, of course, emerge commonly in couples therapy. As Wachtel (1977) emphasized, the patient's transference reactions to the therapist are not solely the result of misplaced and anachronistic interpersonal perceptions; they must be understood as the patient's "idiosyncratic way of construing and reacting to what the therapist is doing—and the therapist is never doing 'nothing', even when he is being silent or reflecting back a question instead of answering it" (p. 112). Thus, transference reactions in a focused marital therapy include important information on each partner's feelings, perceptions, misperceptions, and attributions of intent, motivation, and loyalties concerning specific therapist interventions.

Focusing primary attention on the patient–therapist transference will divert the therapist from what is both the major source of resistance and the major potential source of an individual's growth in marriage. The most powerful transference relationships in couples therapy exist between the husband and wife and between each spouse and his or her family of origin. Indeed, it can be said that working toward the resolution of a limited number of currently relevant, bilateral marital transference patterns is the aim in all efforts to modify a couple's interactional contract (Sager, 1976, 1981). As Sager (1981) also notes, with particular relevance to brief marital therapy, "In the short run, the greatest aid in getting to unconscious material is each spouse's understanding of the other's deepest needs" (p. 115). Thus, regardless of the extent to which marital conflict reflects ongoing transferential reactions to past relationship experiences, current interaction not only may reinforce such reactions but may also produce secondary (but very real and salient) difficulties that must be treated independently of this historical underpinnings. A therapist can change the impact of past experiences on present behavior only by changing present behavior and ways of construing one's experience.

Given this perspective on the nature of the multiple transferences in conjoint marital therapy, two additional guidelines for the therapist's intervention may be specified. First, because time is often quite limited, it is important that the therapist address actively and overtly any significant evidence of negative transference reactions on the part of either spouse. While it is counterproductive in such a brief therapy to address a broad range of such reactions, it is essential that those negative reactions that clearly block progress toward the achievement of the partners' stated goals be addressed as they appear. Some marital therapists have taken the position that when one spouse manifests such negative reactions, he or she is speaking for the other spouse as well, even though the latter may deny any negative feelings about either the therapist or the therapy process. My experience has been that while this is sometimes the case, it is not routinely true.

Two strategies for responding to clear and significant negative transference reactions are useful. First, the feelings and thoughts of the spouse who is presenting negative transference reactions or, for that matter, any important change-blocking resistance must not be disregarded, nor should they lead to the presumptuous interpretation that the patient is speaking for his or her spouse as much as for him- or herself. Early in therapy, especially, offering such a universal interpretation may seriously damage the progress that has been made in establishing a working alliance with that spouse. Still, keeping such an interpretive possibility in mind, the therapist must inquire of the second spouse what his or her thoughts and feelings are regarding what the mate has expressed. In this way, the focus of the therapist's response is not upon the resistance to the therapist's efforts at inducing change, but rather upon the meaning of such resistance for the marital relationship. This emphasis, of course, follows from the position taken earlier that the husband–wife transferences are at the core of both therapeutic change and blocks to such change.

Finally, it must be underscored that the potential for countertransferential acting out is heightened for the marital therapist under such goal-oriented, active, and relatively self-revealing conditions as are inherent in conjoint treatment. As difficult as it is to avoid unconsciously colluding with the patient in individual treatment, it may be more difficult to do so in marital therapy, because it is nearly impossible for most marital therapists not to encounter, in their own current intimate relationships, the painful issues involved in the relationships of patient couples, and because the therapist's level of activity does not allow a great deal of time and opportunity for in-process self-reflection. Because of the power of couples' problems to elicit such reality-focused concerns in therapists, untoward countertransference reactions probably reflect conscious attitudes, beliefs, and values as much as they may reflect unconscious conflict in the therapist.

Intervention Techniques

Elaboration of a truly representative range of specific intervention techniques, consonant with goals of the approach to couples therapy presented here, is beyond the scope of this chapter. Nonetheless, an active, focused, and usually brief course of therapy should be technically characterized by three principles of therapist activity. These are (1) interruption of collusive processes, (2) linking individual experience to the marital relationship, and (3) creating therapeutic tasks.

The therapist must persistently track, label, and interrupt the marital collusive process as it occurs in treatment sessions. When a marital therapist intervenes to change this dysfunctional mutual defensive process, he or she necessarily is involved in implicitly challenging the rules of the relationship. As I have argued elsewhere (Gurman, 1978), collusion requires paradoxical communication for its maintenance and, at the same time, produces paradoxical communication. As suggested earlier, the two major ways in which collusion may be seen to operate are (1) when either spouse fails to see aspects of his or her mate which are quite perceptible to an observer, and (2) when either spouse behaves in a manner aimed at protecting his or her mate from engaging in behaviors and experiences that are inconsistent with the latter's definition of self in intimate relationships, and would therefore be anxiety-arousing.

The marital therapist must consistently translate events or experiences that are of significance to one spouse as an individual into the meaning they carry for the other spouse as an individual and for the relationship in its interactional sense. Consistent with the position taken earlier, a disregard in marital therapy for intrapsychic events is not only arbitrary but also therapeutically limiting. It is quite acceptable and even desirable that a good deal of what may appear to an outside observer to be individual therapy occurs in an integrative couples therapy. The only serious danger in doing such individually focused work in couples therapy is that it might be left unconnected to the marital interaction. The main dangers in so doing are that the therapist may become so fascinated with the experiences of one spouse that he or she begins to implicitly, though unwittingly, identify that spouse as either the "ill" partner or the "attractive" partner in the marriage, so that the second spouse's anxiety is nontherapeutically avoided or diminished, or conversely, that such untranslated individual work alienates the other spouse, who may perceive a special alliance being developed from which he or she feels excluded.

The therapist must sensitively present therapeutic tasks that are in accord with each spouse's behavior change objectives and that simultaneously address each spouse's needs and fears in the marital relationship. The marital therapist, like any psychotherapist, is obliged to attempt to produce symptomatic improvement that is consistent with the patient's expressed goals. Toward such ends, as Freud (1904/1953) stated long ago, in a different context, "there are many ways and means of practicing psychotherapy. All that lead to recovery are good" (p. 259). Thus, both an attitude of technical flexibility and a concrete mastery of a rather broad range of intervention skills are requisite for the marital therapist. Still, marital therapist should be willing to work for change at the content and symptom level only so long as such intervention is not likely to produce negative effects at the metalevel (Gurman & Knudson, 1978), such as when honoring requests for help in producing particular behavior changes may be antagonistic to the psychological growth of women (cf. Gurman & Klein, 1980, in press). Tasks certainly include, but are not limited to, concrete homework "assignments" given to patient couples to be carried out outside the treatment sessions. They also include the creation of experiences within the sessions that have two separable yet synergistic goals: the teaching of adaptive interpersonal skills, and the exposure of spouses to aspects of themselves and of each other which are beyond awareness, yet which are clearly central to the major contractual or collusive impasse to each individual's and the couple's growth. In the terms used here, such tasks may include, but are not limited to:

- encouraging each spouse to differentiate between the experiential impact of one spouse's behavior on the other, on the one hand, and the intent attributed to that person's behavior
- requiring that each spouse interrupt behavior that is aimed toward reducing anxiety in the other spouse, especially when that spouse is behaving in ways that are historically contrary to the couple's collusive interactional contract
- having each spouse attend to concrete evidence in the behavior of his or her partner that denies similarly anachronistic perceptions of that partner, with particular emphasis on behavior that occurs within the therapy hour
- in like fashion, encouraging each spouse to directly acknowledge his or her own behavioral changes that are incompatible with the maladaptive ways in which the patient has tended to see him- or herself and to be seen by the marital partner

Each of these tasks suggests self-evident requirements of the therapist's activity, such that minor rephrasing of these tasks identifies the necessary work to be done by the therapist. Nonetheless, these tasks are viewed here as those of the couple, rather than of the therapist, in that the behavior asked of the patients requires focused effort and purposeful activity that is, initially, emotionally difficult to perform. Note that this emphasis on the patients', as distinct from the therapist's, task is fully in accord with the principle set forth earlier: that the therapist's attention to the bilateral transference within the couple is far more important in marital therapy than is attention to the patient–therapist transference.

The sorts of anticollusive tasks just described are conceived as facilitating change by directly modifying each spouse's self-experiencing and experiencing of his or her mate. In general, it is preferable that such therapist-orchestrated experiences within the therapy session precede, rather than follow, the presentation to the couple of cognitive explanations (i.e., interpretations of the underlying dynamic struggles addressed by these tasks). In most cases, prior explanation of such issues are counterproductive, in that they may be misused by the couple to impose so much structure to the tasks that the level of anxiety potentially associated with engaging in the tasks is quite limited. Thus, the potential for experiencing, rather than talking about, new ways of being with one's self and one's mate is constrained. Moreover, some marital therapists, and even therapists with enormously different views of the therapy process, argue strongly, if not vehemently, that almost any interpretation by the marital therapist is either unnecessary for change (e.g., Stanton, 1981) or even antithetical to it (Whitaker & Keith, 1981).

The view espoused here is that helping patients acquire and develop a cognitive understanding of the developmental forces in their relationship, the current implicit rules that govern some aspects of their relationship, the maritally relevant functions of defenses, and the like is very useful on two levels. First, such cognitive understanding can help couples learn to self-monitor their own internal experiences and to relate these intrapsychic experiences to interpersonal events. Thus, the therapist's interpretative activity serves to integrate the patients' affective, cognitive, and behavioral experiences. This integrative purpose is best achieved by therapist interpretations which "track" the sequences of events in the affective, cognitive, and behavioral spheres, in a manner similar to the behavior therapist's functional analysis of behavior, in which attention is focused on the antecedents to, and consequences of, given behaviors, and which selectively tie together past and present relationship experiences.

The sort of functional analysis referred to here, however, differs from the strict behavioral use of the term in two ways. First, the target behaviors considered in the analysis are not limited to discrete, single behavioral events but may and often do include a sequence of events. The second difference is that in the present approach, the antecedents and consequences of interest need not be limited to overt behavior (or physical stimuli) but may also include cognitive events (e.g., thoughts, attributions, interpretations) and affective events (e.g., feelings of anger, joy, despair, fear).

The second pragmatic value of interpretation is that it helps couples develop a "cognitive map" of multiple levels of their relationship experience, which facilitates the generalization of therapeutic effects and their durability.

The Role and Use of Behavioral Techniques

As should by now be clear, in an integrative marital therapy, the therapist's interventions may center, at different times, on affective, cognitive, or behavioral (including motoric) events. As I have pointed out elsewhere (e.g., Gurman, 1978), all the dominant psychodynamic approaches to marriage therapy (e.g., Martin, 1976; Nadelson, 1978; Sager, 1976, 1981) routinely include the use of techniques which are either usually associated with the practice of behavioral marital and family therapies or clearly derived from developments in that area. I have become convinced, through my own clinical experience, that this has occurred for two reasons. First, that given the constraints in couples therapy in using standard psychoanalytic techniques, the couple's overt behavior and verbal self-reports are the predominant psychological data available for direct intervention. Second and, I believe, even more significant, though rarely discussed in the marital therapy literature (cf. Gurman, 1980a), many commonly used behavioral methods can facilitate the process of helping marital partners to reintegrate denied aspects of themselves and each other, that is, to work toward the fundamental, reintegrative goals of the treatment approach described in this chapter.

Marital partners must be exposed to aspects of themselves and their mates which are blocked from awareness. This exposure can be accomplished—and, in fact, from a technical vantage point, may need to be accomplished—in a manner analogous to the way in which well-known behavioral techniques, such as systematic desensitization or anxiety management training, teach coping and/or mastery of anxiety-eliciting stimuli. This notion of exposure in integrative marital therapy is identical in principle to the use of exposure treatments of fears and phobias (e.g., Marks, 1978). But it differs from its usual use in individual behavior therapy in two ways. First, to set up a formal and systematic hierarchy of anxiety-eliciting stimuli in couples therapy, as would occur in individual behavioral exposure treatment, is unmanageably cumbersome, since there obviously exist multiple hierarchical themes (i.e., each mate has his or her own theme or themes). Moreover, the themes of each spouse do not operate independently of themes of the mate, so that it would be enormously taxing for the therapist to attempt to unite these reciprocal and interactive themes on a single dimension.

The second obvious difference from the usual use of exposure treatment in behavior therapy is that the anxiety-eliciting stimuli of clinical concern are events and experiences that occur within the patient, not outside the patient, as in the exposure treatment of, say, a height phobia. Even in this regard, however, there is a good deal of overlap with the individual behavioral exposure treatment of some disorders, such as agoraphobia, in which it is the private experience, both cognitively and physiologically, of the patient which provides the anxiety-arousing stimuli (Chambless & Goldstein, 1980; Goldstein & Chambless, 1978).

Obviously, then, the tasks set forth by the marital therapist must be sensitive to the idiosyncratic meanings likely to be attached to any important, direct behavior change intervention, so that the level of anxiety aroused is not so great as to lead to rejection of the task (or of the therapist), unless, as Sager (1981) notes, the therapist's aim is to have the task rejected for a predictable therapeutic purpose. Except for the latter such purpose, the therapist's goal in posing such tasks is to have the spouses learn by experience that unacceptable aspects of themselves and their mates need not be overwhelming. As this aim is being achieved, it often becomes progressively easier for couples to negotiate changes in overt behavior.

While many behavioral techniques are quite compatible with the general model and goals of integrative marital therapy, it must be emphasized that, for two reasons, a focus on overt behavior change alone is not in keeping with the major tenets of this approach. First, as should be clear from what has preceded in this chapter, the overt behavioral parameters of marital interaction are viewed as a reflection (not in whole, but to a clinically significant degree) of the interlocking of each spouse's most fundamental self-perceptions and as the vehicle for attempting to adhere to familiar anxiety-reducing defenses.

On a more pragmatic, clinical level, a corollary of this view is that each spouse must come to feel allied with the therapist against the behavior described as undesirable. Since few patients are consciously aware of the change-resistant value of these behaviors or of the value of these behaviors in maintaining a consistent self-perception and self-experiencing, the implementation of direct behavior change interventions very early in therapy may often serve only to increase anxiety at a point in treatment at which these troublesome yet derivative behaviors remain largely egosyntonic.

Here, I briefly illustrate the ways in which some of the most common types of behavioral interventions can help remove the intrapersonal and interpersonal blocks in the way of fuller experiencing of one's self and one's mate.

Communication Training and Problem-Solving Training. These may offer some of the most direct, available antidotes to unconscious collusion and "splitting." Poor marital communication and problem-solving skills are almost routinely predictable from an observed marital pattern of paradoxical communication, and such a communicational style and such skills deficits are required in order to maintain unconscious collusion and, in particular, the use of projective identification. In essence, then, poor social skills in a marital relationship themselves often reflect the more basic rule of minimal intimacy, self-disclosure, and self-exposure. Thus, to challenge these rules by explicit teaching of interpersonal skills is to challenge the collusive defenses, in the service of which the skill deficits exist. Obviously, then, explicit attention to the defensive functions of such skill deficits for individuals and for the stability of their relationship is necessary in order to prevent undermining of therapeutic efforts toward direct behavior change.

While remaining attentive to the defensive functions of poor communication and problem-solving skills, the marital therapist should also more optimistically consider that such behavioral skill-training procedures require that

- the spouses speak only for themselves, not for others
- they assume responsibility for their own thoughts and feelings
- they systematically track their own affective and cognitive experience
- they focus on current intrapersonal and interpersonal events
- they desist from the idealized and defensive stance that the other spouse should be able to know what they want without having to be asked

- they attend to their own interactional contribution to displeasing relationship patterns

Moreover, the teaching of both communication and problem-solving skills implicitly places value on

- an integrated and necessary balance between the cognitive and affective components in intimate relationships

Of course, effective communication training with couples requires that each spouse first be aware of his or her own personal, private experiencing. In the absence of such awareness, implementation of structured communication-training exercises may challenge existing individual and dyadic defenses too much and thus fail. For this reason, a heavy emphasis on enhancing communication skills should not generally characterize very early therapy sessions, just as other direct behavior change techniques are usually contradicted in the first few sessions, as noted earlier.

Teaching Spouses Positive Reinforcement Techniques. This intervention, which aims at increasing the spouse's "desired" behavior, often has the correlated effect on inhibiting the couple's proclivities to engage in projective identification. Spouses often identify as unwanted those behaviors in their mate which stimulate anxiety about their own impulses, needs, desires, or styles of relating, processing information, or responding to conflict. Direct instruction to positively reinforce desired spouse behaviors implicitly requires the partner to acknowledge aspects of the mate which are minimized or discounted, that is, blocked from awareness. When such directive reinforcement methods are consistently complied with, and if the mate's behavior changes as consciously desired, it may be assumed that the level of anxiety aroused in the spouse by this forced reality testing was not severe, so that simple, though unlabeled exposure to the cues usually leading to defensive actions has led to extinction of the associated anxiety. On the other hand, persistent noncompliance with such an approach may signify the intensity of the projective process and allow the therapist to redirect his or her attention to the desperation with which the spouse clings to a negative perception of the mate's behavior. Such a formulation, while not offered as a universal explanation of noncompliance with prosocial behavioral reinforcement methods, can put some conceptual meat on the skeleton of what Gordon and Davidson (1981) atheoretically and rather euphemistically refer to as "interpersonal interference factors," which prevent effective use of reinforcement strategies in parent training, where the same methods are used to teach patients to increase desired behaviors in other family members.

I have shown how the application of some common behavioral marital therapy techniques can indirectly counteract collusive and projective processes in marriage, serve as a rapid means for assessing the interplay between intrapersonal and interpersonal sources of resistance to change, and produce behavior change consistent with the couple's stated goals. Hopefully, this brief discussion has illustrated the potential for rapprochement between a psychodynamic understanding of marital process and a behavioral methodology for producing therapeutic change.

The Role and Use of Paradox

As Stanton (1981) puts it quite clearly, strategic therapists (the marital therapists most likely to use paradoxical intervention) "will employ skill and maneuvering to get covert control of the therapy." These therapists "differ from behavioral therapists in being much more indirect" in their efforts to induce behavior change. Frequent use of such paradoxical interventions in the treatment of a couple assumes that "the family has self-perpetuating properties. Therefore, processes that the therapist initiates within the family will be maintained in his absence by the family's self-regulatory mechanisms" (Minuchin, 1974, p. 14). Stated otherwise, such systems approaches assume, then, that natural reinforcement will take over once the problematic interaction pattern has been changed and will result in extratherapy generalization. Predictably, then, in this view, little or no skill training or interpretation of marital interaction dynamics is required.

In an integrative marital therapy, the concern is with what the couple takes away from therapy in addition to symptom reduction. The integrative marital therapist will also be concerned that the therapist's use of covert and indirect influence may model such style for the couple, which, of course, is antithetical to many of integrative therapy goals discussed earlier in this chapter. In an integrative model, it is believed that durable clinical change is most likely to occur when couples learn new, effective modes of achieving their interpersonal aims and learn them in such a way as to promote self-change after therapy has ended. Hence, paradoxical instructions (e.g., prescribing the symptom, symptom scheduling), while they may be employed very selectively in integrative marital therapy, are rarely the central interventions used to achieve the major clinical changes desired. On the other hand, what may be called "paradoxical commentary," such as "positive connotation" or "ascribing noble intention" (Stanton, 1981) may be used fruitfully and in accord with the major reintegrative goal of therapy, which is to help spouses relate more as whole persons. Skynner (1981) expressed this view exquisitely:

> *All* double-binds and other paradoxical communications are attempts to maintain a fantasy world, different from reality, by expressing *both* fantasy and reality at the same time in a form which conceals the discrepancy between the two, and also by conveying at the same time a "command" to others to collude with the "self-deception" and so preserve the speaker's fantasy world (or the joint fantasy of the marriage or family). Paradoxical *therapeutic* interventions can then be seen not as "tricks" but as expressions of the most essential truth, which subtly break the rule that fantasy and reality must be kept apart, by relating the two in a disguised, seemingly innocent fashion which expresses only the positive aspects. Once the family or couple accept the bait, they cannot avoid seeing more than appeared to be implied in the original paradoxical intervention. (p. 76)

As Papp (1980) noted, "The target of the systemic paradox is this *hidden interaction* that expresses itself in a symptom" (p. 46, italics added). Psychodynamic models also assume that part of the hidden interaction is the complex of unconscious contracts, collusions, and mutual agreements not to emerge as whole persons. Thus, in integrative therapy, paradoxical commentary aims to make explicit the covert interactions which produce symptoms or marital distress, so that they may be better understood, and so that the conflicts they reflect surreptitiously may be handled by the couple overtly.

As noted earlier, the use of paradoxical interventions very early in couples therapy is rarely appropriate. There are two reasons for this. First, paradoxical interventions are not the strategy of choice for couples who comply with the requirements of their patient role; they are to be reserved for situations of major noncompliance (Papp, 1980). Of course, "compliance" is a relativistic notion, and as emphasized earlier, most couples will show at least some resistance to change in therapy. The crucial issue that the therapist must address is, thus, not whether noncompliance exists, but whether and how readily it can be overcome, especially by the use of more direct interventions, such as further development of the therapeutic alliance, confrontation or interpretation, or instructional reiteration of the importance of the couple's following the therapist's ground rules for therapy, especially those subsumed under any of the types of tasks discussed earlier. As any experienced therapist knows, direct dealing with the couple's resistance to change often yields more therapeutic change and improvement than a single-minded focus on presenting problems, target complaints, and the like. Except in rare circumstances, it is unwise and probably countertherapeutic for the therapist to assume (based, for example, on the couple's previous treatment history or identified patient diagnosis) that noncompliance both is and will remain severe. Rather, a more experimental attitude is called for, whereby assessments and/or predictions of major noncompliance are tested in response to interventions aimed at overcoming such resistance. In general, at least a few treatment sessions are required in order to gather concrete, experiential evidence to either support or refute such predictions.

The second reason why paradoxical intervention is rarely appropriate in very early sessions is that, in order for the therapist to formulate accurately the paradoxical intervention, he or she must develop a penetrating understanding of the hidden dynamics and functions of the major presenting symptom or, where one spouse is not initially a symptom bearer, of the most salient distressing interaction patterns. While such a rich formulation may be easier to come by when a therapist operates as part of a therapeutic team (e.g., Papp, 1980; Selvini-Palazzoli, Boscolo, Cecchin, & Prata, 1978), most marital therapists are not fortunate enough to have this advantage. Except in those rare cases of a very gifted therapist or in the presence of a couple whose dynamics are immediately obvious, such an understanding of the most basic hidden interaction underlying a symptom or interaction pattern is not achieved readily. Indeed, except in the infrequent circumstances just mentioned, it is probably a useful rule of thumb for the therapist to assume that when such a fundamental appreciation of the couple's hidden dynamics appears in the first session or two, it is probably either quite inaccurate or incomplete.

An additional issue in the timing of paradoxical interventions may be considered. Coopersmith (1980) usefully outlined the components and steps in the proper delivery of a paradoxical prescription in family therapy:

1. overt identification of the functions of a symptom (which, as noted, can also include the functions of a dominant interaction pattern)
2. positive connotation of the recurrent behaviors of concern
3. attribution volitional control of those behaviors
4. the prescription to continue those behaviors, or some variation thereof (e.g., to increase their rate, frequency, intensity)

The first two components comprise the essence of what I referred to before as paradoxical commentary. The use of these two components in tandem calls for no observable behavioral action or change by the couple. Thus, even while the therapist's understanding of the hidden interactions and dynamics is still being formulated, as in very early therapy sessions, such paradoxical commentary may be offered tentatively, with a quality of working collaboratively with the couple to generate useful hypotheses about what maintains their dysfunctional and distressing behavior. But, as noted, progressing to using the third and fourth components, defined by Coopersmith (1980), should generally be delayed a while longer.

THE TERMINATION OF MARITAL THERAPY

The termination of marital therapy in clearly unsuccessful cases may occur abruptly and with a good deal of intensity and even anger on the part of the couple or, more often, of one spouse. Successful cases, however, will end more gradually and with greater equanimity. Since the transference involvement from couple to therapist is not usually very intense, as emphasized at numerous points in this chapter, and is not a major focus of the therapeutic experience, the patients' loss of the therapist is felt much less profoundly than in most psychodynamically oriented brief individual therapies (e.g., Malan, 1976; Mann, 1973). The task for the couple at this point, of course, is to continue the integration of what has been experienced and learned in treatment into their everyday lives, without the help of a therapist.

Still, it has been the experience of many experienced marital therapists that it is not unusual for a terminated couple to return for help anywhere from several months to several years after the initial termination of their therapy. While such an occurrence may signal either an ineffective or an incomplete initial course of treatment, this generally is not the case. Quite the contrary, such a return more often indicates not only that a positive working alliance has been established, but also that the couple derived benefit from their initial therapeutic experience. Since marriage is a developmental process and not merely a demographic fact, a couple's return for further work is often quite appropriate.

CONCLUSION

In this chapter, I have argued that if marital therapy is likely to achieve durable and generalizable outcomes in the brief time usually available for the therapeutic work, it needs to address multiple levels and domains of the marital relationship. Moreover, I have argued that the most appropriate theoretical foundation for an integrative understanding of marital interaction, dynamics, and change is to be found in psychodynamic thinking, especially in a focused use of certain concepts originating in object relations theory. On the other hand, these dynamic models have, in the past, suggested few guides to the necessary technical aspects of the work. It has been argued that such technical guidelines can, in fact, be derived from thinking in an interpersonal–psychodynamic framework, and that, moreover, an impressive number of techniques historically associated with methods of therapy that pay little attention to psychodynamic issues can be used to facilitate both direct behavior change and changes in the structural dynamics of the married couple.

Finally, it can be suggested that the use of an integrative approach to marital therapy may also serve to help marital therapists integrate their own professional skills and knowledge and, in so doing, help keep them open to thinking flexibly, incorporating new information and understanding, and perhaps even broadening their own personal schemata for intimate relationships.

ACKNOWLEDGMENTS

I am grateful to several colleagues for their critical reading of a first draft of this chapter. Thanks are extended to Simon Budman, Howard Dichter, Sharon Foster, Laura Giat, David Rice, and Dorothea Torstenson.

REFERENCES

Ables, B., & Brandsma, J. *Therapy for couples.* San Francisco: Jossey-Bass, 1977.

Alexander, F., & French, T. M. *Psychoanalytic therapy: Principles and applications.* New York: Ronald Press, 1946.

Andolfi, M. Personal communication, 1978.

Andolfi, M. *Family therapy: An interactional approach.* New York: Plenum Press, 1979.

Aponte, H., & VanDeusen, J. M. Structural family therapy. In A. Gurman & D. Kniskern (Eds.), *Handbook of family therapy.* New York: Brunner/Mazel, 1981.

Barnett, J. Narcissism and dependency in the obsessional–hysteric marriage. *Family Process,* 1971, *10,* 75–83.

Beck, A. T., Rush, A. J., Shaw, B. F., & Emery, G. *Cognitive therapy of depression.* New York: Guilford Press, 1979.

Bentovim, A. The rejected scapegoated child. In A. Gurman (Ed.), *Questions and answers in the practice of family therapy.* New York: Brunner/Mazel, 1981.

Bentovim, A., & Kinston, W. Brief focal family therapy when the child is the referred patient: I. Clinical. *Journal of Child Psychology and Psychiatry,* 1978, *19,* 1–12.

Bergin, A. E. The evaluation of therapeutic outcomes. In A. Bergin & S. Garfield (Eds.), *Handbook of psychotherapy and behavior change.* New York: Wiley, 1971.

Bergin, A. E., & Lambert, M. The evaluation of therapeutic outcomes. In S. Garfield & A. Bergin (Eds.), *Handbook of psychotherapy and behavior change* (2nd ed.). New York: Wiley, 1978.

Berman, E. M., & Lief, H. I. Marital therapy from a psychiatric perspective: An overview. *American Journal of Psychiatry,* 1975, *132,* 583–592.

Berman, E., Lief, H., Williams, A. M., & Green, S. A model of marital interaction. In G. P. Sholevar (Ed.), *Marriage is a family affair.* New York: Spectrum Press, 1980.

Birchler, G. R., & Spinks, S. Behavioral-systems marital and family therapy: Integration and clinical application. *American Journal of Family Therapy,* 1980, *8,* 6–28.

Bodin, A. The family therapy approaches of the Mental Research Institute. In A. Gurman & D. Kniskern (Eds.), *Handbook of family therapy.* New York: Brunner/Mazel, 1981.

Bowen, M. The use of family theory in clinical practice. *Comprehensive Psychiatry,* 1966, *7,* 345–374.

Bowen, M. Theory in the practice of psychotherapy. In P. Guerin (Ed.), *Family therapy.* New York: Gardner, 1976.

Broderick, C. B., & Shrader, S. The history of professional marriage and family therapy. In A. Gurman & D. Kniskern (Eds.), *Handbook of family therapy.* New York: Brunner/Mazel, 1981.

Butcher, J., & Koss, M. Research on brief and crises-oriented therapies. In S. Garfield & A. Bergin (Eds.), *Handbook of psychotherapy and behavior change* (2nd ed.). New York: Wiley, 1978.

Chambless, D., & Goldstein, A. The treatment of agoraphobia. In A. Goldstein & E. Foa (Eds.), *Handbook of behavioral interventions.* New York: Wiley, 1980.

Coopersmith, E. *Strategic family therapy: A team approach.* Workshop presented at the annual meeting of the Ontario Association for Marriage and Family Therapy, London, Ontario, April 1980.

Dicks, H. V. *Marital tensions.* New York: Basic Books, 1967.

Duhl, B., & Duhl, F. Integrative family therapy. In A. Gurman & D. Kniskern (Eds.), *Handbook of family therapy.* New York: Brunner/Mazel, 1981.

Feldman, L. Marital conflict and marital intimacy: An integrative psychodynamic–behavioral–systemic model. *Family Process,* 1979, *18,* 69–78.

Ferenczi, S. *Further contribution to the theory and technique of psychoanalysis.* London: Hogarth Press, 1950. (Originally published, 1920.)

Framo, J. Integration of marital therapy with sessions family of origin. In A. Gurman & D. Kniskern (Eds.), *Handbook of family therapy.* New York: Brunner/Mazel, 1981.

Freud, S. On psychotherapy. In J. Strachey (Ed.), *The standard edition of the complete psychological works of Sigmund Freud* (Vol. 7). London: Hogarth Press, 1953. (Originally published, 1904.)

Garfield, S. L. Research on client variables in psychotherapy. In A. Bergin & S. Garfield (Eds.), *Handbook of psychotherapy and behavior change.* New York: Wiley, 1971.

Garfield, S. L., & Kurtz, R. A study of eclectic values. *Journal of Consulting and Clinical Psychology,* 1977, *45,* 78–83.

Goldstein, A., & Chambless, D. A reanalysis of agoraphobia. *Behavior Therapy,* 1978, *9,* 47–59.

Gordon, S., & Davidson, N. Behavioral parent training. In A. Gurman & D. Kniskern (Eds.), *Handbook of family therapy:* New York: Brunner/Mazel, 1981.

Guerin, P. Family therapy: The first twenty-five years. In P. Guerin (Ed.), *Family therapy.* New York: Gardner Press, 1976.

Gurman, A. S. Group marital therapy: Clinical and empirical implications for outcome research. *International Journal of Group Psychotherapy*, 1971, *21*, 174-189.

Gurman, A. S. Some therapeutic implications of marital therapy research. In A. Gurman & D. Rice (Eds.), *Couples in conflict*. New York: Jason Aronson, 1975.

Gurman, A. S. The patient's perception of the therapeutic relationship. In A. Gurman & A. Razin (Eds.), *Effective psychotherapy: A handbook of research*. New York: Pergamon Press, 1977.

Gurman, A. S. Contemporary marital therapies: A critique and comparative analysis of psychoanalytic, behavioral and systems theory approaches. In T. Paolino, Jr., & B. McCrady (Eds.), *Marriage and marital therapy*. New York: Brunner/Mazel, 1978.

Gurman, A. S. Dimensions of marital therapy: A comparative analysis. *Journal of Marital and Family therapy*, 1979, *5*, 5-16.

Gurman, A. S. Behavioral marriage therapy in the 1980's: The challenge of integration. *American Journal of Family Therapy*, 1980, 86-96.(a)

Gurman, A. S. Creating a therapeutic alliance in marital therapy. *American Journal of Family Therapy*, 1980, in press. (b)

Gurman, A. S., & Klein, M. H. Marital and family conflict. In A. M. Brodsky & R. T. Hare-Mustin (Eds.), *Women and psychotherapy: An assessment of research and practice*. New York: Guilford Press, 1980.

Gurman, A. S., & Klein, M. H. Women and behavioral marriage and family therapy: An unconscious male bias? In E. Blechman (Ed.), *Current issues in behavior modification with women*. New York: Guilford Press, in press.

Gurman, A. S., & Kniskern, D. P. Behavioral marriage therapy: II. Empirical perspective. *Family Process*, 1978, *17*, 139-148. (a)

Gurman, A. S., & Kniskern, D. P. Research on marital and family threapy: Progress, perspective and prospect. In S. L. Garfield & A. E. Bergin (Eds.), *Handbook of psychotherapy and behavior change* (2nd ed.). New York: Wiley, 1978. (b)

Gurman, A. S., & Kniskern, D. P. Family therapy outcome research: Knowns and unknowns. In A. Gurman & D. Kniskern (Eds.), *Handbook of family therapy*. New York: Brunner/Mazel, 1981.

Gurman, A. S., & Knudson, R. M. Behavioral marriage therapy: I. A psychodynamic-systems analysis and critique. *Family Process*, 1978, *17*, 123-138.

Gurman, A. S., Knudson, R. M., & Kniskern, D. P. Behavioral marriage therapy: IV. Take two aspirin and call us in the morning. *Family Process*, 1978, *17*, 165-180.

Haley, J. *Strategies of psychotherapy*. New York: Grune & Stratton, 1963.

Heard, D. Keith: A case study of structural family therapy. *Family Process*, 1978, *17*, 338-332.

Jackson, D. D. The study of the family. *Family Process*, 1965, *4*, 1-20.

Jacobson, N. S. A review of the research on the effectiveness of marital therapy. In T. Paolino, Jr., & B. McCrady (Eds.), *Marriage and marital therapy*. New York: Brunner/Mazel, 1978.

Jacobson, N. S. Behavioral marriage therapy. In A. Gurman & D. Kniskern (Eds.), *Handbook of family therapy*. New York: Brunner/Mazel, 1981.

Jacobson, N. S., & Margolin, G. *Marital therapy: Strategies based on social learning and behavior exchange principles*. New York: Brunner/Mazel, 1979.

Jacobson, N. S., & Weiss, R. L. Behavioral marriage therapy: III. The contents of Gurman *et al.* may be hazardous to our health. *Family Process*, 1978, *17*, 149-163.

Kanfer, F. Self-management methods. In F. Kanfer & A. Goldstein (Eds.), *Helping people change*. New York: Pergamon Press, 1975.

Karoly, P. Operant methods. In F. Kanfer & A. Goldstein (Eds.), *Helping people change*. New York: Pergamon Press, 1975.

Kazdin, A. *History of behavior modification*. Baltimore: University Park Press, 1979.

Kelley, G. *The psychology of personal constructs.* New York: Norton, 1955.

Kerr, M. Family systems theory and therapy. In A. Gurman & D. Kniskern (Eds.), *Handbook of family therapy.* New York: Brunner/Mazel, 1981.

Klein, M. H., Dittman, A. T., Parloff, M. B., & Gill, M. M. Behavior therapy: Observations and reflections. *Journal of Consulting and Clinical Psychology, 1969, 33,* 259–266.

Kniskern, D. P., & Gurman, A. S. Advances and prospects for family therapy research. In J. P. Vincent (Ed.), *Advances in family intervention, assessment and theory* (Vol. 2). Greenwich: JAI Press, 1980.

Knudson, R. M., Gurman, A. S., & Kniskern, D. P. Behavioral marriage therapy: A treatment in transition. In C. M. Franks & G. T. Wilson (Eds.), *Annual review of behavior therapy* (Vol. 7). New York: Brunner/Mazel, 1980.

Koss, M. P. Length of psychotherapy for clients seen in private practice. *Journal of Consulting and Clinical Psychology, 1979, 47,* 210–212.

Lederer, W., & Jackson, D. *The mirages of marriage.* New York: Norton, 1958.

Lorion, R. P. Socioeconomic status and traditional treatment approaches reconsidered. *Psychological Bulletin, 1973, 79,* 263–270.

Lorion, R. P. Patient and therapist variables in the treatment of low income patients. *Psychological Bulletin, 1974, 81,* 344–354.

Mahoney, M. Psychotherapy and the structure of personal revaluations. In M. Mahoney (Ed.), *Psychotherapeutic process.* New York: Plenum Press, 1979.

Malan, D. *The frontier of brief psychotherapy.* New York: Plenum Press, 1976.

Mann, J. *Time-limited psychotherapy.* Cambridge: Harvard University Press, 1973.

Marks, I. Behavior therapy of adult neuroses. In S. Garfield & A. Bergin (Eds.), *Handbook of psychotherapy and behavior change* (2nd ed.). New York: Wiley, 1978.

Martin, P. *A manual of marital therapy.* New York: Brunner/Mazel, 1976.

Matarazzo, J. Psychotherapeutic processes. *Annual Review of Psychology, 1965, 16,* 181–224.

Meissner, W. The conceptualization of marriage and family dynamics from a psychoanalytic perspective. In T. Paolino, Jr., & B. McCrady (Eds.), *Marriage and marital therapy.* New York: Brunner/Mazel, 1978.

Minuchin, S. *Families and family therapy.* Cambridge: Harvard University Press, 1974.

Nadelson, C. C. Marital therapy from a psychoanalytic perspective. In T. Paolino, Jr., & B. McCrady (Eds., *Marriage and marital therapy.* New York: Brunner/Mazel, 1978.

Paolino, T., Jr. Introduction: Some basic concepts of psychoanalytic psychotherapy. In T. Paolino, Jr., & B. McCrady (Eds.), *Marriage and marital therapy.* New York: Brunner/Mazel, 1978.

Papp, P. The Greek chorus and other techniques of family therapy. *Family Process, 1980, 19,* 45–57.

Rank, O. *Will therapy.* New York: Knopf, 1947.

Raush, H. L., Barry, W. A., Hertel, R. K., & Swain, M. A. *Communication, conflict and marriage.* San Francisco: Jossey-Bass, 1974.

Sager, C. J. *Marriage contracts and couple therapy.* New York: Brunner/Mazel, 1976.

Sager, C. J. Couples therapy and marriage contracts. In A. Gurman & D. Kniskern (Eds.), *Handbook of family therapy.* New York: Brunner/Mazel, 1981.

Selvini-Palazzoli, M., Boscolo, L., Cecchin, G., & Prata, G. *Paradox and counterparadox.* New York: Jason Aronson, 1978.

Sifneos, P. E. *Short-term psychotherapy and emotional crisis.* Cambridge: Harvard University Press, 1972.

Skynner, A. C. R. *Systems of family and marital psychotherapy.* New York: Brunner/Mazel, 1976.

Skynner, A. C. R. An open systems, group-analytic approach to family therapy. In A. Gurman & D. Kniskern (Eds.), *Handbook of family therapy*. New York: Brunner/Mazel, 1981.

Stanton, M. D. Marital therapy from a structural/strategic viewpoint. In G. P. Sholevar (Ed.), *Marriage is a family affair*. New York: Spectrum Press, 1980.

Stanton, M. D. Strategic approaches to family therapy. In A. Gurman & D. Kniskern (Eds.), *Handbook of family therapy*. New York: Brunner/Mazel, 1981.

Stewart, R. H., Peters, T. C., Marsh, S., & Peters, M. J. An object-relations approach to psychotherapy with marital couples, families and children. *Family Process*, 1975, *14*, 161–178.

Stuart, R. B. *Behavioral marital therapy*. Workshop presented at the meeting of the Association for the Advancement of Behavior Therapy, San Francisco, December 1979.

Stuart, R. B. *Helping couples change: A social learning approach to marital therapy*. New York: Guilford Press, 1980.

Thibaut, J. W., & Kelley, H. H. *The social psychology of groups*. New York: Wiley, 1959.

Wachtel, P. L. *Psychoanalysis and behavior therapy: Toward an integration*. New York: Basic Books, 1977.

Watzlawick, P., Weakland, J., & Fisch, R. *Change: Principles of problem resolution*. New York: Norton, 1974.

Weakland, J. H., Fisch, R., Watzlawick, P., & Bodin, A. Brief therapy: Focused problem resolution. *Family Process*, 1974, *13*, 141–168.

Weeks, G., & L'Abate, L. A compilation of paradoxical methods. *American Journal of Family Therapy*, 1979, *7*, 61–76.

Weiss, R. L. Contracts, cognitions and change: A behavioral approach to marital therapy. *The Counseling Psychologist*, 1975, *5*, 15–26.

Weiss, R. L. The conceptualization of marriage from a behavioral perspective. In T. Paolino, Jr., & B. McCrady (Eds.), *Marriage and marital therapy*. New York: Brunner/Mazel, 1978.

Weiss, R. L., A systems behavioral approach to marital therapy. In J. Vincent (Ed.), *Advances in family intervention, assessment and theory* (Vol. I). Greenwich: JAI Press, 1979.

Whitaker, C. A., & Keith, D. V. Symbolic–experiential family therapy. In A. Gurman & D. Kniskern (Eds.), *Handbook of family therapy*. New York: Brunner/Mazel, 1981.

Wolberg, L. R. *Short-term psychotherapy*. New York: Grune & Stratton, 1965.

SECTION VI
CONCLUSION

CHAPTER 17
LOOKING TOWARD THE FUTURE

Simon H. Budman

This volume has sought to acquaint the reader with some of the new and significant trends in the area of brief therapy. Using as my base the contributions here, other materials appearing in the literature, and my and my colleagues' past ten years of experience at the Harvard Community Health Plan (HCHP), I hope to do some consolidation and crystal-ball gazing in this final chapter.

What are the important elements which unify the various forms of brief therapy, and what will be the future refinements and trends in this most significant area?

UNIFYING ELEMENTS IN BRIEF THERAPIES

Butcher and Koss (1978) listed nine elements which they call "common technical characteristics of crisis-oriented and brief psychotherapy systems." Summarized briefly, these are:

1. *Utilization of Time.* Most brief therapies have an upper limit of 25 sessions and an emphasis on brevity of treatment.

2. *Limited Goals.* Specific symptoms, problems, sectors of disturbance and the like become the focus of the treatment; a wide-ranging "character" change does not.

3. *Focused Interviewing and Present Centeredness.* There is an attempt to keep the patient dealing in a focal way with the problem at hand rather than free association, open-ended interviewing and so on. A recent study seems to support the belief that clients feel considerably more improvement in regard to those target problems which are focused upon than those which are not focused upon (Blizinsky & Reid, 1980).

SIMON H. BUDMAN. Harvard Community Health Plan and Department of Psychiatry, Harvard Medical School, Boston, Massachusetts.

4. *Activity and Directiveness.* The therapist in brief treatment tends to talk more and interpret more, may give advice and suggestions, and, as Wilson (Chapter 6, this volume) so clearly describes for the behavior therapist, assign homework, tasks, and so forth.

5. *Rapid, Early Assessment.* For the most part, assessment and treatment in brief therapy begin almost simultaneously. In Bloom's (Chapter 7, this volume) focused single-session approach, for example, assessment and treatment are inextricably interwoven and are one and the same. In short-term group psychotherapy (Chapter 12, this volume; Budman, Clifford, Bader, & Bader, in press) with young adults in particular, the assessment procedure itself is a group experience. Because of the press of time in most brief approaches, one cannot provide a lengthy and extensive evaluation, which would, in and of itself, require as much time as many such brief therapies!

6. *Therapeutic Flexibility.* Although flexibility is seen as quite central to brief therapy, Strupp's (1980) work in the Vanderbilt project and that of Sloane and his colleagues (Sloane, Staples, Cristol, Yorkston, & Whipple, 1975) raise some doubts (at least regarding dynamically oriented therapists) as to whether, indeed, such flexibility is practiced. Both Strupp and Sloane *et al.* found that the psychotherapists in their studies showed a strong disinclination toward modifying their technique when practicing time-limited treatment. This was not as true of the behavior therapists in the Sloane study. It may be that, in general, behavior therapists are becoming more open to the use of cognitive approaches (Wilson, Chapter 6, this volume) than are analytically oriented therapists to the use of behavioral interventions (Wachtel, 1977). The entire field of psychotherapy, however, may be headed toward a great ecumenism, with eclecticism becoming the dominant theoretical affiliation for most therapists (Garfield, 1980).

7. *Ventilation.* Most major proponents of brief therapy believe that the opportunity to express and ventilate emotional tension is an important element in the treatment.

8. *Therapeutic relationship.* It is of the essence that the therapist and patient quickly develop a therapeutic alliance in brief therapy, lest the treatment end before such a fulcrum develops. Strupp (Chapter 8, this volume) indicates that the formation of such an alliance either occurs quickly or is unlikely to occur at all.

9. *Selection of Patients.* This is probably the most important single element in brief therapy. In spite of Gustafson's (Chapter 5, this volume)

description of Balint's (Balint, Ornstein, & Balint, 1973) brilliant work with more disturbed patients and Davanloo's (1978) treatment of characterological problems in brief therapy, the weight of the evidence thus far implies that brief therapy is more suitable to less disturbed patients (Strupp, Chapter 8, this volume). This appears to be true regardless of whether the treatment is short-term individual or short-term group therapy (Budman, Demby, & Randall, 1980).

OTHER FORMS OF BRIEF THERAPY

Although Butcher and Koss (1978) referred, in the main, to short-term, individual, dynamic approaches to therapy, much of what they described applies equally well to brief, behaviorally oriented therapy, to short-term group therapy, and to the brief treatment of couples and families. For example, a short-term group psychotherapy is, in many ways, a melding of brief individual treatment principles and group dynamics (Budman, Bennett, & Wisneski, Chapter 12, this volume). The brevity of couples therapy may, in part, be predicated on the fact that couples are, by definition, made up of people who are not total social isolates, have some reasonable ability to relate to others, and enter treatment with a clear and focal problem—the marriage (Gurman, Chapter 16, this volume). Similarly, behavior therapy carries the seeds of a brief therapy modality, in that the therapist is direct, focal, active, and flexible.

THE FUTURE OF BRIEF THERAPY

Most clinicians currently see most patients for a relatively limited period. It seems that brief therapy is the norm in this country, certainly not the exception (Pardes & Pincus, Chapter 2, this volume). What is probably exceptional, however, is *planned* brief therapy, that is, treatment which is organized in such a way as to be maximally beneficial in a brief period. We are now moving into an age of increased consumerism in all areas of health care, and most certainly as regards psychotherapy. For the most part, it is not the vast majority of psychotherapy consumers who wish or come in seeking open-ended, time-unlimited treatment. The proponents of such a viewpoint are, in the main, psychotherapists, who are desirous of what Malan (1963) called "psychotherapeutic perfectionism." As the informed public, legislative groups, and third-party payers become increasingly concerned with the cost effectiveness of mental health treatment, brief therapies will be demanded with greater and greater frequency.

DEVELOPMENTS IN BRIEF THERAPY

I believe that two interrelated areas will prove most important in the future refinements of brief treatment. The first is the increased understanding of human growth and development throughout the life cycle, and the second is the knowledge, in the part of therapists and patients, that therapy cannot cure.

My colleagues and I at HCHP (Budman, Bennett, & Wisneski, 1980, Chapter 12, this volume; Daley & Koppenaal, Chapter 13, this volume), as well as Burke, White, and Havens (1979, Chapter 9, this volume), have begun to address the issues of treatment specificity and life stage development. It is becoming more obvious to all informed clinicians that humans change, grow, and develop throughout the life cycle, and that to assume that all of life's ups and downs are predicated upon infantile fixations is to take an exceedingly narrow viewpoint in any form of psychotherapeutic endeavor. The understanding and thoughtful application of a life cycle developmental perspective is of particular importance when practicing brief therapy. The reason for this is that such a perspective may allow for more rapid clarification of a treatment focus and can aid the therapist in a flexible application of technique. Although no one, to my knowledge, has applied such a life stage developmental perspective to the differential treatment of couples, it is a task which can and should be tackled.

For analytically oriented therapists, Freud's (1933/1964) often quoted dictum, "where id was, there ego shall be," stands like a beacon. One imagines a therapist, like an explorer of old, conquering the wilderness once and for all. Thus, in his early writing, Freud appeared quite convinced of the prophylactic qualities of analysis. For example, in 1917 (Freud, 1916–1919/1964), discussing the value of analytic therapy, he wrote, "through the overcoming of these resistances the patient's mental life is *permanently changed* . . . and *remains protected* against fresh possibilities of falling ill" (p. 451, italics added). It was only later in his life, after having observed a number of patients return to treatment periodically, that Freud began to reconsider his position and raised the possibility that fresh neuroses could occur in a treated patient, or that even a previously analyzed neurosis could recur (Freud, 1933/1964). It seems that, by this time, it was too late; the attitude underlying psychotherapy was already established as one of seeking prophylaxis as well as cure. That is, by definition, successful outcome leads to a cure, and if one needs to return to treatment, the previous therapy has been unsuccessful. This striving for perfection became and remains a dominant attitude amongst individual and group therapists. For a variety of historical reasons (Gurman, Chapter 16, this volume), however, those doing marital and family therapy were mercifully spared this bias.

Rather than a contrast between long-term and short-term therapies, I believe that we will move toward evaluating a patient's needs for continuous psychotherapy (Bennett & Wisneski, 1979) as opposed to his or her ability to use discontinuous psychotherapy. As Rabkin (1977) wrote:

> Under the best of conditions, relationships with professionals other than psychotherapists are not regarded as terminating at all. They are seen as intermittent. For example, the accountant, lawyer, family doctor, or barber may have permanent relationships with clients and perhaps their families, although the actual face-to-face contacts occur only for specific tasks or problems . . . [such a] tie may last a lifetime. (p. 211)

Thus, the approaches and models which have been described and discussed in this book may be used at various points with a given patient and need not be viewed as the definitive treatment for that patient. Cummings and Vandenbos (1979) provided an excellent case illustration of the discontinuous application of such approaches. Rather than the onus being placed upon those who apply short-term therapies to prove that such therapy is "good treatment," the clinical and research burden will eventually fall also to those who insist that the application of long-term (i.e., continuous) therapy is a prerequisite for improvement in a given patient.

TRAINING IN BRIEF THERAPIES

In the next decade, I believe that research evidence will accumulate indicating that good brief therapists are made and not born. Evidence already exists that when one takes highly experienced therapists, unfamiliar with brief treatment, and asks them to do time-limited therapy, their therapeutic outcomes are no better than untrained "natural helpers" (Gomes-Schwartz, 1978; Strupp & Hadley, 1979). Such findings should not be too terribly surprising. Indeed, many of the behaviors most encouraged for those trained as long-term therapists (e.g., low therapist-activity level, a nondirective stance) run counter to some of the nine common elements in brief therapy, described previously.

Brief therapy is more than truncated long-term treatment. The therapist, in order to make a maximal contribution, needs a basic familiarity with such approaches and, perhaps, closely supervised experience in this area. It is doubtful that one can simply "do" brief therapy just because one has done long-term therapy (or even behavioral therapy).

This has implications for the training of therapists. Few training programs provide more than a single course or seminar (if that) in short-term treatment. It is assumed that with a firm grounding in open-ended psychotherapy or behavior therapy, the student will enter the world able to do whatever brief therapy he or she is later called upon to do. Specialized skills, such as rapid clarification of focus, the use of structured interviews, and so on may be singularly important to the well-trained "brief therapist." Eventually, we may need to provide clearly specialized training in briefer therapies both to our trainees and to highly trained "long-term therapists."

CONCLUSIONS

The next decade will undoubtedly bring with it increased consumer demand for brief therapy approaches. To this observer, at least, it is unlikely that major technological advances of a radical nature will occur, since most of the basic and central principles of effective brief treatment are presumably now in existence. It is of major importance that we judiciously apply current theory and research regarding short-term therapy in order to improve and refine existing approaches. It is also essential that training programs in psychiatry, psychology, social work, and so on provide students with a basic understanding of brief treatment, and that continuing education in mental health emphasize such approaches. It is only by breaking down old prejudices and providing a newer, more realistic perspective that we can effectively meet the challenges ahead of us.

REFERENCES

Balint, M., Ornstein, P. H., & Balint, E. *Focal psychotherapy.* London: Tavistock Publications, 1973.

Bennett, M. J., & Wisneski, M. J. Continuous psychotherapy within an HMO. *American Journal of Psychiatry,* 1979, *136,* 1283–1287.

Blizinsky, M. H., & Reid, W. J. Problem focus and change in a brief treatment model. *Social Work,* 1980, *25,* 89–93.

Budman, S. H., Bennett, M. J., & Wisneski, M. J. Short-term group psychotherapy: An adult developmental model. *International Journal of Group Psychotherapy,* 1980, *30,* 63–76.

Budman, S. H., Clifford, M., Bader, L., & Bader, B. Experiential pre-group preparation and screening. *Group,* in press.

Budman, S. H., Demby, A., & Randall, M. Short-term group psychotherapy: Who succeeds and who fails? *Group,* 1980, *4,* 3–16.

Burke, J. D., White, H. S., & Havens, L. L. Which short-term therapy? Matching patient and method. *Archives of General Psychiatry,* 1979, *35,* 177–186.

Butcher, J. N., & Koss, M. P. Research on brief and crisis-oriented therapies. In S. L. Garfield & A. E. Bergin (Eds.), *Handbook of psychotherapy and behavior change.* New York: Wiley, 1978.

Cummings, N. A., & Vandenbos, F. The general practice of psychology. *Professional Psychology,* 1979, *10,* 430–440.

Davanloo, H. (Ed.). *Basic principles and techniques in short-term dynamic psychotherapy.* New York: Spectrum Press, 1978.

Freud, S. Introductory lectures. In J. Strachey (Ed.), *The standard edition of the complete psychological works of Sigmund Freud* (Vol. 16). London: Hogarth Press, 1964. (Originally published, 1916-1917.)

Freud, S. Introductory lectures. In J. Strachey (Ed.), *The standard edition of the complete psychological works of Sigmund Freud* (Vol. 22). London: Hogarth Press, 1964. (Originally published, 1933.)

Garfield, S. L. *Psychotherapy: An eclectic approach.* New York: Wiley, 1980.

Gomes-Schwartz, B. Effective ingredients in psychotherapy: Prediction of outcomes from process variables. *Journal of Consulting and Clinical Psychology,* 1978, *46,* 1023–1035.

Malan, D. H. *A study of brief psychotherapy.* London: Tavistock Publications, 1963.

Rabkin, R. *Strategic psychotherapy.* New York: Basic Books, 1977.

Sloane, R. B., Staples, F. R., Cristol, A. H., Yorkston, N. J., & Whipple, K. *Psychotherapy versus behavior therapy.* Cambridge: Harvard University Press, 1975.

Strupp, H. H. Success and failure in time-limited psychotherapy. *Archives of General Psychiatry,* 1980, *37,* 595–603.

Strupp, H. H., & Hadley, S. W. Specific versus non-specific factors in psychotherapy: A controlled study of outcome. *Archives of General Psychiatry,* 1979, *36,* 1125–1136.

Wachtel, P. *Psychoanalysis and behavior therapy: Toward an integration.* New York: Basic Books, 1977.

INDEX

Abandonment fears, 119
Ables, B., 424, 453n.
Abramowitz, S., 343, 344, 347, 357n.
Addictive disorders, 138–140, 148, 150 *(see also* Alcohol abuse; Drugs, abuse of)
Addington, H. J., 140, 162n.
Adolescence, developmental approach to, 254–256
Aggression, 103
  defense against, 106
Agoraphobic disorders, 13, 133, 134, 143, 151, 446 *(see also* Phobias)
Agras, W. S., 141, 145, 148, 161n., 162n.
Al-Anon, 191, 192, 204, 207–209
Alcohol abuse, 20, 94, 138–140, 148, 150, 151, 179, 207–209, 324, 348, 406
Alcohol, Drug Abuse and Mental Health Administration (ADAMHA), 11
Alcoholics Anonymous (AA), 191, 204
Alexander, F., 2, 4n., 45, 80n., 83, 85, 87, 101, 102, 106, 109, 119, 120, 127n., 156, 158, 161n., 220, 233, 239, 241n., 245, 251–253, 263, 264, 267n., 415, 453n.
Alexander, J. A., 411, 412n.
Allen, D., 170, 176, 215n., 216n.
Allgeyer, J. M., 287, 288, 300, 303n.
American Psychologist, 157
Amitriptyline, 137
Amnesia, 29
Anderson, E. A., 400, 413n.
Andolfi, M., 417, 427, 453n.
Anorexia nervosa, 365
Antidepressant drugs, 8, 136
Antisocial behavior, 223
Anxiety, 2, 37, 41, 70, 91, 100, 101, 124n., 224, 290, 295, 309, 314, 317, 319, 325, 327, 331, 334, 339, 347 *(see also* Short-term anxiety-provoking psychotherapy)
  analysis of, 98, 111
  anticipatory, 13
  avoidance of, 72

Anxiety *(continued)*
  and central issue, 33
  confrontation of, 144
  about control, 38, 106
  disabling, 92
  and emotional confrontation, 258
  and groups, 309, 314, 317, 319, 325, 327, 331, 334, 339
  management of, 445, 446
  and marital/family therapy, 366, 446, 448
  and meaning in therapy, 378
  and rejection, 404
  separation, 31, 245, 322, 327, 328
  sexual, 138
  and somatization, 336, 337
  and time, 27, 30, 32
  and unconscious, 423
  and women, 346
Aponte, H., 418, 427, 428, 453n.
Appelbaum, A., 229, 242n.
Aries, E. J., 343–345, 356n.
Arkin, A., 123n.
Armstrong, S., 367, 381, 385n.
Asher, S. J., 391, 412n.
Assertion training, 136
Assessment, 408, 434
  behavioral, 156
  and ongoing process, 142
  and treatment, 462
Asthma, 20
Attention-placebo control condition, 133
Authority figure, therapist as, 50–53
Aved, B. M., 391, 414n.
Azrin, N. H., 140, 162n., 397, 400, 409, 412n.

Bacal, H. A., 102, 127n., 175, 215n.
Bachrach, H. M., 221, 241n.
Bader, B., 311, 341n., 462, 467n.
Bader, L., 311, 341n., 462, 467n.
Baer, D. M., 149, 165n.
Balfour, F. H. G., 102, 127n., 174, 215n.
Balint, E., 84–87, 114, 121, 123n., 127n., 182, 214n., 362, 385n., 463, 467n.

Balint, M., 1, 83–89, 91, 102, 112–121, 122*n*., 123*n*., 126*n*., 127*n*., 182, 184, 214*n.,* 305, 362, 385*n.,* 463, 467*n.*
Balter, M. B., 20, 21*n.*
Bancroft, J. H. J., 133, 138, 163*n*., 164*n.*
Bandura, A., 132, 133, 145, 148, 149, 157–159, 162*n.*
Barlow, D. H., 145, 162*n.*
Barnett, J., 423, 453*n.*
Barnett, L. W., 150, 163*n.*
Barron, F., 289, 290, 295, 303*n.*
Barry, W. A., 433, 456*n.*
Barten, H. H., 174, 214*n*., 307, 341*n.*
Barton, C., 411, 412*n.*
Basic Skills Training Group (BST), 276–278
Beavers, W. R., 376, 385*n.*
Bechtel, R., 400, 412*n.*
Beck, A. T., 136, 159, 162*n*., 165*n*., 228, 241, 246, 253, 263, 264, 267*n*., 432, 453*n.*
Beck, D. B., 387, 412*n.*
Becker, J., 137, 162*n.*
Beech, R. P., 172, 216*n.*
Behavioral marital therapy (BMT), 4, 136, 387–415, 421, 425, 426, 445–449 *(see also* Behavior therapy, individual)
  approaches to, 396–408
    appropriateness in, 405–407
    empirical basis of, 396–405
    training, 407, 408
  behavioral rehearsal, 398, 399
  as brief therapy by design, 408–412
  resistance to, 394, 411
  targets of, 391–395
  and therapeutic approaches, 388–395
Behavior therapy, individual, 13, 31, 131–168 *(see also* Behavioral marital therapy)
  applicability of, 140, 141
  clinical illustrations of, 133–140
    addictive disorders, 138–140, 148, 150
    depression, 136, 137
    obsessive–compulsive disorders, 135, 136, 143
    phobic disorders, 133, 134, 141, 159
    sexual dysfunction, 137, 138, 146, 147, 151, 157
  evaluation of, 151–161
    behavioral practice, 155–159
    criteria broadening for, 153–155
    multiple strategies, 153

Behavior therapy, individual, evaluation of *(continued)*
    and nonbehavioral treatments, 155
    therapeutic relationship, 159–161
  multimodal, 133
  and psychoanalysis, 156, 157, 160
  summary on, 161
  technical aspects of, 141–151
    brief versus longer-term, 141–143
    and change, 149–151
    and difficulty/treatment length, 143–145
    individualization, 147, 148
    therapy format, 145–147
Benjamin Rush Center, 170
Benne, K. D., 275, 277, 281*n.*
Bennett, M. J., 4, 272, 277, 283–303, 305–342, 346, 356*n*., 357*n*., 463–465, 466*n*., 467*n.*
Benson, H., 28, 42*n.*
Bentovim, A., 4, 361–386, 385*n*., 420, 424, 453*n*., 454*n.*
Bergin, A. E., 152, 162*n*., 229, 238, 241*n*., 422, 454*n.*
Berkowitz, R., 141, 161*n.*
Berman, E. M., 421, 428, 454*n.*
Bernard, H., 343, 357*n.*
Besalel, V. A., 400, 412*n.*
Beth Israel Hospital of Boston, 47
Bienvenu, J., 311, 342*n.*
Birchler, G. R., 391, 397, 411, 412*n*., 414*n*., 421, 454*n.*
Blake, R. B., 278, 281*n.*
Blind psychiatric ratings, 134
Blizinsky, M. H., 461, 466*n.*
Bloom, B. L., 2, 3, 167–216, 214*n*., 391, 412*n*., 462
Blos, P., 254, 267*n.*
Bloxom, A. L., 239, 242*n.*
Blue Cross/Blue Shield program, 16
Bodin, A. M., 367, 386*n*., 419, 421, 427, 429, 454*n*., 457*n.*
Bond, G., 312, 341*n.*
Borderline conditions, 235, 236, 300, 348
Borkovec, T. D., 141, 146, 162*n*., 165*n.*
Boscolo, L., 362, 386*n*., 451, 456*n.*
Boszormenyi-Nagy, I., 362, 385*n.*
Boulougouris, J. C., 136, 146, 164*n.*
Bowen, M., 420, 423, 454*n.*
Brady, J. P., 138, 162*n.*
Brainstorming, 275

Branch, L. G., 150, 163n.
Brandsma, J., 424, 453n.
Breuer, J., 83, 127n., 175, 214n.
Briddell, D. W., 140, 164n.
Brigham, T., 141, 162n.
Broderick, C. B., 420, 421, 454n.
Brodsky, A., 344, 345, 347, 356n.
Budman, S. H., ix, x, 1–5, 272, 277, 281n.,
    305–343, 341n., 348, 356n., 461–
    467, 467n.
Burck, C., 366, 385n.
Burke, J. D., Jr., 3, 4, 17, 21n., 122n.,
    127n., 238, 241n., 243–267, 267n.,
    464, 467n.
Burstein, E. D., 229, 242n.
Butcher, J. N., 2, 5n., 131, 155, 159, 162n.,
    221, 222, 236, 241n., 307, 341n.,
    416, 418, 454n., 461, 463, 467n.

Caddy, G. R., 140, 162n.
Cameron, R., 132, 164n.
Carlock, C., 344, 345, 356n.
Carroll, D., 400, 412n.
Carter, J., 11
Carter, R., 11
Caston, 101, 128n.
Catania, A. C., 141, 162n.
Cecchin, G. F., 362, 386n., 451, 456n.
Central issue in therapy, 25–43 (see also
    Focal psychotherapy)
  conclusion on, 42
  defining of, 25, 33–42
    case example of, 39–41
    and patient selection, 42
    and termination phase, 41, 42
Chambless, D., 432, 446, 454n.
Chemotherapy, 8
Chicago Institute of Psychoanalysis, Sec-
    ond Brief Psychotherapy Council,
    275
Child abuse, 365
Childbearing, deferred, 346
Chodorow, N., 345, 356n.
Ciba Foundation Research Conference, 46
Classification, development of, 13, 14
Clifford, M., 311, 312, 341n., 343, 356n.,
    462, 467n.
Cognitive behavior therapy, 13, 132, 136,
    415
Cohen, F., 169, 215n.
Colarusso, C. A., 266, 267n.

Coleman, J. V., 168, 214n.
Community mental health centers, devel-
    opment of, 9–11
Community Mental Health Centers Act, 9,
    11
Compulsions, 144, 150, 370
Conaway, L., 170, 216n.
Confession in groups, 328
Conflict, focal/nuclear, 97, 98
Connecticut State Interracial Commission,
    275
Connolly, J., 134, 164n.
Consciousness-raising groups, 347, 348
Contracts, therapeutic, 239, 396, 397, 402
Control–mastery theory, 124n.–126n.
Coopersmith, E., 451, 454n.
Core conflict, 229
Corporal punishment, 70–72
Corrective approach to therapy, 251–254
Cost of medical care, 15, 16
Cotherapy
  behavioral, 134
  in groups, 302
Counterintrojection, 118, 119
Counteroffer, 85–89
Counterprojection, 119
Countertransference, 41, 42, 229, 432,
    439–441 (see also Transference)
Cox, J., 400, 412n.
Coyne, L., 229, 242n.
Crassweller, K. D., 28, 42n.
Crisis psychotherapy, 174, 271
  in groups, 283–303
Cristol, A. H., 143, 160, 165n., 227, 242n.,
    307, 342n., 462, 467n.
Cross-validation of theory, 111, 112, 124n.
Cummings, N. A., 177–179, 214n., 465,
    467n.

Daley, B. S., 4, 343–357, 464
Dallas, M., 399, 413n.
Darrow, C. N., 306, 341n.
Davanloo, H., 80, 80n., 220, 229, 241n.,
    463, 467n.
Davidson, N., 448, 454n.
Davison, G. C., 144, 146, 158, 159, 162n.,
    163n., 165n.
Debbane, E. G., 311, 342n.
Decompensation, 26
  acute manic/schizophrenic, 36
  and time, 28

Demby, A., 272, 281n., 311, 325, 341n., 463, 467n.
Denial, 33, 262, 382
Department of Health and Human Services (HHS), 11
Dependency, 90, 96, 102, 222 *(see also* Separation/individuation)
  and ambiguity in treatment time, 31
  in case example, 193–195, 200, 201
  in groups, 316, 318
  and narcissism, 423
  and parents, 206, 207
  of women, 352, 356
Depersonalization and time, 28
Depression, 36, 89, 94, 126n., 151, 224, 262–264, 290, 295, 436
  behavioral approach to, 136, 137
  and central issue, 33
  depressive position, 322
  and groups, 317, 320, 332, 334, 339
  and inadequacy feelings, 32
  and infancy, 321
  and marriage, 391
  and psychosis, 31
  and self-esteem, 323
  and time, 27, 30
Derealization and time, 28
Desensitization, systematic, 133–135, 148, 445
Detroit Community Health Association Program, 170
Developmental approaches to short-term therapy, 4, 243–267
  conclusion on, 266
  corrective, 251–253
  empathic, 249–251
  interpretive, 247–249
  matching patient to, 253–266
    adolescence, 254–256
    adulthood, 265
    early adulthood, 256–259
    midlife, 261–265
    old age, 265
    settling down, 259–261
Dewees, S., 171, 216n.
Dicks, H. V., 421, 423, 424, 428, 433, 454n.
DiMascio, A., 17, 22n.
Discrimination training, 396
Dittman, A. T., 416, 456n.
Divorce, 406
  and health status, 391

Doctor, His Patient and the Illness, The (Balint), 83, 85–89, 113, 120, 121
Donovan, J. M., 283–303
Double binds, 361
Dreams, time in, 29
Dressler, D. M., 307, 367, 342n., 396n.
Drugs
  abuse of, 94, 323, 324, 348
  and time, 27, 28
DSM-III, 224
Duhl, B., 430, 454n.
Duhl, F., 430, 454n.
D'Zurilla, T. J., 391, 412n.

Edwards, G., 176, 177, 179, 214n.
Egert, S., 176, 214n.
Ego, 124n.
  boundaries of, 345
  and duration of therapy, 174
  expansion of, 41
  functioning of, 254
  ideal of, 259
  identity of, 255, 256
  integration of, 255
  integrity/despair of, 265, 332
  maturation of, 254, 255
  in midlife, 321
  and problem solving, 286
  resources of, 221, 233–235
  strength of, 3, 182, 183, 290, 291, 295
    scale for, 289
  and time, 27, 32
Eitington, M., 184
Electroconvulsive therapy (ECT), 7, 94
Elwood, R., 399, 413n.
Emery, G., 432, 453n.
Empathy, 119, 229, 243, 249–251, 345, 347
Encounter groups, 273, 275–281
Encounter Groups: First Facts (Lieberman et al.), 279, 281
Epstein, L. J., 333, 342n.
Erikson, E. H., 253, 256, 257, 263, 267n., 308, 321, 332, 341n.
Ersner-Heshfeld, R., 147, 162n.
Esalen, 276
Ethnicity and community health care, 170
Evans, I. M., 142, 144, 158, 159, 165n.
Ewalt, P. L., 170, 214n.
Ewing, C. P., 174, 214n.
Existentialism, 87, 88
Eysenck, H. E., 132, 162n.
Ezriel, H., 378, 385n.

Fallacy of misplaced objectivity, 244
Family myths, 376
Family Service Association of America, 169
Family therapy *(see* Marital/family therapy, focus for)
Fantasy
  time in, 29
  range of, 38
Fay, A., 158, 163*n.*
Federal Employee Health Benefits Program, 16
Feedback in group therapy, 157, 292, 313
Feldman, J., 305, 341*n.*
Feldman, L., 421, 423, 428, 454*n.*
Fenichel, O., 157, 162*n.*
Ferenczi, S., 45, 80*n.*, 83, 127*n.*, 415, 454*n.*
Field theory, 273
Fiester, A. R., 169, 170, 172, 214*n.*
Fisch, R., 367, 386*n.*, 394, 414*n.*, 419, 427, 457*n.*
Fishman, S., 142, 145, 162*n.*
Fixation
  on beauty, 53, 54
  infantile, 464
  pregenital, 258
Flexibility of therapeutic technique, 231, 232
Flooding, 135, 136, 148
Focal issue *(see* Central issue in therapy; Focal psychotherapy)
Focal psychotherapy, 84, 112–120, 122, 123*n. (see also* Focused single-session therapy)
  accounts of, 116–120
  case of, 113–115
  clinical outlines in, 114, 115
  conflict in, 222
  context of, 112, 113
  hypothesis on, 365–368, 380, 381
  treatment outline for, 115
Focal Psychotherapy (Balint *et al.),* 112–121, 123*n.*
Focused single-session therapy (FSST), 3, 167–216 *(see also* Focal psychotherapy)
  case example of, 190–213
  conclusion on, 213, 214
  early termination and client satisfaction, 171–173
  effectiveness of, 173–180
  frequency of, 164–171
  preliminary report on, 180–190
    and affect encouragement, 185

Focused single-session therapy, preliminary report on *(continued)*
  ambitiousness of, 187, 188
  and client self-awareness, 190
  and client strengths, 182, 183
  and detours, 189, 190
  factual questions for, 188, 189
  interpretation in, 184, 185
  and precipitating event, 189
  problem identification, 182
  and problem solving, 186, 187
  prudent activity for, 183, 184
Follette, W. T., 177, 179, 214*n.*
Foreyt, J., 132, 162*n.*
Fowles, J., 123*n.*, 127*n.*
Framington Youth Guidance Center, 170
Framo, J., 417, 420, 421, 429, 454*n.*
Frank, J. D., 160, 162*n.*, 229, 240, 241*n.*, 280, 281*n.*
Franks, C. M., 138, 141, 163*n.*
French, T. M., 2, 4*n.*, 45, 80*n.*, 83, 85, 87, 101, 102, 106, 109, 119, 120, 127*n.*, 156, 158, 161*n.*, 220, 233, 239, 241*n.*, 245, 251, 252, 263, 264, 267*n.*, 415, 453*n.*
Freud, A., 89
Freud, S., 14, 83, 85, 86, 88, 89, 97, 123*n.*, 127*n.*, 157, 163*n.*, 175, 214*n.*, 221, 226, 228, 241*n.*, 415, 443, 454*n.*, 464, 467*n.*
Frings, J., 169, 214*n.*
Frontier of Brief Psychotherapy, The (Malan), 96, 100–103, 111, 116, 121, 124*n.*
Fujita, B. N., 176, 215*n.*

Gajdos, E., 149, 162*n.*
Garant, J., 311, 342*n.*
Garfield, S. L., 168, 215*n.*, 415, 416, 454*n.*, 462, 467*n.*
Gassner, S., 101, 128*n.*
Gath, D., 133, 138, 163*n.*, 164*n.*
Gauthier, J., 146, 163*n.*
Gelder, M. G., 133, 163*n.*
Gendrich, J. C., 170, 215*n.*
Generalization in therapy, 149
General practitioner (GP) workshops, 85, 87, 88
Generativity, 321
Gestalt therapy, 1, 157, 273, 415
Getz, W. L., 176, 215*n.*
Gill, M. M., 416, 456*n.*

Gilligan, C., 345, 350, 356n.
Gillman, R. D., 175, 215n.
Giovacchini, P., 236, 241n.
Glasgow, R. E., 154, 163n.
Glass, G. V., 1, 5n., 18, 20, 22n.
Glover, E., 84, 98, 127n.
GLS Associates, 16, 21n.
Goldberg, A., 245, 251–253, 260, 261, 267n.
Goldberg, D., 20, 21n., 22n.
Goldberg, I. D., 19, 22n., 167, 177–179, 215n., 334, 341n.
Goldfried, M. R., 157, 159, 163n., 391, 412n.
Goldstein, A., 432, 446, 454n.
Gomes-Schwartz, B., 19, 22n., 222, 241n., 465, 467n.
Gordon, J. R., 150, 158, 159, 164n.
Gordon, S., 448, 454n.
Gossett, J. T., 376, 385n.
Gottman, J. M., 390, 399, 400, 413n.
Gould, R. L., 253, 257, 262, 265, 267n.
Gould Academy, 276
Grandiosity, 259–261
Great society programs, 9
Green, L., 157, 163n.
Green, S., 421, 454n.
Greenson, R. R., 228, 241n., 246, 267n.
Greenwood, M. M., 28, 42n.
Grief, delayed, 33
Groddeck, G., 175, 215n.
Group for Research in Psychotherapy (GRIP), x
Group Health Association of America, 17, 178
Group psychotherapy, 3, 13, 271–357
  adult developmental model of, 305–342
    conclusions on, 340
    later midlife groups, 332–340
    midlife groups, 320–332
    young adult groups, 308–320
  crisis groups, 283–303
    curative parameters of, 297–301
    format/management of, 284–286
    limitations/strengths of, 301, 302
    literature on, 287–289
    outcome study on, 289–296
  curative parameters of, 297–301
  historical introduction on, 271–273
  National Training Laboratories, 275–277

Group psychotherapy (continued)
  T-groups/encounters, 273–275, 277–281
  of women, 343–357
    conclusion on, 355
    literature on, 344–346
    process in, 351–355
    referrals for, 348–351
    psychotherapy/consciousness raising, 347, 348
    short-term, 349
Guerin, P. H., 362, 385n., 421, 454n.
Guerney, B., 397, 400, 413n.
Gurman, A. S., 4, 5n., 361, 385n., 387, 394, 411, 413n., 415–457, 455n., 463, 465
Gustafson, J. P., 1, 83–128, 462
Guthrie, S., 176, 214n.
Gutmann, D. G., 321, 341n.

Hackmann, A., 138, 164n.
Hadley, S. W., 18, 19, 22n., 222, 227, 229, 236, 241n., 242n., 465, 467n.
Hakstian, A. R., 137, 164n.
Halas, C., 344, 345, 357n.
Haley, J., 159, 160, 163n., 363, 385n., 411, 413n., 420, 421, 455n.
Hallam, R. S., 134, 164n.
Hand, I., 134, 163n.
Hankin, J., 334, 341n.
Hare, N., 146, 163n.
Harrell, J., 400, 413n.
Harrington, J. A., 311, 342n.
Harris, L., 368, 385.
Hartley, D., 307, 341n., 367, 385n.
Harvard Community Health Plan (HCHP), ix, x, 17, 271, 272, 277, 279, 281, 283–303, 305–341, 343, 344, 348, 349, 354, 461, 464
Harwood Manufacturing Company, 274
Havens, L. L., 3, 4, 17, 21n., 86, 97, 117, 118, 120, 123n., 127n., 238, 241n., 243–267, 267n., 464, 467n.
Hawker, A., 176, 214n.
Health Maintenance Organizations (HMOs), 16, 17, 272, 281, 283, 305
  (see also Harvard Community Health Plan)
Heard, D., 427, 455n.
Heath, E. S., 102, 127n., 174, 215n.
Hensman, C., 176, 214n.

Hertel, R. K., 433, 456n.
Hildebrand, 94, 97
Hitler, A., 274
Hodgson, R., 135, 136, 163n., 164n.
Hoeper, E. W., 334, 341n.
Hoffman, D. L., 168, 170, 175, 215n.
Hollon, S., 136, 165n.
Homosexuality, 94
Hops, H., 396, 414n.
Horwitz, L., 229, 242n.
Hospital for Sick Children, The, London, 362
Hospitalization, 8, 168, 178, 287, 300, 375
Hoyt, M. F., 265, 267n.
Hunt, W. A., 150, 163n.
Hyperventilation, 309
Hypnotic suggestion and groups, 290
Hypochondriasis, 290, 308
Hypomania, 300

Identification with parents, 264
Identity and separation, 255, 256, 258
Illinois State Psychiatric Institute, 288
Imipramine, 137
Individual Psychotherapy and the Science of Psychodynamics (Malan), 111, 121, 126n.
Infantile wishes and ambiguity in treatment time, 31
Inhibited sexual desire (ISD), 138 (see also Sexuality)
Institute of Behavior Therapy, 142
Insulin shock treatment, 7
Integrative marital therapy, 415–457
    behavioral approaches to, 425, 426, 445–449
    and brief individual therapy, 416, 417
    and brief marital therapy, 417–419
    conceptual/technical principles for, 428–432
    conclusion on, 452, 453
    conjoint, 429, 430, 433
    development of, 420–422
    goals/assessment in, 432–435
    intervention in, 442–445
    midphase issues, 429–452
    and paradox, 449–452
    and psychodynamic approaches, 423–425
    structural–strategic approaches to, 427, 428

Integrative marital therapy (continued)
    termination of, 452
    therapeutic alliance in, 435–438
    and time-limited marital therapy, 419, 420
International Congress of Psychotherapy, 46
Interpretive approach to short-term therapy, 247–249
    time-limited, 229–233
Intimacy, 256, 308
Introjection, 119, 256
Intuition
    and conceptual mastery, 83–85
    and reinterpretation, 107–112

Jackson, D. D., 421, 425, 431, 455n., 456n.
Jacobson, A., 169, 215n., 334, 341n.
Jacobson, G. F., 170, 174, 215n.
Jacobson, N. S., 4, 387–414, 413n., 419–421, 425, 426, 429, 430, 435, 439, 455n.
Jameson, J., 177, 215n.
Jaques, E., 262, 267n., 308, 321, 332, 341n.
Jeffrey, R. W., 149, 150, 162n., 163n.
Johnson, L., 9
Johnson, R. F., 171, 216n.
Johnson, V., 137, 146, 157, 164n.
Johnston, D. W., 133, 134, 163n., 164n.
Jones, J., 28
Jones, K. R., 20, 22n.
Jones, R., 396, 412n.
Jonestown, 28
Julier, D., 138, 164n.
Jung, C. J., 321, 341n.

Kaiser Foundation Health Plan of Southern California, 170
Kanfer, F., 432, 455n.
Kaplan, H., 138, 163n.
Karoly, P., 434, 455n.
Kazdin, A. E., 13, 22n., 140, 141, 148, 149, 151–153, 161, 161n., 163n., 415, 455n.
Keith, D. V., 444, 457n.
Keithly, L. H., 222, 241n.
Kellert, S. R., 13, 22n.
Kelley, G., 396, 414n., 424, 456n.
Kelly, H. H., 425, 457n.

Keniston, K., 257, 260, 267n.
Kenmore Center, 305 *(see also* Harvard Community Health Plan)
Kennedy, J. F., 9
Kernberg, O. F., 126n., 127n., 229, 236, 241, 242n.
Kerr, M., 420, 456n.
Kinston, W., 4, 361–386, 385n., 420, 454n.
Kirch, B., 346, 357n.
Klein, E. B., 306, 341n.
Klein, M. H., 88, 113, 126n., 127n., 321, 322, 341n., 416, 443, 455n., 456n.
Klein, R. H., 343, 357n.
Klerman, G. L., 17, 22n.
Kniskern, D. P., 4, 5n., 361, 385n., 387, 394, 413n., 417, 422, 427, 431, 439, 455n., 456n.
Knudson, R. M., 411, 413n., 422, 423, 430, 435, 443, 455n.
Koffman, M., 175, 215n.
Kogan, L. S., 169, 171, 215n.
Kohut, H., 99, 102, 127n., 236, 242n., 251, 260, 267n.
Kopel, S., 147, 162n.
Koppenaal, G. S., 4, 343–357, 464
Kornreich, M., 18, 22n.
Kosloski, K. D., 170, 215n.
Koss, M. P., 2, 5n., 131, 155, 159, 162n., 221, 222, 236, 241n., 307, 341n., 416, 418, 454n., 456n., 461, 463, 467n.
Kotch, J. B., 28, 42n.
Kovacs, M., 136, 165n.
Krantz, G., 177, 179, 215n.
Kravetz, D., 348, 357n.
Kurtz, R., 415, 454n.

L'Abate, L., 428, 457n.
Lambert, M. J., 152, 162n., 229, 238, 241n., 422, 454n.
Lamontagne, Y., 134, 163n.
Lazare, A., 169, 215n.
Lazarus, A. A., 133, 157, 158, 163n., 166n.
Leaff, L. A., 221, 241n.
Learning theory *(see* Social learning theory)
Lederer, W., 425, 456n.
Lever, J., 345, 357n.
Levine, J., 400, 413n.

Levinson, D. J., 253, 255, 257, 259, 260, 262, 265, 267n., 306, 321, 341n.
Levinson, M. H., 306, 341n.
Levis, D. J., 146, 163n.
Lewin, K. K., 174, 175, 215n., 273–276, 281n.
Lewis, J. M., 376, 385n.
Ley, P., 20, 22n.
Liberman, R. P., 400, 413n.
Lieberman, M. A., 279, 281n., 312, 341n.
Lief, H., 421, 428, 454n.
Lifton, R. J., 262, 267n.
Lithium, 18
Littlepage, G. E., 170, 172, 215n.
Lloyd, G., 288, 303n.
Loader, P., 366, 385n.
Locke, B. Z., 177, 179, 215n.
Loevinger, J., 266, 267n.
Lorion, R. P., 168, 215n., 416, 456n.
LSD, 28
Lubetkin, B., 142, 145, 162n.
Lubin, B., 289, 303n.
Luborsky, L., 3, 5n., 18, 22n., 148, 229, 163n., 242n.
Lynch, C., 344, 345, 357n.

MacIver, J., 13, 22n.
Madanes, C., 362, 385n.
Mahler, G., 14
Mahoney, M. J., 158, 164n., 429, 456n.
Malan, D. H., 1, 4, 80, 80n., 83–85, 88–116, 120, 121, 122n.–127n., 174, 176, 215n., 220, 222, 223, 229, 235, 236, 239, 242n., 258, 267n., 279, 280, 281n., 305, 307, 341n., 362, 364, 385n., 419, 420, 434, 452, 456n., 463, 467n.
Mancera, M., 400, 412n.
Manic–depression, 18 *(see also* Depression)
Mann, J., 2, 25–43, 43n., 80, 81n., 85, 96, 127n., 220, 229, 242n., 245, 249–251, 255, 267n., 272, 277, 280, 281n., 305, 319, 322, 323, 326, 341, 341n., 417–420, 452, 456n.
Mantra and time, 27
Margolin, G., 387, 390, 391, 394, 396, 397, 399–401, 405, 408, 409, 411, 413n., 414n., 419–421, 425, 426, 429, 430, 435, 439, 455n.
Marijuana and time, 27

Marital/family therapy, focus for, 13, 136,
    361–386 *(see also* Behavioral marital
    therapy; Integrative marital therapy)
  conclusion on, 383
  focal hypothesis on, 365–368, 380–381
  and individual therapy, 363–365
  initial attempt at, 363–365
  meaning in, 369–383
    avoidance of, 378, 379
    common meanings, 273–276
    depth structure, 371–373
    intersubjective meanings, 376, 382
    surface action, 369–371
Marks, I. M., 133–136, 138, 146, 148,
    163n.–165n., 446, 456n.
Marlatt, G. A., 150, 158, 159, 164n.
Marmor, J., 2, 5n., 13–15, 22n., 240,
    242n.
Marrow, A. J., 273, 281n.
Marsh, S., 424, 457n.
Marshall, W. L., 146, 163n.
Martin, P., 344, 345, 356n., 455, 456n.
Masochism, 222, 259
Massarik, F., 278, 282n.
Masters, W., 137, 146, 157, 164n.
Masturbation, 247
Matarazzo, J., 416, 456n.
Mathews, A. M., 133, 134, 138, 163n.,
    164n.
McCord, E., 174, 215n.
McElroy, C. M., 283–303
McGuire, M., 175, 215n.
McKee, B., 306, 341n.
McLean, P. D., 137, 164n.
McMullen, S., 138, 164n.
McNees, M. P., 170, 215n.
Medicaid, 16
Medical Care, 20
Medical Psychology Outpatient Clinic, 178
Medicare, 16
Meditation and time, 27, 28
Meichenbaum, D., 132, 164n.
Meissner, W. W., 388, 414n., 438, 456n.
Meltzoff, J., 18, 22n.
Memory and time in therapy, 27
Menninger, K., 84, 127n.
Menninger Project, 229
Menopause, 263
Mental Health Systems Act, 11
Mental Research Institute, 419

Michalicek, A., 400, 412n.
Midlife, groups for, 320–340
  later midlife, 332–340
  and theories of midlife development,
    321, 322
  and time, 322, 323
Mignone, R. J., 169, 215n.
Miles, M. D., 279, 281n.
Miller, T. I., 1, 5n., 18, 22n.
Miller, W. R., 138, 164n.
Minuchin, S., 427, 449, 456n.
MIT, 273
Mitchell, C., 180, 216n.
Mitcheson, M., 176, 214n.
MMPI, 225, 290
Modeling, participant, 133–136, 146, 149,
    400
Mogul, K., 345, 346, 357n.
Moore, D., 395, 413n.
Morley, W. E., 170, 215n.
Mouton, J. S., 278, 281n.
Multiple Affect Adjective Checklist, 289
Mumford, E., 20, 22n.
Munby, M., 134, 164n.
Muslin, H., 333, 342n.
Myers, E. D., 311, 342n.
Myers, E. S., 170, 215n.

Nadelson, C. C., 346, 357n., 420, 421,
    424, 445, 456n.
Narcissism, 236, 251, 259–261, 266, 300,
    333, 337
  and dependency, 423
  and time, 28, 29
Nassi, A., 343, 344, 347, 357n.
Naster, B., 397, 412n.
Nathan, P. E., 140, 164n.
National Institute of Mental Health
    (NIMH), 8, 10–12, 15, 22n.
National mental health issues, 7–22
  and brief treatment development, 12–17
  future developments, 17–21
  historical context of, 7–12
National Training Laboratory (NTL), 277,
    278, 280
Navy, U. S., Department of Research, 276
Nemiroff, R. A., 266, 267n.
Neugarten, B. L., 253, 262, 263, 265,
    267n., 322, 333, 342n.
Neurosis, 121, 157, 226, 278

Neurosis *(continued)*
  complex, alternative hypothesis for,
      107–111
  in groups, 285, 286, 302
  and psychoanalysis, 90–93
  roots of, 90
Newman, L., 288, 303*n*.
New York Community Service Society,
      Division of Family Services, 169
Nightmares, 69, 70
Norell, J. S., 86, 123*n*., 127*n*.
Normand, W. D., 288, 303*n*.
Notman, M. T., 260, 263, 267*n*., 346,
      357*n*.
Nuclear conflict, 182
Nurses as primary therapists, 134
Nyez, G. R., 334, 341*n*.

Obesity, 138, 142, 150, 374
Object relations theory, 337, 423, 424, 433,
      453
Obsessive-compulsive disorders, 29, 94,
      135, 136, 143, 146, 148, 229, 423, 438
Oedipal conflicts, 2, 31, 47, 57, 58, 88, 92,
      115, 229, 243, 247–249, 254, 257,
      259, 266
Offset studies, 20
Olbrisch, M. E., 179, 180, 215*n*.
O'Leary, K. D., 132, 133, 142, 145, 159,
      164*n*., 166*n*.
O'Leary, V., 346, 356*n*.
Operant conditioning, 132 *(see also* Behav-
      ior therapy, individual)
Oppenheimer, E., 176, 214*n*.
Orford, J., 176, 214*n*.
Ornstein, P. H., 84, 114, 121, 127*n*., 182,
      214*n*., 362, 385*n*., 463, 467*n*.
Outpatient treatment, short-term, 178
Overdetermination, 90
Overeating, 148

Panic, 13
Paolino, T., 429, 456*n*.
Papp, P., 362, 386*n*., 450, 456*n*.
Paradox and marital therapy, 449–452
Paranoia, 89, 114, 115, 126*n*.
Pardes, H., 1, 7–22, 463
Parloff, M. B., 18, 22*n*., 152, 164*n*., 238,
      242*n*., 415, 456*n*.
Passivity, 110

Patterson, G. R., 396, 397, 414*n*.
Paul, G. L., 148, 164*n*.
Paykel, E. S., 17, 22*n*.
Perkins, D., 140, 162*n*.
Peters, M. J., 424, 457*n*.
Peters, T. C., 424, 457*n*.
Phillips, V. A., 376, 385*n*.
Philpott, R., 134, 164*n*.
Phobias, 13, 33, 36, 92, 133, 134, 141, 143,
      148, 151, 159, 224, 238, 434, 446
Pincus, H. A., 1, 7–22, 463
Piper, W. E., 311, 342*n*.
Planning of brief therapy, 94–102
  and complexity, unexplained, 98–102
  and stages of therapy, 96, 97
  and unified therapy conception, 98
Polster, E., 157, 164*n*.
Polster, M., 157, 164*n*.
Popper, K., 111, 127*n*.
Prata, G., 362, 386*n*., 451, 456*n*.
Prejudice
  of depth, 305
  racial/religious, 275
  and women, 346–348
Premature ejaculation, 157 *(see also* Sex-
      uality)
President's Commission on Mental Health,
      11, 14
Principle of contemporaneity, 273
Problem solving, 186, 187, 393, 399, 400,
      404, 405, 447–449
Projection, 308, 314, 335, 423, 434
Projective identification, 447, 448
Projective tests, 96
Prusoff, B., 17, 22*n*.
Psychoanalysis, 249 *(see also* Unconscious)
  assessment in, 434
  and behavior therapy, 156, 157, 160
  Chicago School of, 175, 275
  and conflict, 97
  counteroffer in, 86
  and duration of treatment, 14
  in focal therapy, 116
  hermeneutic approach in, 371
  and marital therapy, 361, 362, 420, 421,
      423, 424
  and neurosis, 90–93
  and patient selection, 221, 223
  scope of work in, 244
  as term, 429

Psychoanalysis *(continued)*
  as theoretical base, 1
  and time, 31
  traditional bonds in, breaking of, 90–93, 120
    context for, 90
    described, 90–92
    outcome of, 92
    overall conception, 93
    technique/selection for, 92, 93
"Psychodynamic" as term, 429
Psychodynamicism and social learning theory, 430–432
Psychopharmacology, introduction of, 8
Psychosis, 28, 29, 31, 36
Psychosurgery, 7
Public health programs, single sessions in, 172, 173
Public Health Service, 11

Rabavilas, A. D., 146, 164*n.*
Rabkin, J. G., 236, 242*n.*
Rabkin, R., 213, 215*n.*, 465, 467*n.*
Rachman, S., 133, 135, 136, 138, 141, 148, 151, 152, 161, 163*n.*, 164*n.*
Randall, M., 272, 281*n.*, 311, 325, 341*n.*, 463, 467*n.*
Rank, O., 45, 81*n.,* 83, 127*n.,* 415, 456*n.*
Rathjen, D., 132, 162*n.*
Raush, H. L., 433, 456*n.*
Rayner, E., 123*n.*
Redlich, F. C., 13, 22*n.*
Reed, L. S., 170, 215*n.*
Referrals of women to groups, 348–351
Regier, D. A., 19, 22*n.*, 167, 215*n.*, 334, 341*n.*
Regression
  and ambiguity in treatment time, 31
  and development, 254
  and groups, 286, 297, 331
  and long-term therapy, 106
  and marital therapy, 439, 440
Reid, J. B., 396, 414*n.*
Reid, W. J., 409, 414*n.*, 461, 466*n.*
Reider, N., 175, 216*n.*
Reinforcement, 396, 398
Reinterpretation and intuition, 107–112
Relaxation training, 135, 144
Remmel, M. L., 168, 170, 175, 215*n.*

Repression, 182, 262
Research Center for Group Dynamics, 273
Resistance, 42, 75, 76, 90, 144, 231, 246
  to adaptive change, 274, 275
  and behavioral marital therapy, 394, 411 ·
  to change, 159
  to marital therapy, 439–441
  to therapy, 229
Reynolds, E. J., 145, 162*n.*
Ricoeur, P., 371, 386*n.*
Role models, 260, 275, 345
Rolfing, 1
Romancyzk, R. G., 157, 165*n.*
Rosen, G. M., 154, 163*n.*
Rosen, J. C., 177–179, 216*n.*
Rosen, R. C., 138, 164*n.*
Rosenbaum, C. P., 175, 216*n.*
Rosenthal, T. L., 133, 159, 165*n.*
Rosser, R., 381, 385*n.*
Rubin, Z., 180, 216*n.*
Rudestam, K. E., 169, 170, 172, 214*n.*
Rush, A. J., 136, 137, 165*n.*, 432, 453*n.*

Sabin, J. E., 271–282, 282*n.*
Sadock, B., 288, 303*n.*
Sager, C. J., 421, 423, 424, 429, 430, 433, 434, 440, 445, 456*n.*
Samples, S. J., 222, 241*n.*
Sampson, H., 101, 108, 112, 120, 124*n.,* 125*n.,* 128*n.*
Sanders, N., 400, 413*n.*
Sarvis, M. A., 171, 216*n.*
Schafer, R., 246, 267*n.*
Scheidemandel, P. L., 170, 215*n.*
Schizoid characters, 235, 308
Schizophrenia, 323, 324, 365
Schlesinger, H. J., 20, 22*n.*
Schneider, S., 170, 215*n.*
Schnelle, J. F., 170, 215*n.*
Schrader, S., 420, 421, 454*n.*
Schuckit, M. A., 137, 162*n.*
Schutz, W. C., 157, 165*n.*
Screen memories, 29 *(see also* Unconscious)
Selection in therapy, 97, 102–104
Selective service system, 8
Self-centeredness, 222
Self-esteem, 48, 194, 209, 251, 290, 293, 301, 323, 324, 331, 333, 378, 406
"Self in Process, The," 278

Self-monitoring, 157, 158
Self-ratings, 134, 137
Selvini-Palazzoli, M., 362, 386n., 451, 456n.
Seminars for the Separated, 287
Senate Finance Committee, 16
Sensitivity training, 278
Separation/individuation, 31, 41, 42, 92, 245, 249–251, 255, 256, 258, 266, 322, 327, 328, 331, 345, 374 *(see also* Anxiety, separation; Dependency)
Sethna, E. R., 311, 342n.
Settling down, 259–261
Seven Per Cent Solution, The, 123n.
Sexuality
    behavioral treatment of, 134–138, 146, 147, 151, 157
    discussed, in short-term anxiety-provoking psychotherapy, 49ff.
    exhibitionism, 148
    potency problem, 14
    problems in, delineated, 13
    sex therapy, 157
Shaping, 396
Shapiro, D., 249, 267n.
Shapiro, R., 361, 386n.
Shaw, B. F., 432, 453n.
Shaw, P., 133, 134, 138, 163n., 164n.
Short-term anxiety-provoking psychotherapy (STAPP), 45–81
    conclusion on, 79, 80
    instruction of, 49
    interviews for, 49–79
    outcome of, 48, 49
    patient selection criteria for, 46, 47
    technique in, 47, 48
Shuford, D., 400, 412n.
Shuman, L. J., 177, 215n.
Shyne, A. W., 169, 216n., 409, 414n.
Sifneos, P. E., 2, 45–81, 81n., 175, 216n., 220, 229, 234, 239, 242n., 245–249, 258, 259, 267n., 277, 280, 282n., 305, 418–420, 456n.
Silberschatz, G., 101, 128n.
Silverman, W. H., 172, 216n.
Simon, K. M., 157, 162n.
Singer, B., 3, 5n., 18, 22n., 148, 163n.
Skilback, C. E., 20, 22n.
Skill practice supervision, 278

Skinner, B. F., 132, 165n.
Skynner, A. C. R., 421, 423, 429, 438, 450, 456n., 457n.
Sloane, R. B., 143, 151, 152, 156, 160, 165n., 227, 229, 242n., 307, 342n., 462, 467n.
Small, L., 25, 26, 43n., 266, 267n., 307, 342n.
Smith, M. L., 1, 5n., 18, 22n.
Smoke-Enders, 287
Smoking, behavioral treatment of, 138, 150
Sobell, L. C., 138, 140, 165n.
Sobell, M. B., 138, 140, 165n.
Social learning theory, 132, 146, 425, 430–432
Socioeconomic class and treatment, 10, 169, 416
Somatization and anxiety, 336, 337
Sommer, G. J., 170, 215n.
Spark, G. M., 362, 385n.
Speers, R. W., 171, 216n.
Spinks, S. H., 411, 412n., 421, 454n.
Spoerl, O. H., 170, 174, 216n.
S-R approach, 132
Stanford University, 279
Stanton, M. D., 419–421, 427–429, 432, 435, 439, 444, 449, 450, 457n.
Staples, F. R., 143, 160, 165n., 227, 244n., 307, 342n., 462, 467n.
Steele, R. S., 371, 386n.
Stefanis, C., 146, 164n.
Stereotyped roles of women, 344
Stern, R., 146, 165n.
Stewart, R. H., 424, 429, 457n.
Stokes, T. F., 149, 165n.
Stone, M., 146, 165n.
Strachey, J., 84, 124n., 128n.
Stratford, J., 366, 385n.
Stress
    and family therapy, 381–383
    maladaptive response to, 223
Strickler, M., 170, 215n., 287, 303n.
Structural–strategic approaches to marital therapy, 427, 428
Strupp, H. H., 3, 19, 22n., 219–242, 241n., 242n., 281, 307, 311, 342n., 462, 463, 465, 467n.
Stuart, R. B., 147, 150, 165n., 396, 397,

Stuart, R. B. *(continued)*
    409, 414*n.*, 419–421, 425, 426, 427*n.*,
    429, 435, 438, 439, 455*n.*, 457*n.*
Study of Brief Psychotherapy, A (Malan),
    83, 88, 94, 120, 123*n.*
Stunkard, A. J., 150, 163*n.*
Sue, S., 170, 216*n.*
Suicide, 31, 94, 300, 312, 348
Superego, 124*n.*
    lessening of demands of, 41
Swain, M. A., 433, 456*n.*
Symptoms
    and behavioral marital therapy, 389, 390
    and family therapy, 449
    hysterical, 92
    obsessional, 94
    relief of as by-product, 36
    and short-term anxiety-provoking psy-
        chotherapy, 48
    substitution of, 151
    and surface action, 369
    and therapeutic goals, 225, 226
Systems theory and marital therapy, 430–
    432, 439

Tannenbaum, R., 278, 282*n.*
Tannenbaum, S. A., 175, 216*n.*
Taube, C. A., 19, 22*n.*, 167, 215*n.*
Tavistock Clinic, London, 1, 83, 89, 102,
    120, 229, 362
Taylor, C., 176, 214*n.*
Teasdale, J., 134, 164*n.*
Temple Study, 229
Termination of therapy, 90, 418
T-groups, 273–281
Therapeutic alliance, 228, 234
Thibaut, J. W., 396, 414*n.*, 425, 457*n.*
Thorpe, G. L., 157, 165*n.*
Time-limited dynamic psychotherapy, 219–
    242, 322, 323, 419, 420
    future directions in, 233–240
    patient selection for, 221–225, 239
    therapeutic goals in, 225, 226, 239
    therapeutic technology for, 227–233
        and interpretation, 229–233
        and patient–therapist relationship,
            228, 229, 240
    time in, 239
        and commonalities in brief therapy,
            25, 26

Time-limited dynamic psychotherapy,
        time in *(continued)*
    importance of, 27–32
    model for time-limited therapy, 26
Time-Limited Psychotherapy (Mann), 25
*Toward the Validation of Dynamic Psy-
        chotherapy* (Malan), 99, 102, 121,
    124*n.*
Tracey, D. A., 157, 165*n.*
Trakos, D. A., 288, 303*n.*
Tranquilizers, 8
Transactional Analysis (TA), 1, 415
Transference, 39–42, 80, 90, 97, 100, 102,
        106, 111, 221, 432 *(see also* Counter-
        transference)
    acknowledgment of, 50, 51
    avoidance, 90, 91
    and behavioral therapy, 160
    and central issue, 33, 35
    confrontation of, 237
    expectations of, 85, 101, 109
    and fee, 193
    and groups, 286, 297, 315
    and intuition, 83
    for lessons, 247, 248
    management of, 228, 230, 240, 243,
        246
    in marital therapy, 439–441, 452
    and neurosis, 91, 92
    passive/active, 118
    radical interpretation of, 93
    and termination of therapy, 90
    and time, 28, 29
    use/nonuse of, 25, 26
Transsexual, 145
Transvestitism, 148
Tuckman, B. W., 316, 342*n.*

UCLA School of Industrial Management,
    278
Unconscious *(see also* Psychoanalysis)
    and anxiety, 423, 441
    and central issues, 37
    and childhood wishes, 39
    and interpersonal behavior, 429
    and learning theory, 430
    and marital therapy, 423
    and primal reunions, 35
    and time, 25, 30, 31
    and trauma repetition, 109

United Auto Workers Health Insurance
Program, 16
University of Berlin, 273
University of Michigan, 273
University of Oregon Health Sciences Center, 178
Ursano, R. J., 307, 367, 342n., 386n.

Vaillant, G. E., 253, 255, 256, 259, 263, 267n., 306, 308, 321, 322, 342n.
Vandenbos, F., 465, 467n.
Vanderbilt Psychotherapy Project, 222, 225, 227, 229–231, 235, 238
VanDeusen, J. M., 418, 427, 428, 453n.
Video taping in therapy, 133, 361, 400
Vincent, J. P., 397, 412n., 414n.
Vischi, T. R., 20, 22n.
Voth, H., 229, 242n.

Wachtel, P. L., 2, 5n., 13, 22n., 440, 457n., 462, 467n.
Waldron, H., 395, 413n.
Wallace, C., 400, 413n.
Walter, B., 14
Waskow, I., 18, 22n.
Watergate, 10
Watzlawick, P., 367, 386n., 394, 414n., 419, 421, 427, 439, 457n.
Waxer, P. H., 343, 357n.
Weakland, J. H., 367, 386n., 394, 414n., 419–421, 427, 457n.
Weeks, G., 428, 457n.
Weiss, J., 101, 108, 110, 112, 118–120, 124n.–126n., 128n.
Weiss, R. L., 158, 159, 165n., 387–414, 413n., 414n., 419–421, 425, 430, 455n., 457n.
Weissman, M., 17, 22n.
Weschler, I. R., 278, 282n.
Wheatly, D., 20, 22n.
Wheeler, E., 400, 413n.
Whipple, K., 143, 160, 165n., 227, 242n., 307, 342n., 462, 467n.

Whitaker, C. A., 444, 457n.
White, H., 3, 4, 17, 21n., 122n., 127n., 238, 241n., 243–267, 267n., 464, 467n.
White, S. W., 391, 412n.
Whitehead, A., 138, 164n.
Whitworth, M. A., 20, 22n.
Wiens, A. N., 177–179, 216n.
Williams, A. M., 421, 454n.
Williams, M. W., 169, 215n.
Wills, T. A., 397, 414n.
Wilner, D. M., 170, 215n.
Wilson, G. T., 2, 131–168, 161n., 163n.–166n., 462
Wing, R. R., 150, 163n.
Winnicott, 89
Wisneski, M. J., 272, 277, 305–343, 341n., 356n., 463–465, 466n., 467n.
Withdrawal, 308
Wolberg, L. R., 25, 43n., 174, 216n., 298, 299, 303n., 305, 307, 342n., 434, 457n.
Wolfe, B., 18, 22n.
Wolpe, J., 131, 132, 157, 166n., 168n.
Wolpin, M., 168, 215n.
Working through, 90, 116

Yale University Student Health Service, 246
Yalom, I. D., 271, 279, 280, 281n., 282n., 287, 303n., 305, 324, 342n.
Yasuna, A., 367, 385n.
Yorkston, N. J., 143, 160, 165n., 227, 242n., 307, 342n., 462, 467n.
Young, W. W., 177, 215n.
Young adulthood, groups for, 308–320

Zeiss, R. A., 138, 154, 166n.
Zinner, J., 361, 386n.
Zisook, S., 169, 215n.
Zuckerman, M., 289, 290, 303n.
Zuckerman scales, 290, 295